Atlas of Ultrasound-Guided Procedures in Interventional Pain Management

Samer N. Narouze, MD, MSc, DABPM, FIPP

Atlas of Ultrasound-Guided Procedures in Interventional Pain Management

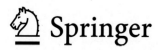 Springer

Editor
Samer N. Narouze, MD, MSc, DABPM, FIPP
Chairman, Pain Management Department
Summa Western Reserve Hospital
Clinical Professor of Anesthesiology
and Pain Medicine, NEOUCOM
1900 23rd Street
Cuyahoga Falls, OH 44223
USA

Cover Illustration Credits (left to right)

Front Cover Illustrations
Figure 10.2 (first two images)
Figure 23.3(b). Courtesy of Joseph Kanasz BFA.
Image courtesy of Samer N. Narouze, MD.
Figure 23.10(b). Courtesy of Joseph Kanasz BFA.

Back Cover Illustrations
Figure 29.6. Reprinted with permission from Ohio Pain and Headache Institute.
Figure 13.2, Figure 8.5, and Figure 15.9. Reprinted with permission, Cleveland Clinic Center for
    Medical Art & Photography© 2008–2010. All rights reserved.
Image courtesy of Samer N. Narouze, MD.
Figure 28.2. Reprinted with permission, Cleveland Clinic Center for Medical Art & Photography©
    2010. All rights reserved.

ISBN 978-1-4419-1679-2   e-ISBN 978-1-4419-1681-5
DOI 10.1007/978-1-4419-1681-5
Springer New York Dordrecht Heidelberg London

To my wife, Mira, and my children, John, Michael,
and Emma – the true love and joy of my life.
Without their continued understanding and support,
I could not have completed this book.

This book is dedicated to the memory of my father who always had
faith in me and to my mother for her ongoing love and guidance.

Foreword

For much of the past decade, fluoroscopy held sway as the favorite imaging tool of many practitioners performing interventional pain procedures. Quite recently, ultrasound has emerged as a "challenger" to this well-established modality. The growing popularity of ultrasound application in regional anesthesia and pain medicine reflects a shift in contemporary views about imaging for nerve localization and target-specific injections. For regional anesthesia, ultrasound has already made a marked impact by transforming antiquated clinical practice into a modern science. No bedside tool ever before has allowed practitioners to visualize needle advancement in real time and observe local anesthetic spread around nerve structures. For interventional pain procedures, I believe this radiation-free, point-of-care technology will also find its unique role and utility in pain medicine and can complement some of the imaging demands not met by fluoroscopy, computed tomography, and magnetic resonance imaging. And over time, practitioners will discover new benefits of this technology, especially for dynamic assessment of musculoskeletal pain conditions and improving accuracy of needle injection for small nerves, soft tissue, tendons, and joints.

Ultrasound application for pain medicine is an evolving subspecialty area. Most conventional pain interventionists skilled in fluoroscopy will find it necessary to undertake some special learning and training to acquire a new set of cognitive and technical skills before they can optimally integrate ultrasound into their clinical practices. Although continuing medical educational events help to facilitate the learning process and skill development, they are often limited in breadth, depth, and training duration. This is why the arrival of this comprehensive text, *Atlas of Ultrasound-Guided Procedures in Interventional Pain Management*, is so timely and welcome. To my knowledge, this is the first illustrative atlas of its kind that addresses the educational void for ultrasound-guided pain interventions.

Preparation of this atlas, containing 6 parts and 30 chapters and involving more than 30 authors, is indeed a huge undertaking. The broad range of ultrasound topics selected in this book provides a good, solid educational foundation and curriculum for pain practitioners both in practice and in training. Included is the current state of knowledge relating to the basic principles of ultrasound imaging and knobology, regional anatomy specific to interventional procedures, ultrasound scanning and image interpretation, and the technical considerations for needle insertion and injection. The ultrasound-guided techniques are described step-by-step in an easy-to-follow, "how to do it" manner for both acute and chronic pain interventions. The major topics include somatic and sympathetic neural blockade in the head and neck, limbs, spine, abdomen, and pelvis. Using a large library of black-and-white images and colored illustrative artwork, the authors elegantly impart scientific knowledge through the display of anatomic cadaveric dissections, sonoanatomy correlates, and schematic diagrams showing essential techniques for needle insertion and injection. The information in the last two chapters of this book is especially enlightening and unique and is not commonly found in other standard pain textbooks. One chapter describes how ultrasound can be applied as an extension of physical examination to aid pain physicians in the diagnosis of musculoskeletal pain conditions. With ultrasound as a screening tool, pain physicians now have new opportunities to become both a diagnostician and an interventionist. The last chapter discussing advanced ultrasound techniques for cervicogenic headache, stimulating lead placement, and cervical disk injection gives readers a glimpse of future exciting applications.

This book is a distinguished product carefully prepared by Dr. Samer Narouze, the editor, and his hand-picked group of contributors from all over the world. The authors are all recognized opinion leaders in anesthesiology, pain medicine, anatomy, and radiology. I believe this quick reference book containing useful practical information will become a standard resource for any practitioner who seeks to learn ultrasound-guided interventional pain procedures for relief of acute, chronic noncancer, and cancer pain. I am sure the readers will find this atlas comprehensive, inspiring, practical, and easy to follow.

Vincent W. S. Chan, MD, FRCPC
Professor, Department of Anesthesia
University of Toronto, ON, Canada

Preface

Ultrasonography is a very welcome addition to fluoroscopy and other imaging techniques in interventional pain practice. Over the past few years, interest in ultrasonography in pain medicine (USPM) has been fast growing, as evidenced by the plethora of published papers in peer-reviewed journals as well as presentations at major national and international meetings. This has prompted the creation of a special interest group on USPM within the American Society of Regional Anesthesiology and Pain Medicine, of which I am honored to be chair.

The major advantages of ultrasonography (US) over fluoroscopy include the absence of radiation exposure for both patient and operator, and the real-time visualization of soft tissue structures, such as nerves, muscles, tendons, and vessels. The latter is why US guidance of soft tissue and joint injections brings great precision to the procedure and why ultrasound-guided pain nerve blocks improve its safety. That said, USPM is not without flaws. Its major shortcomings are the limited resolution at deep levels, especially in obese patients, and the artifacts created by bone structures.

While the evidence points to the superiority of US over fluoroscopy in peripheral nerves, soft tissue, and joint injections, it also suggests that we should not abandon fluoroscopy in favor of US in spine injections and should instead consider combining both imaging modalities to further enhance the goal of a successful and safer spine injection.

When I first started using US in pain blocks a few years ago, there was no single text on the subject, and that remains true today. Most of my knowledge on the subject was gained from traveling overseas to learn from expert sonographers, radiologists, and anatomists. The rest was worked out by trial and error using dissected cadavers and confirming appropriate needle placement with fluoroscopy or CT scan. When I started teaching courses on USPM, the overwhelmingly enthusiastic response from students persuaded me of the need for a comprehensive and easy-to-follow atlas of US-guided pain blocks. That is how this book – the first to cover this exciting new field – was born.

Not surprisingly, an extensive learning curve is associated with US-guided pain blocks. The main objective of this atlas is to enable physicians managing acute and chronic pain syndromes who are beginning to use US-guided pain procedures to shorten their learning curve and to make their learning experience as enjoyable as possible. Among the target groups are pain physicians, anesthesiologists, physiatrists, rheumatologists, neurologists, orthopedists, sports medicine physicians, spine specialists, and interventional radiologists.

I was fortunate to gather almost all of the international experts in US-guided pain blocks to contribute to this book, each one writing about his or her area of subspecialty expertise, and for this reason, I am very proud of the book. Its central focus is on anatomy and sonoanatomy. The clinical section begins with a chapter devoted to anatomy and sonoanatomy of the spine written by a dear friend, Professor Dr. Moriggl, who is a world-class anatomist from Innsbruck, Austria, with special expertise in sonoanatomy. He is the only one who could have written such a chapter. Each clinical chapter follows this format: description of sonoanatomy accompanied by illustrations; detailed description of how to perform the procedure, beginning with the choice and application of the transducer, to how the needle is introduced, and finally, to how to confirm appropriate needle placement. This stepwise description of the technique is enhanced by sonograms both without labels and – to better understand the images – with labels.

The book comprises 30 chapters, organized into 6 parts, covering US-guided pain blocks in the acute perioperative and chronic pain clinic settings as well as US-guided MSK applications.

Part I reviews the imaging modalities available to perform pain procedures and the basics of ultrasound imaging. Two important clinical chapters cover the essential knobology of the ultrasound machine and how to improve needle visibility under US.

Part II is also the largest and covers the sonoanatomy of the entire spine and spine injection techniques in the cervical, thoracic, lumbar, and sacral areas. All the different applications are well documented with simple illustrations and labeled sonograms to make it easy to follow the text.

Part III focuses on abdominal and pelvic blocks. It covers the now famous transversus abdominis plane (TAP) block, celiac plexus block, and various pelvic and perineal blocks.

Part IV addresses peripheral nerve blocks and catheters in the acute perioperative period as well as peripheral applications in chronic pain medicine. Ultrasound-guided stellate and cervical sympathetic ganglion blocks are presented, as are peripheral nerve blocks commonly performed in chronic pain patients (e.g., intercostals, suprascapular, ilioinguinal, iliohypogastric, and pudendal).

Part V is devoted to the most common joint and bursa injections and MSK applications in pain practice. The chapters are written by *world experts* in the area of MSK ultrasound.

Part VI covers advanced and new applications of ultrasound in neuromodulation and pain medicine and looks ahead to its future. Ultrasound-guided peripheral nerve stimulation, occipital, and groin stimulation are presented as innovative applications of US in the cervical spine area, namely, atlantoaxial joint injection and cervical diskography. Given the multitude of vessels and other vital soft tissue structures compacted in a limited area, ultrasonography seems particularly relevant in the cervical area.

A couple of notes about the book: the text has been kept to a minimum to allow for a maximal number of instructive illustrations and sonograms, and the procedures described here are based on a review of the techniques described in the literature as well as the authors' experience.

The advancement of ultrasound technology and the range of possible clinical circumstances may give rise to other, more appropriate approaches in USPM. Until then, mastering the current approaches will take preparation, practice, and appropriate mentoring before the physician can comfortably perform the procedures independently. It is my hope that this book will encourage and stimulate all physicians interested in interventional pain management.

Samer N. Narouze, MD, MSc, DABPM, FIPP
Cleveland, OH, USA

Acknowledgments

In preparing *Atlas of Ultrasound-Guided Procedures in Interventional Pain Management*, I had the privilege of gathering highly respected international experts in the field of ultrasonography in pain medicine. I thank Dr. Chan, professor of Anesthesiology at the University of Toronto and President of the American Society of Regional Anesthesiology and Pain Medicine (ASRA), for agreeing to contribute a chapter to this book. I also extend my sincere thanks to the founding members of the ASRA special interest group on ultrasonography in pain medicine, who are also my friends and colleagues, for contributing essential chapters in their area of expertise: Dr. Eichenberger (Switzerland), Dr. Gofeld (Seattle), Dr. Morrigl (Austria), Dr. Peng (Canada), and Dr. Shankar (Wisconsin).

My sincere thanks to Dr. Galiano and Dr. Gruber of Austria for contributing two chapters to the book – and for introducing me to ultrasound-guided pain blocks when I visited their clinic in Innsbruck in 2005. I also acknowledge my esteemed colleagues from the University of Toronto for their help and support: Dr. Brull, Dr. McCartney, Dr. Perlas, Dr. Awad, Dr. Bhatia, and Dr. Riazi. I cannot thank enough my friends Dr. Huntoon (Mayo Clinic) and Dr. Karmakar (Hong Kong) for agreeing to contribute essential chapters despite their busy schedules. A special thank you to Dr. Ilfeld and Dr. Mariano (UCSD) for their help with the regional anesthesia section and to Dr. Bodor (UCSF), Dr. Hurdle (Mayo Clinic), and Dr. Schaefer (CWRU) for their help with the musculoskeletal (MSK) section.

I express my sincere thanks to all the Springer editorial staff for their expertise and help in editing this book and making it come to life on time.

I am very blessed that these experts agreed to contribute to my book, and I am very grateful to everyone.

Contents

II   Spine Sonoanatomy and Ultrasound-Guided Spine Injections

5   Spine Anatomy and Sonoanatomy for Pain Physicians 79

Bernhard Moriggl

6   Ultrasound-Guided Third Occipital Nerve and Cervical Medial Branch Nerve Blocks 107

Andreas Siegenthaler and Urs Eichenberger

III   Ultrasound-Guided Abdominal and Pelvic Blocks

V Musculoskeletal (MSK) Ultrasound

24   Ultrasound-Guided Hip Injections............................ 325

Hariharan Shankar and Swetha Simhan

25   Ultrasound-Guided Knee Injections 331

Mark-Friedrich B. Hurdle

VI   Advanced and New Applications of Ultrasound in Pain Management

26   Ultrasound-Guided Peripheral Nerve Stimulation 337

Marc A. Huntoon

Contributors

Imad T. Awad, MBChB, FCA, RSCI
Department of Anesthesia, Sunnybrook Health Sciences Center, University of Toronto,
2075 Bayview Avenue,
Toronto, ON, Canada M4N 3M5

Anuj Bhatia, MBBS, MD, DNB, MNAMS, FRCA, FFPMRCOA
Department of Anesthesia and Pain Management, University of Toronto, Toronto
Western Hospital, McL 2-405, 399 Bathurst Street, Toronto, ON, Canada M5T 2S8

Marko Bodor, MD
Department of Neurological Surgery, University of California San Francisco, and
Physical Medicine and Rehabilitation, Sports Medicine, Electrodiagnostic Medicine,
3421 Villa Lane 2B, Napa, CA, USA
mbodormd@sbcglobal.net

Richard Brull, MD, FRCPC
Department of Anesthesia, University of Toronto, Toronto Western Hospital, 399
Bathurst Street, MP 2-405, Toronto, ON, Canada M5T 2S8
Richard.Brull@uhn.on.ca

Chin-Wern Chan, MBBS, BMedSci, FANZCA
Wasser Pain Management Center and Department of Anesthesia, University Health
Network and Mount Sinai Hospital, 600 University Avenue, Toronto, ON, Canada
M5G 1X5

Vincent Chan, MD, FRCPC
Department of Anesthesia, University of Toronto, Toronto Western Hospital, 399
Bathurst Street, MP 2-405, Toronto, ON, Canada M5T 2S8
mail2vincechan@aol.com

Sean Colio, MD
Physical Medicine and Rehabilitation, Sports Medicine, Electrodiagnostic Medicine,
University of California San Francisco, 3421 Villa Lane 2B, Napa, CA 94558, USA

Urs Eichenberger, MD
Department of Anesthesiology and Pain Therapy, University Hospital of Bern,
Inselspital, Bern, Switzerland
Urs.Eichenberger@insel.ch

Kermit Fox, MD
Case Western Reserve University, Metro Health Rehabilitation Institute of Ohio, 2500 Metro Health Dr, Cleveland, OH 44109, USA

Klaus Galiano, MD, PhD
Department of Neurosurgery, Innsbruck Medical University, TILAK, Anichstrasse 35, Innsbruck 6020, Austria
klaus.galiano@i-med.ac.at

Michael Gofeld, MD
Department of Anesthesia and Pain Medicine, University of Washington School of Medicine, 4225 Roosevelt Way NE, Seattle, WA 98105, USA
gofeld@u.washington.edu

Hannes Gruber, MD, PhD
Department of Radiology, Innsbruck Medical University, TILAK, Anichstrasse 35, Innsbruck 6020, Austria
hannes.gruber@i-med.ac.at

Thomas M. Halaszynski, DMD, MD, MBA
Department of Anesthesiology, Yale University School of Medicine, 333 Cedar Street, TMP-3, P.O. Box 208051, New Haven, CT 06520-8051, USA
thomas.halaszynski@yale.edu

Marc A. Huntoon, M.D
Department of Anesthesiology, Division of Pain Medicine, Mayo Clinic, 200 1st street SW, Rochester, MN 55905, USA
Huntoon.Marc@mayo.edu

Mark-Friedrich B. Hurdle, M.D
Department of Anesthesiology and Pain Medicine, Mayo Clinic, 200 First Street SW, Rochester, MN 55905, USA
Hurdle.MarkFriedrich@mayo.edu

Brian M. Ilfeld, MD, MS
University of California San Diego, 9300 Campus Point Drive, MC 7651, San Diego, CA 92037-7651, USA
bilfeld@ucsd.edu

David M. Irwin, DO
Department of Anesthesia and Pain Medicine, University of Washington, 4225 Roosevelt Way NE, Seattle, WA 98105, USA

Manoj Kumar Karmakar, MD, FRCA, FHKCA, FHKAM
Department of Anaesthesia and Intensive Care, The Chinese University of Hong Kong, Prince of Wales Hospital, 32 Ngan Shing Street, Shatin, New Territories, Hong Kong
karmakar@cuhk.edu.hk

Imanuel Lerman, MD, MS
Yale New Haven Hospital, 69 Beacon Avenue, New Haven, CT 06512, USA
lerman2@gmail.com

John M. Lesher, MD, MPH
Carolina Neurosurgery and Spine Associates 9735 Kincey Avenue, Suite 301 Huntersville, NC 28078

Alan J. R. Macfarlane, BSc (Hons), MBChB, MRCP, FRCA
Glasgow Royal Infirmary, 84 Castle Street, Glasgow G4 0SF, UK

Edward R. Mariano, MD, MAS
Anesthesiology and Perioperative Care Service, Veterans Affairs Palo Alto Health
Care System, Stanford University School of Medicine, 3801 Miranda Avenue (112A),
Palo Alto, CA 94304, USA
emariano@stanford.edu

Colin J. L. McCartney, MBChB, FRCA, FCARCSI, FRCPC
Department of Anesthesia, Sunnybrook Health Sciences Center, University of Toronto,
2075 Bayview Avenue, Toronto, ON, Canada M4N 3M5
cjlmccartney@sympatico.ca

Bernhard Morrigl, MD
Department of Anatomy, Histology and Embryology, Division of Clinical and Functional
Anatomy, Innsbruck Medical University, Muellerstrasse 59, Innsbruck A-6020, Austria
bernhard.moriggl@i-med.ac.at

Haresh Mulchandani, MBChB, FRCA
Department of Anesthesia, Sunnybrook Health Sciences Center, University of Toronto,
2075 Bayview Avenue, Toronto, ON, Canada M4N 3M5

Samer N. Narouze, MD, MSc, DABPM, FIPP
Center for Pain Management, Summa Western Reserve Hospital, 1900 23rd Street,
Cuyahoga Falls, OH 44223, USA
narouzs@ccf.org

Philip W. H. Peng, MBBS, FRCPC
Department of Anesthesia, University of Toronto, Toronto Western Hospital, McL
2-405, 399 Bathurst Street, Toronto, ON, Canada M5T2S8
Philip.Peng@uhn.on.ca

Anahi Perlas, MD, FRCPC
Department of Anesthesia, University of Toronto, Toronto Western Hospital,
399 Bathurst Street, MP 2-405, Toronto, ON, Canada M5T 2S8
anahi.perlas@uhn.on.ca

Sheila Riazi, MD, FRCPC
Department of Anesthesia, University of Toronto, Toronto Western Hospital,
399 Bathurst Street, MP 2-405, Toronto, ON, Canada M5T 2S8

Michael P. Schaefer, MD
Case Western Reserve University, Metro Health Rehabilitation Institute of Ohio,
2500 Metro Health Dr, Cleveland, OH 44109, USA
mschaefer@metrohealth.org

Hariharan Shankar, MBBS
Department of Anesthesiology, Clement Zablocki VA Medical Center & Medical
College of Wisconsin, 5000 West National Avenue, Milwaukee, WI 53295, USA
hshankar@mcw.edu

Andreas Siegenthaler, MD
Department of Anesthesiology and Pain Therapy, University Hospital of Bern,
Inselspital, Bern, Switzerland

Swetha Simhan, MD
Department of Anesthesiology, Medical College of Wisconsin, 5000 West National
Avenue, Milwaukee, WI 53295, USA

Dmitri Souzdalnitski, MD, PhD
Department of Anesthesiology, Yale New Haven Hospital, TMP-3, 333 Cedar Street, New Haven, CT 06510, USA
dmitri.souzdalnitski@yale.edu

Cyrus C. H. Tse, BSc
Department of Anesthesia, University of Toronto, 399 Bathurst Street, MP 2-405, Toronto, ON, Canada M5T 2S8

Amaresh Vydyanathan, MD, MS
Department of Pain Medicine, Cleveland Clinic, 9500 Euclid Avenue, C25, Cleveland, OH 44195, USA
VYDYANA@ccf.org

I

Imaging in Interventional Pain Management and Basics of Ultrasonography

1

Imaging in Interventional Pain Management

Marc A. Huntoon

Introduction

Interventional pain procedures are commonly performed either with image-guidance fluoroscopy, computed tomography (CT), or ultrasound (US) or without image guidance utilizing surface landmarks. Recently, three-dimensional rotational angiography (3D-RA) suites, also known as flat detector computed tomography (FDCT) or cone beam CT (CBCT) and digital subtraction angiography (DSA) have been introduced as imaging

M.A. Huntoon(✉)
Department of Anesthesiology, Division of Pain Medicine, Mayo Clinic,
200 First Street SW, Rochester, MN 55905, USA
e-mail: Huntoon.Marc@mayo.edu

S.N. Narouze (ed.), *Atlas of Ultrasound-Guided Procedures in Interventional Pain Management*,
DOI 10.1007/978-1-4419-1681-5_1, © Springer Science+Business Media, LLC 2011

adjuncts. These systems are indicative of a trend toward increased use of specialized visualization techniques. Pain medicine practice guidelines suggest that most procedures require image guidance to improve the accuracy, reproducibility (precision), safety, and diagnostic information derived from the procedure.[1] Historically, pain medicine practitioners were slow adopters of image-guidance techniques, largely because the most common parent specialty (anesthesiology) had a culture of using surface landmarks to aid the perioperative performance of various nerve blocks and vascular line placements.[2] Indeed, some pain medicine practitioners in the 1980s and early 1990s felt that studies advocating the inaccuracy of epidural steroid injections performed with surface landmarks[3] were published more for specialty access than to increase patient safety or improve outcomes.

Ultrasound has recently exploded in popularity for perioperative regional blockade, but utilization of other imaging modalities in the perioperative arena, e.g., fluoroscopy, has lagged behind, despite more accurate placements compared to surface landmark-driven placements.[2] Technology acquisition costs and the physician learning required to master the new technologies are significant barriers to full implementation of many advanced imaging systems. However, the increasing national focus on safety in clinical medicine may ultimately mandate the use of optimal image guidance for selected procedures. In most cases, studies are lacking to compare the various types of image guidance in terms of patient outcomes, safety, and cost value for specific procedures. This is further complicated by the fact that many procedures in pain medicine have been considered poorly validated for the conditions being treated.[4-6] Thus, it may not matter if a particular image-guidance technique improves the reliability of a given procedure, if that procedure ultimately loses favor due to poor evidence or lack of evidence. Whether high-technology imaging brings safety and/or cost savings to the performance of evidence-based pain procedures is, thus, of paramount importance. The risks of the image guidance must also be considered as part of any imaging technology that is felt to be necessary for routine use. For example, a risk/benefit ratio of CT scanning relative to an equally suitable alternative technique may force physicians to use the lesser technology in some cases. CT as a diagnostic tool has come under greater scrutiny with the recent publication of several trials depicting the meteoric rise in the annual performance of CT scans (now over 72 million per year) and the large doses of radiation received by adults and particularly children.[7] Cancer risk from CT radiation has been modeled after longitudinal studies of cancer occurrences in atomic bomb survivors.[8] Now, it seems that the risk of cancer is something that should be more actively considered when CT is utilized. Radiation risks are not trivial, and likely amount to about 14,000 or more future cancer deaths as a consequence of year 2007 CT scans.[7] For those treating patients with chronic pain, one needs to merely consider how many patients with an elusive diagnosis receive advanced imaging in efforts to find the cause of that pain. Thus, repeating imaging studies with a fairly low yield may actually be harming our patients. Ultrasound guidance, the focus of this atlas, has many advocates for these same radiation safety issues.[9] The use of ultrasound, however, is limited in many obese or larger adults,[10] and the cost of some advanced systems capable of rendering deeper structures with high clarity can surpass the cost for fluoroscopes in some cases. The use of imaging modalities such as 3D-RA and DSA are being advocated by others. While a FDCT suite is extremely expensive, DSA is actually a relatively inexpensive add-on to a conventional fluoroscope that may have a substantial role in the safe performance of transforaminal epidural steroid injections.[11] For example, when performing injections or other procedures in critical areas, such as the left T11 and 12, the territory of the great segmental medullary artery of Adamkiewicz, digital subtraction can demonstrate vascular uptake more clearly (Figure 1.1). Chap. 2 focuses on the limited studies currently present in the literature, with suggestions for areas where one imaging modality may have certain advantages over another. Ultimately, further study will be necessary to ascertain the most safe, accurate, and cost-effective practices for image-guided procedures.

Figure 1.1. A digital subtraction image of a thoracic dorsal root ganglion contrast injection at T11 prior to pulsed radiofrequency. Note that the contrast spreads medial to the pedicle. Below, a second needle has been placed at the pedicle of T12 just inferior to the sagittal bisector.

C-Arm FDCT

Most pain procedures require cross-sectional or 3D soft tissue imaging to accurately target structures in a complex anatomical landscape. Very few procedures are intended to target bony structures, with the exception of such procedures as vertebral and sacral augmentation, bone biopsies, and a few others. Yet, fluoroscopy remains the most popular imaging method, for primarily soft tissue targets, despite its limitations. Intradiskal procedures, vertebral augmentation, neuromodulation procedures, and deep abdominopelvic and head and neck blocks may be examples of some procedures where a limited CT scan capability (FDCT) would enhance the accuracy and safety of the procedure as compared to plain fluoroscopy. C-arm FDCT or C-arm CBCT utilize different gantries, but are nearly synonymous terms for a modern 3D imaging system that can also integrate 2D data from fluoroscopy, sometimes US, and DSA in a single suite. Interventional radiologists and some pain physicians are using these advanced image-guidance systems to aid procedural performance in certain cases, with an expanding list of potential indications. FDCT is accomplished via a single rotation of the fluoroscope gantry, rendering a complete volumetric data set using a flat panel detector. These flat panel detectors have significantly better resolution than older image intensifiers. This is in contrast to conventional CT which uses multiple detectors and requires several rotations of the gantry, with the patient being moved into the CT scanner.[12] With FDCT, the patient is stationary through the imaging cycle. CT images do take approximately 5–20 s to be acquired, thus this is not a true real-time CT fluoroscopy procedure. Images from FDCT scanning have lower resolution due to scattered radiation, but in many cases the lower resolution images are more than adequate for the intended procedure. However, during the 200° gantry rotation of a FDCT system, experiments have shown that radiation doses are less than that for a single helical CT.[12] Carefully limiting the field of scanning will decrease radiation dose to the patient and improve image contrast. CBCT units may have significant application for intraoperative minimally invasive surgical applications. Surgeons using CBCT for mini-

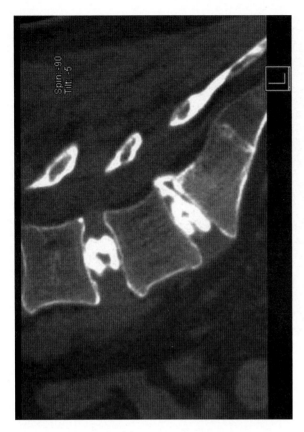

Figure 1.2. A sagittal CT view of a two level diskogram. Note an annular tear at L5/S1 with epidural extravasation.

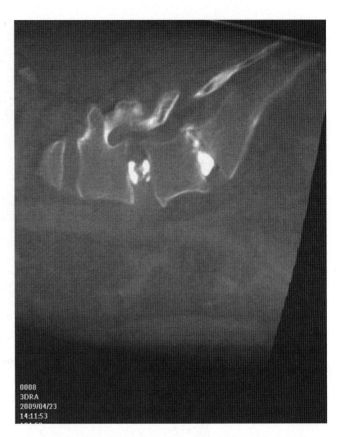

Figure 1.3. Compare similar FDCT/3D-RA sagittal diskogram in same patient as above. The epidural extravasation is seen again.

mally invasive spine procedures tended to want to utilize the higher technology of the CBCT in their cases in an escalating fashion with increasing exposure to the new technology.[13]

Many creative interventionalists are adapting the FDCT capability to new procedures, such as diskography, without the need for a postprocedural standard CT (Figures 1.2 and 1.3). In diskography, it is usual and customary to perform contrast injections into the presumed diseased disk as well as a control disk. A postprocedural delayed CT image to better quantitate annular tears and contrast leak into the spinal canal is considered standard. CBCT technology may allow these CT images to be performed in the same suite, saving time and expense. This "single-suite" concept for specific blocks can also save on radiation exposure for both the patient and the physicians.

Deep plexus blocks such as celiac or superior hypogastric plexus blocks may benefit from the ability to better quantitate the spread of injected contrast in multiple planes. Potentially, factors such as local tumor burden or lymphadenopathy that limit the spread of the contrast and neurolytic solution may be noted earlier with these advanced imaging techniques. For example, Goldschneider et al [14] performed celiac plexus blocks in children utilizing 3D-RA to show the benefits of examining contrast spread in three dimensions. Similarly, superior hypogastric blocks (Figure 1.4a–c) have added detail when a 3D image is rendered. In another recent report,[15] Knight et al performed vertebroplasty in a patient with a retropulsed bone fragment in the spinal canal, normally at least a relative contraindication. The authors utilized FDCT technology to visualize these areas during injection of the polymethylmethacrylate cement and avoid spinal cord injury.[15] Neuromodulation, particularly spinal cord stimulation, may be more easily targeted in some cases with FDCT technology. The anterior or lateral movement of the electrodes could more easily be seen, eliminating the need for multiple repositionings of the electrode

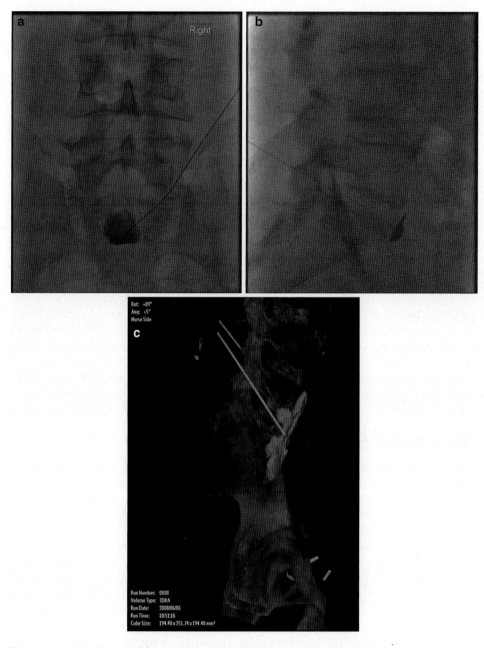

Figure 1.4. (a) AP view of fluoroscopic superior hypogastric plexus block, (b) lateral view of superior hypogastric plexus block, and (c) 3D-RA view of contrast in three dimensions.

and needle in the epidural space. The utilization of FDCT/CBCT/3D-RA technology to better treat patients seems to be limited only by one's imagination.

Ultrasound

Ultrasound has become extremely popular in acute pain block procedures, and chronic pain practitioners are slowly adopting ultrasound as both a diagnostic and image-guided block aid. Chronic pain procedures may include nerve blocks (such as the brachial or lumbar plexus) commonly performed in an acute perioperative nerve block suite, but also may require image-guided injection of more distal branches of the plexus, or at less common locations (proximal to sites of trauma or entrapment or neuroma formation). Blockade of various small sensory or mixed nerves, such as the ilioinguinal,[16,17] lateral femoral cutaneous,[18] suprascapular,[19] pudendal,[20] intercostal,[21] and various other sites have been performed. In addition, many spinal procedures including epidurals, selective spinal nerve blocks,[22,23] facet joint, medial branch blocks, and third occipital nerve blocks,[24,25] as well as sympathetic blocks (stellate ganglion)[26] may be performed. Finally, a broad array of possible applications for peripheral neuromodulation electrode placement may be possible with ultrasound guidance[27] (see Chapter 26).

Intra-Articular Injections

Intra-articular injections of medications (primarily corticosteroids) are extremely common procedures performed by physicians from primary care disciplines as well as specialists. While few would dispute that these procedures are easy to do and very accurate, whether image guidance can improve the outcome of intra-articular procedures was not specifically known. A recent study of intra-articular injections suggests that these may be one area where the use of image guidance is useful.[28] The study of 148 painful joints (shoulder, knee, ankle, wrist, hip) compared the use of US guidance to a surface landmark-based injection. The authors found that the use of US led to a 43% decrease in procedural pain, a 25.6% increase in the rate of responders, and a 62% decrease in the nonresponder rate. Sonography also increased the rate of detection of effusion by 200% as compared to use of surface landmarks. None would dispute that the use of image guidance would add to the cost of the actual procedures. However, health care economics studies would be required to ascertain whether the improved outcomes would lead to better health care value viewed through a long-term perspective.

Trigger Point and Muscular Injections

The performance of most deep muscular and trigger point injections has been relegated to a trivial office-based procedure, generating little enthusiasm from the interventional pain community. Image guidance (fluoroscopy) for these soft-tissue structures was not helpful, and many physicians considered the performance of the procedures to be "the art of medicine." However, the addition of ultrasound may be changing the way one views these procedures. Certainly, it is easy to see how a target such as the piriformis muscle could be identified more accurately using US. It is likely that fluoroscopic techniques may actually mistake the gluteal or quadratus femoris muscles on occasion. In addition, the anatomic variability and proximity of neurovascular structures, including the sciatic nerve, make visualization important. US also allows the use of a diagnostic exam (hip rotation) to aid in the proper identification of the muscle (Figure 1.5). Studies to date suggest that the piriformis muscle is easily injected using this modality.[29] Other muscular targets such as trigger points have been targeted using US guidance.[30] Pneumothorax is an all too frequent complication of thoracic area trigger points. In the 2004 ASA Closed Claims Project, 59 pneumothorax claims were filed. Of this 59, fully half (23 intercostal blocks and 1 costochondral injection) would likely have been preventable under US guidance. Additionally, 15 of the cases were trigger point muscular injections which would likely be preventable as well. Together, at least 2/3 of the pneumothorax claims (and likely even more) could be prevented with better imaging.[31]

Whether the use of US or another imaging technique is justified in all cases by the avoidance of complications may depend on a more accurate depiction of the true incidence of complications and better outcome data. Certainly, it may be true that positive responses could be more accurately replicated in some cases.

Zygapophyseal and Medial Branch Blocks

One of the better studies of ultrasound guidance in pain medicine evaluated third occipital nerve block procedures and peaked interest in US for many in the pain medicine

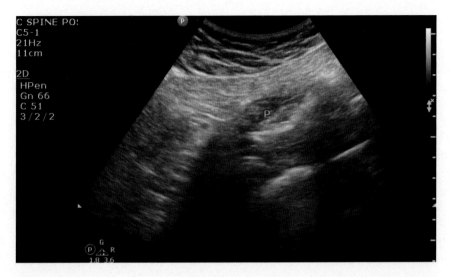

Figure 1.5. A dynamic exam is depicted wherein the piriformis muscle (P) is contracted.

community.[24] The third occipital nerve had been suggested as a therapeutic target for conditions, including high-cervical spondylosis and cervicogenic headaches, and as a predictor of success for radiofrequency ablative procedures. In that study, the accuracy of US guidance compared to that of fluoroscopy was good, with 23 of 28 needles demonstrating accurate radiographic positioning.[24] Fluoroscopic procedures targeting the third occipital nerve around the C2/3 zygapophyseal joint have been performed utilizing three sequential needle placements. These fluoroscopy-guided placements have been very accurate, but suffer from the inability to actually see the targeted nerve. Whether US is superior in some way to standard fluoroscopy remains to be tested.

Epidural Blocks

Epidural techniques including interlaminar, caudal, and selective spinal root blocks have been studied in limited fashion utilizing ultrasound guidance. Fluoroscopy techniques are extremely easy and generally use small amounts of radiation, thus the advocates for US will need to perform comparative studies to demonstrate any particular advantages. Caudal procedures are perhaps most promising in this regard.

Caution should be exercised until mechanisms of ischemic injury during transforaminal epidural procedures are better understood. Lack of a contrast control in US in spite of "extraforaminal" vascular structure visibility is the most significant drawback. Even CT scanning is not foolproof for cervical transforaminal corticosteroid injections.[11,22,23]

Sympathetic Blocks

Sympathetic blocks have been studied in limited fashion with ultrasound guidance. Stellate ganglion block (SGB) was performed at C6 anterior to Chassaignac's tubercle based on surface landmarks for years prior to modern fluoroscopy techniques which have become the standard of care in most regions. A recent analysis of 27 previously reported cases of retropharyngeal hematoma after SGB emphasized the potential for delayed bleeding and hematoma formation.[32] Although image-guided techniques were not described in this review, aspiration of blood was negative in all but four cases requiring needle redirection. One of the earliest papers examining US guidance was by Kapral et al.[26] In this study, the nonultrasound group had three hematomas. The authors theorized that the vertebral artery might be more likely to be involved in left-sided injections. They and other researchers have raised the possibility of other arteries at risk, specifically, the ascending cervical branch off the inferior thyroid artery, which commonly passes over the C6 anterior tubercle.[33] No head to head comparison studies of ultrasound vs. CT or fluoroscopy for SGB have yet been performed. The advantages of ultrasound would seem to be avoidance of vascular or soft tissue injuries. Advantages of fluoroscopy or CT would appear to be ease of interpreting contrast spread patterns, and better representation of 3D anatomy in the case of CT.

Combined US and CT/Fluoroscopy

The use of combinations of these imaging modalities has had limited study to date, but may have some indications as time and experience accumulates. For example, peripheral nerve stimulation may be best accomplished with US and FDCT, or US and fluoroscopy.[27] It is possible that combined imaging techniques of US-fluoroscopy, CT-fluoroscopy, and US/CT and other combined techniques may become normalized in particularly complicated procedures.

Conclusion

The future of image guidance for pain medicine interventions must balance risk to the patient and clinician from ionizing radiation, risks of procedural complications, outcomes, and relative value. Although ultrasound imaging is feasible in many instances, best practice may favor fluoroscopy or CT in some cases. Ultrasound appears to have advantages for musculoskeletal diagnosis and therapy for some joint and soft tissue conditions, procedures where the peritoneum or pleura may be punctured, deep muscle injections, most peripheral nerve procedures, possibly SGB, possibly caudal epidurals, and perhaps equivalency for sacroiliac joint and some medial branch blocks. Other uses will require ongoing comparison to other image-guidance techniques. The following table compares the relative attributes of various imaging techniques, and points out areas where one image-guidance modality may have unique advantages relative to another (Table 1.1).

Table 1.1. Comparison of relative attributes of various imaging techniques.

Procedure	Guidance	+Attributes	Problems
Sympathetic blocks			
Stellate ganglion	Fluoroscopy	Contrast use	Soft tissues not seen
	US	Visualize vessels, fascia/ muscle	Advanced skills needed
Celiac plexus	CT, FDCT	3D anatomy in cross section	Delayed contrast, increased radiation
	Fluoroscopy	Real-time contrast	No 3D imaging
Epidurals			
Caudal	Fluoroscopy	Lateral view	Minimal, radiation
	US	Real-time contrast Needle visualization No radiation	Contrast flow
Lumbar TF	Fluoroscopy	Real-time contrast	Missed vascular injection
	DSA	Vessel detection	Equipment availability
	US	No role	Obesity Poor visualization
Lumbar IL	Fluoroscopy	Contrast use	Minimal radiation
	US	Needle entry	Poor contrast

(Continued)

Table 1.1. (Continued)

Procedure	Guidance	+Attributes	Problems
Cervical TF	Fluoroscopy	Real-time contrast	Miss vascular injection
	DSA	Vessel detection	Equipment availability
	US	Vessel detection	Contrast flow
	CT	3D anatomy	Radiation increased
		Vertebral artery visible	Small vessels missed
Lumbar medial branch block	Fluoroscopy	Easy, contrast use	Small
	US	Fair visual	Obese patient technically difficult
Cervical medial branch block	Fluoroscopy	Easy, contrast use	Small
	US	Fair visual	Obese, technically difficult
Lumbar facet joint	Fluoroscopy	Easy, contrast use	Small
	US	Feasible	Obesity
Cervical facet joint	Fluoroscopy	Contrast	Difficult
	US	Feasible	Advanced

CT computed tomography, *DSA* digital subtraction angiography, *FDCT* flat detector computed tomography, *US* ultrasound, TF transforaminal epidural

References

1. Manchikanti L, Boswell MV, Singh V, et al. Comprehensive evidence-based guidelines for interventional techniques in the management of chronic spinal pain. *Pain Physician.* 2009,12: 699–802.
2. Huntoon MA. Ultrasound in pain medicine: advanced weaponry or just a fad? *Reg Anesth Pain Med.* 2009;34:387–388.
3. el-Khoury GY, Ehara S, Weinstein JN, Montgomery WJ, Kathol MH. Epidural steroid injection: a procedure ideally performed with fluoroscopic control. *Radiology.* 1988;168:554–557.
4. American College of Occupational and Environmental Medicine. *Low Back Disorders. Occupational Medicine Practice Guidelines.* 2nd ed. Elk Grove Village, IL: American College of Occupational and Environmental Medicine; 2008 [chapter 12].
5. Manchikanti L, Singh V, Derby R, et al. Review of occupational medicine practice guidelines for interventional pain management and potential implications. *Pain Physician.* 2008;11:271–289.
6. Manchikanti L, Singh V, Helm S II, Trescot A, Hirsch JA. A critical appraisal of 2007 American College of Occupational and Environmental Medicine practice guidelines for interventional pain management: an independent review utilizing AGREE, AMA, IOM, and other criteria. *Pain Physician.* 2008;11:291–310.
7. Berrington de Gonzalez A, Mahesh M, Kim K-P, et al. Projected cancer risks from computed tomographic scans performed in the United States in 2007. *Arch Intern Med.* 2009;169: 2071–2077.
8. Brenner DJ, Hall EJ. Computed tomography – an increasing source of radiation exposure. *N Engl J Med.* 2007;357:2277–2284.
9. Gofeld M. Ultrasonography in pain medicine: a critical review. *Pain Pract.* 2008;8:226–240.
10. Galiano K, Obwegeser AA, Walch C, et al. Ultrasound-guided versus computed tomography-controlled facet joint injections in the lumbar spine: a prospective randomized clinical trial. *Reg Anesth Pain Med.* 2007;32:317–322.
11. Huntoon MA. Anatomy of the cervical intervertebral foramina: vulnerable arteries and ischemic neurologic injuries after transforaminal epidural injections. *Pain.* 2005;117:104–111.
12. Orth RC, Wallace MJ, Kuo MD. C-arm cone-beam CT: general principles and technical considerations for use in interventional radiology. *J Vasc Interv Radiol.* 2008;19:814–821.

13. Siewerdsen JH, Moseley DJ, Burch S, et al. Volume CT with flat-panel detector on a mobile, isocentric C-arm: pre-clinical investigation in guidance of minimally invasive surgery. *Med Phys.* 2005;32:241–254.

14. Goldschneider KR, Racadio JM, Weidner NJ. Celiac plexus blockade in children using a three-dimensional fluoroscopic reconstruction technique: case reports. *Reg Anesth Pain Med.* 2007;32: 510–515.

15. Knight JR, Heran M, Munk PL, Raabe R, Liu DM. C-arm cone-beam CT: applications for spinal cement augmentation demonstrated by three cases. *J Vasc Interv Radiol.* 2008;19:1118–1122.

16. Eichenberger U, Greher M, Kirchmair L, et al. Ultrasound-guided blocks of the ilioinguinal and iliohypogastric nerve: accuracy of a selective new technique confirmed by anatomical dissection. *Br J Anaesth.* 2006;97:238–243.

17. Gofeld M, Christakis M. Sonographically guided ilioinguinal nerve block. *J Ultrasound Med.* 2006;25:1571–1575.

18. Hurdle M-F, Weingarten TN, Crisostomo RA, et al. Ultrasound-guided blockade of the lateral femoral cutaneous nerve: technical description and report of 10 cases. *Arch Phys Med Rehabil.* 2007;88:1362–1364.

19. Harmon D, Hearty C. Ultrasound guided suprascapular nerve block technique. *Pain Physician.* 2007;10:743–746.

20. Rofaeel A, Peng P, Louis I, Chan V. Feasibility of real-time ultrasound for pudendal nerve block in patients with chronic perineal pain. *Reg Anesth Pain Med.* 2008;33:139–145.

21. Byas-Smith MG, Gulati A. Ultrasound-guided intercostal nerve cryoablation. *Anesth Analg.* 2006;103:1033–1035.

22. Galiano K, Obwegeser AA, Bodner G, et al. Real-time sonographic imaging for periradicular injections in the lumbar spine: a sonographic anatomic study of a new technique. *J Ultrasound Med.* 2005;24:33–38.

23. Narouze S, Vydyanathan A, Kapural L, Sessler DI, Mekhail N. Ultrasound-guided cervical selective nerve root block: a fluoroscopy-controlled feasibility study. *Reg Anesth Pain Med.* 2009;34(4): 343–348.

24. Eichenberger U, Greher M, Kapral S, et al. Sonographic visualization and ultrasound-guided block of the third occipital nerve: prospective for a new method to diagnose C2/3 zygapophysial joint pain. *Anesthesiology.* 2006;104:303–308.

25. Galiano K, Obwegeser AA, Bodner G, et al. Ultrasound-guided facet joint injections in the middle to lower cervical spine: a CT-controlled sonoanatomic study. *Clin J Pain.* 2006;22: 538–543.

26. Kapral S, Krafft P, Gosch M, Fleischmann M, Weinstabl C. Ultrasound imaging for stellate ganglion block: direct visualization of puncture site and local anesthetic spread. A pilot study. *Reg Anesth.* 1995;20:323–328.

27. Hayek SM, Jasper J, Deer TR, Narouze S. Occipital neurostimulation-induced muscle spasms: implications for lead placement. *Pain Physician.* 2009;12(5):867–876.

28. Sibbitt WL Jr, Peisajovich A, Michael AA, et al. Does sonographic needle guidance affect the clinical outcome of intraarticular injections? *J Rheumatol.* 2009;36:1892–1902.

29. Smith J, Hurdle M-F, Locketz AJ, Wisnewski SJ. Ultrasound-guided piriformis injection: technique description and verification. *Arch Phys Med Rehabil.* 2006;87:1664–1667.

30. Botwin KP, Sharma K, Saliba R, Patel BC. Ultrasound-guided trigger point injections in the cervicothoracic musculature: a new and unreported technique. *Pain Physician.* 2008;11:885–889.

31. Fitzgibbon DR, Posner KL, Domino KB, et al. Chronic pain management: ASA Closed Claims Project. *Anesthesiology.* 2004;100:98–105.

32. Higa K, Hirata K, Hirota K, Nitahara K, Shono S. Retropharyngeal hematoma after stellate ganglion block. *Anesthesiology.* 2006;105:1238–1245.

33. Narouze S. Beware of the "serpentine" inferior thyroid artery while performing stellate ganglion block. *Anesth Analg.* 2009;109(1):289–290.

2

Basics of Ultrasound Imaging

Vincent Chan and Anahi Perlas

Introduction

Ultrasound has been used to image the human body for over half a century. Dr. Karl Theo Dussik, an Austrian neurologist, was the first to apply ultrasound as a medical diagnostic tool to image the brain.[1] Today, ultrasound (US) is one of the most widely used imaging technologies in medicine. It is portable, free of radiation risk, and relatively inexpensive when compared with other imaging modalities, such as magnetic resonance and computed tomography. Furthermore, US images are tomographic, i.e., offering a "cross-sectional" view of anatomical structures. The images can be acquired in "real time," thus providing instantaneous visual guidance for many interventional procedures including those for regional anesthesia and pain management. In this chapter, we describe some of the fundamental principles and physics underlying US technology that are relevant to the pain practitioner.

V. Chan (✉)
Department of Anesthesia, University of Toronto, Toronto Western Hospital,
399 Bathurst Street MP 2-405, Toronto, ON, Canada M5T 2S8
e-mail: mail2vincechan@aol.com

S.N. Narouze (ed.), *Atlas of Ultrasound-Guided Procedures in Interventional Pain Management*,
DOI 10.1007/978-1-4419-1681-5_2, © Springer Science+Business Media, LLC 2011

Basic Principles of B-Mode US

Modern medical US is performed primarily using a pulse-echo approach with a brightness-mode (B-mode) display. The basic principles of B-mode imaging are much the same today as they were several decades ago. This involves transmitting small pulses of ultrasound echo from a transducer into the body. As the ultrasound waves penetrate body tissues of different acoustic impedances along the path of transmission, some are reflected back to the transducer (echo signals) and some continue to penetrate deeper. The echo signals returned from many sequential coplanar pulses are processed and combined to generate an image. Thus, an ultrasound transducer works both as a speaker (generating sound waves) and a microphone (receiving sound waves). The ultrasound pulse is in fact quite short, but since it traverses in a straight path, it is often referred to as an ultrasound beam. The direction of ultrasound propagation along the beam line is called the axial direction, and the direction in the image plane perpendicular to axial is called the lateral direction.[2] Usually only a small fraction of the ultrasound pulse returns as a reflected echo after reaching a body tissue interface, while the remainder of the pulse continues along the beam line to greater tissue depths.

Generation of Ultrasound Pulses

Ultrasound transducers (or probes) contain multiple piezoelectric crystals which are interconnected electronically and vibrate in response to an applied electric current. This phenomenon called the piezoelectric effect was originally described by the Curie brothers in 1880 when they subjected a cut piece of quartz to mechanical stress generating an electric charge on the surface.[3] Later, they also demonstrated the reverse piezoelectric effect, i.e., electricity application to the quartz resulting in quartz vibration.[4] These vibrating mechanical sound waves create alternating areas of compression and rarefaction when propagating through body tissues. Sound waves can be described in terms of their frequency (measured in cycles per second or hertz), wavelength (measured in millimeter), and amplitude (measured in decibel).

Ultrasound Wavelength and Frequency

The wavelength and frequency of US are inversely related, i.e., ultrasound of high frequency has a short wavelength and vice versa. US waves have frequencies that exceed the upper limit for audible human hearing, i.e., greater than 20 kHz.[3] Medical ultrasound devices use sound waves in the range of 1–20 MHz. Proper selection of transducer frequency is an important concept for providing optimal image resolution in diagnostic and procedural US. High-frequency ultrasound waves (short wavelength) generate images of high axial resolution. Increasing the number of waves of compression and rarefaction for a given distance can more accurately discriminate between two separate structures along the axial plane of wave propagation. However, high-frequency waves are more attenuated than lower frequency waves for a given distance; thus, they are suitable for imaging mainly superficial structures.[5] Conversely, low-frequency waves (long wavelength) offer images of lower resolution but can penetrate to deeper structures due to a lower degree of attenuation (Figure 2.1). For this reason, it is best to use high-frequency transducers (up to 10–15 MHz range) to image superficial structures (such as for stellate ganglion blocks) and low-frequency transducers (typically 2–5 MHz) for imaging the lumbar neuraxial structures that are deep in most adults (Figure 2.2).

Ultrasound waves are generated in pulses (intermittent trains of pressure) that commonly consist of two or three sound cycles of the same frequency (Figure 2.3). The pulse

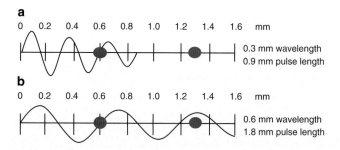

Figure 2.1. Attenuation of ultrasound waves and its relationship to wave frequency. Note that higher frequency waves are more highly attenuated than lower frequency waves for a given distance. Reproduced with permission from ref.[6]

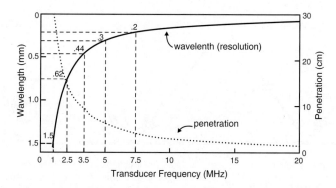

Figure 2.2. A comparison of the resolution and penetration of different ultrasound transducer frequencies. This figure was published in ref.[3] Copyright Elsevier (2000).

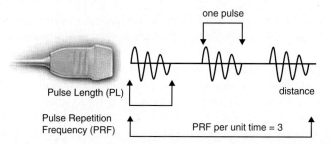

Figure 2.3. Schematic representation of ultrasound pulse generation. Reproduced with permission from ref.[6]

repetition frequency (PRF) is the number of pulses emitted by the transducer per unit of time. Ultrasound waves must be emitted in pulses with sufficient time in between to allow the signal to reach the target of interest and be reflected back to the transducer as echo before the next pulse is generated. The PRF for medical imaging devices ranges from 1 to 10 kHz.

Ultrasound – Tissue Interaction

As US waves travel through tissues, they are partly transmitted to deeper structures, partly reflected back to the transducer as echoes, partly scattered, and partly transformed to heat. For imaging purposes, we are mostly interested in the echoes reflected back to the transducer. The amount of echo returned after hitting a tissue interface is determined by a tissue property called acoustic impedance. This is an intrinsic physical property of a medium defined as the density of the medium times the velocity of US wave propagation in the

Table 2.1. Acoustic impedances of different body tissues and organs.

Body tissue	Acoustic impedance (10^6 Rayls)
Air	0.0004
Lung	0.18
Fat	1.34
Liver	1.65
Blood	1.65
Kidney	1.63
Muscle	1.71
Bone	7.8

Reproduced with permission from ref.[6]

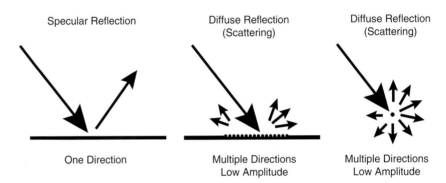

Figure 2.4. Different types of ultrasound wave–tissue interactions. Reproduced with permission from ref.[6]

medium. Air-containing organs (such as the lung) have the lowest acoustic impedance, while dense organs such as bone have very high-acoustic impedance (Table 2.1). The intensity of a reflected echo is proportional to the difference (or mismatch) in acoustic impedances between two mediums. If two tissues have identical acoustic impedance, no echo is generated. Interfaces between soft tissues of similar acoustic impedances usually generate low-intensity echoes. Conversely interfaces between soft tissue and bone or the lung generate very strong echoes due to a large acoustic impedance gradient.[7]

When an incident ultrasound pulse encounters a large, smooth interface of two body tissues with different acoustic impedances, the sound energy is reflected back to the transducer. This type of reflection is called specular reflection, and the echo intensity generated is proportional to the acoustic impedance gradient between the two mediums (Figure 2.4). A soft-tissue–needle interface when a needle is inserted "in-plane" is a good example of specular reflection. If the incident US beam reaches the linear interface at 90°, almost all of the generated echo will travel back to the transducer. However, if the angle of incidence with the specular boundary is less than 90°, the echo will not return to the transducer, but rather be reflected at an angle equal to the angle of incidence (just like visible light reflecting in a mirror). The returning echo will potentially miss the transducer and not be detected. This is of practical importance for the pain physician, and explains why it may be difficult to image a needle that is inserted at a very steep direction to reach deeply located structures.

Refraction refers to a change in the direction of sound transmission after hitting an interface of two tissues with different speeds of sound transmission. In this instance, because the sound frequency is constant, the wavelength has to change to accommodate the difference in the speed of sound transmission in the two tissues. This results in a redirection of the sound pulse as it passes through the interface. Refraction is one of the important causes of incorrect localization of a structure on an ultrasound image. Because the speed of sound is low in fat (approximately 1,450 m/s) and high in soft tissues (approximately 1,540 m/s), refraction artifacts are most prominent at fat/soft tissue interfaces.

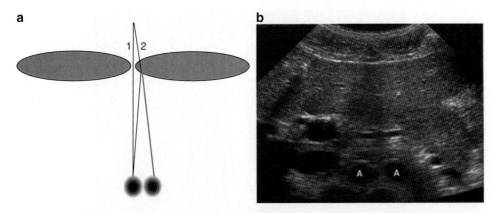

Figure 2.5. Refraction artifact. Diagram (**a**) shows how sound beam refraction results in duplication artifact. (**b**) is a transverse midline view of the upper abdomen showing duplication of the aorta (A) secondary to rectus muscle refraction. This figure was published in ref.[8] Copyright Elsevier (2004).

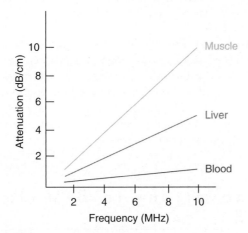

Figure 2.6. Degrees of attenuation of ultrasound beams as a function of the wave frequency in different body tissues. Reproduced with permission from ref.[6]

The most widely recognized refraction artifact occurs at the junction of the rectus abdominis muscle and abdominal wall fat. The end result is duplication of deep abdominal and pelvic structures seen when scanning through the abdominal midline (Figure 2.5). Duplication artifacts can also arise when scanning the kidney due to refraction of sound at the interface between the spleen (or liver) and adjacent fat.[8]

If the ultrasound pulse encounters reflectors whose dimensions are smaller than the ultrasound wavelength, or when the pulse encounters a rough, irregular tissue interface, scattering occurs. In this case, echoes reflected through a wide range of angles result in reduction in echo intensity. However, the positive result of scattering is the return of some echo to the transducer regardless of the angle of the incident pulse. Most biologic tissues appear in US images as though they are filled with tiny scattering structures. The speckle signal that provides the visible texture in organs like the liver or muscle is a result of interface between multiple scattered echoes produced within the volume of the incident ultrasound pulse.[2]

As US pulses travel through tissue, their intensity is reduced or attenuated. This attenuation is the result of reflection and scattering and also of friction-like losses. These losses result from the induced oscillatory tissue motion produced by the pulse, which causes conversion of energy from the original mechanical form into heat. This energy loss to localized heating is referred to as absorption and is the most important contributor to US attenuation. Longer path length and higher frequency waves result in greater attenuation. Attenuation also varies among body tissues, with the highest degree in bone, less in muscle and solid organs, and lowest in blood for any given frequency (Figure 2.6). All ultrasound

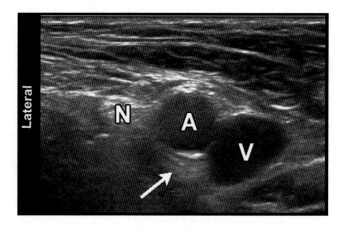

Figure 2.7. Sonographic image of the femoral neurovascular structures in the inguinal area. A hyperechoic area can be appreciated deep to the femoral artery (*arrowhead*). This well-known artifact (known as posterior acoustic enhancement) is typically seen deep to fluid-containing structures. *N* femoral nerve, *A* femoral artery, *V* femoral vein.

equipment intrinsically compensates for an expected average degree of attenuation by automatically increasing the gain (overall brightness or intensity of signals) in deeper areas of the screen. This is the cause for a very common artifact known as "posterior acoustic enhancement" that describes a relatively hyperechoic area posterior to large blood vessels or cysts (Figure 2.7). Fluid-containing structures attenuate sound much less than solid structures so that the strength of the sound pulse is greater after passing through fluid than through an equivalent amount of solid tissue.

Recent Innovations in B-Mode Ultrasound

Some recent innovations that have become available in most ultrasound units over the past decade or so have significantly improved image resolution. Two good examples of these are tissue harmonic imaging and spatial compound imaging.

The benefits of tissue harmonic imaging were first observed in work geared toward imaging of US contrast materials. The term harmonic refers to frequencies that are integral multiples of the frequency of the transmitted pulse (which is also called the fundamental frequency or first harmonic).[9] The second harmonic has a frequency of twice the fundamental. As an ultrasound pulse travels through tissues, the shape of the original wave is distorted from a perfect sinusoid to a "sharper," more peaked, sawtooth shape. This distorted wave in turn generates reflected echoes of several different frequencies, of many higher order harmonics. Modern ultrasound units use not only a fundamental frequency but also its second harmonic component. This often results in the reduction of artifacts and clutter in the near surface tissues. Harmonic imaging is considered to be most useful in "technically difficult" patients with thick and complicated body wall structures.

Spatial compound imaging (or multibeam imaging) refers to the electronic steering of ultrasound beams from an array transducer to image the same tissue multiple times by using parallel beams oriented along different directions.[10] The echoes from these different directions are then averaged together (compounded) into a single composite image. The use of multiple beams results in an averaging out of speckles, making the image look less "grainy" and increasing the lateral resolution. Spatial compound images often show reduced levels of "noise" and "clutter" as well as improved contrast and margin definition. Because multiple ultrasound beams are used to interrogate the same tissue region, more time is required for data acquisition and the compound imaging frame rate is generally reduced compared with that of conventional B-mode imaging.

Conclusion

US is relatively inexpensive, portable, safe, and real time in nature. These characteristics, and continued improvements in image quality and resolution have expanded the use of US to many areas in medicine beyond traditional diagnostic imaging applications. In particular, its use to assist or guide interventional procedures is growing. Regional anesthesia and pain medicine procedures are some of the areas of current growth. Modern US equipment is based on many of the same fundamental principles employed in the initial devices used over 50 years ago. The understanding of these basic physical principles can help the anesthesiologist and pain practitioner better understand this new tool and use it to its full potential.

References

1. Edler I, Lindstrom K. The history of echocardiography. *Ultrasound Med Biol.* 2004;30: 1565–1644.
2. Hangiandreou N. AAPM/RSNA physics tutorial for residents: topics in US. B-mode US: basic concepts and new technology. *Radiographics.* 2003;23:1019–1033.
3. Otto CM. Principles of echocardiographic image acquisition and Doppler analysis. In: *Textbook of Clinical Ecocardiography.* 2nd ed. Philadelphia, PA: WB Saunders; 2000:1–29.
4. Weyman AE. Physical principles of ultrasound. In: Weyman AE, ed. *Principles and Practice of Echocardiography.* 2nd ed. Media, PA: Williams & Wilkins; 1994:3–28.
5. Lawrence JP. Physics and instrumentation of ultrasound. *Crit Care Med.* 2007;35:S314–S322.
6. Chan VWS. *Ultrasound Imaging for Regional Anesthesia.* 2nd ed. Toronto, ON: Toronto Printing Company; 2009.
7. Kossoff G. Basic physics and imaging characteristics of ultrasound. *World J Surg.* 2000;24: 134–142.
8. Middleton W, Kurtz A, Hertzberg B. Practical physics. In: *Ultrasound, the Requisites.* 2nd ed. St Louis, MO: Mosby; 2004:3–27.
9. Fowlkes JB, Averkiou M. Contrast and tissue harmonic imaging. In: Goldman LW, Fowlkes JB, eds. *Categorical Courses in Diagnostic Radiology Physics: CT and US Cross-Sectional Imaging.* Oak Brook: Radiological Society of North America; 2000:77–95.
10. Jespersen SK, Wilhjelm JE, Sillesen H. Multi-angle compound imaging. *Ultrason Imaging.* 1998;20:81–102.

3

Essential Knobology for Ultrasound-Guided Regional Anesthesia and Interventional Pain Management

Alan J.R. Macfarlane, Cyrus C.H. Tse, and Richard Brull

R. Brull (✉)
Department of Anesthesia, University of Toronto, Toronto Western Hospital,
399 Bathurst Street, MP 2-405, Toronto, ON, Canada M5T 2S8
e-mail: Richard.Brull@uhn.on.ca

S.N. Narouze (ed.), *Atlas of Ultrasound-Guided Procedures in Interventional Pain Management*,
DOI 10.1007/978-1-4419-1681-5_3, © Springer Science+Business Media, LLC 2011

Introduction

The safety and efficacy of ultrasound (US)-guided nerve blockade relies heavily upon a comprehensive understanding of machine "knobology."[1,2,3] Despite differences in appearance and layout, all US machines share the same basic operative functions that users must appreciate in order to optimize the image. While modern US machines offer an abundance of features, the basic functions that all operators should be familiar with are frequency and probe selection, depth, gain, time gain compensation (TGC), focus, preprogrammed presets, color Doppler, power Doppler, compound imaging, tissue harmonic imaging (THI) (on some models), and image freeze and acquisition. Once the physical principles of US are understood, it becomes clear that creating the "best" image is often a series of trade-offs between improving one function at the expense of another. Each of the aforementioned functions is presented in turn below, following the sequence we use when performing any US-guided intervention.

Frequency and Probe Selection

Selecting the appropriate frequency of the emitted US wave is perhaps the most crucial of all adjustments. Ultrasound waves are characterized by a specific frequency (f) and wavelength (λ), as described by the equation $v = f \times \lambda$, where v is the speed at which the wave travels (all machines assume that US waves travel through soft tissue at 1,540 m/s). The range of frequencies used for nerve blocks is between 3 and 15 MHz. Higher frequencies provide superior axial resolution (Figure 3.1). Conceptually, axial resolution enables differentiation between structures lying close together at different depths (y-axis) within the ultrasound image, that is, above and below one another. Poor axial resolution, or inappropriately low frequency, may mislead by producing only one structure on the US image when in reality, there are two structures lying immediately above and below each other (Figure 3.2).

Unfortunately, higher frequency waves are attenuated more than lower frequency waves. Attenuation, which is described in more detail below (see "Time Gain Compensation"), refers to the progressive loss of energy (i.e. signal intensity) as the US wave travels from the probe to the target tissue and back to the probe again for processing into an image (Figure 3.3).[1] The end result of excess attenuation is an indiscernible image. The operator must therefore choose the highest possible frequency while still being able to penetrate to the appropriate depth in order to visualize the target. High-frequency transducers are best for depths of up to 3–4 cm; thereafter, a lower frequency probe is often necessary.

Probe categories can be divided into high (8–12 MHz), medium (6–10 MHz), and low (2–5 MHz) frequency ranges. On some machines, a variety of probes are always connected

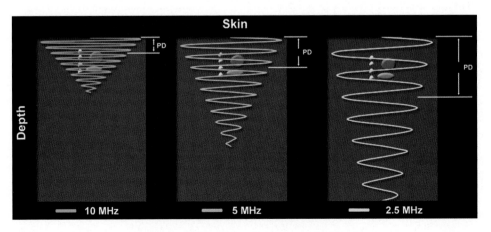

Figure 3.1. Higher ultrasound frequencies produce shorter pulse durations which promote improved axial resolution. The opposite is true when lower frequencies are used.

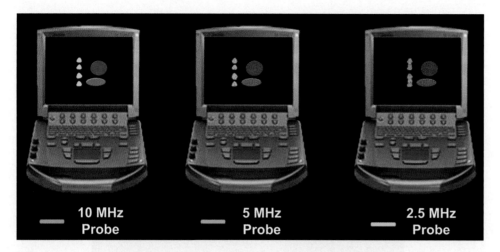

Figure 3.2. Axial resolution denotes the ability of the ultrasound machine to visually separate two structures lying atop one another (y-axis) in a direction parallel to the beam. As frequency increases, axial resolution increases but depth of penetration decreases. Low-frequency waves penetrate deeper at the expense of axial resolution. Note how the ultrasound machine is increasingly unable to resolve distinct structures as separate as the frequency decreases.

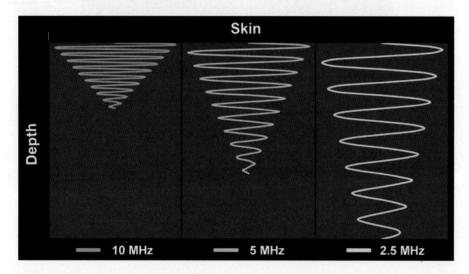

Figure 3.3. Attenuation varies directly with the frequency of the ultrasound wave and the distance traveled by the ultrasound wave. Note how the higher frequency (10 MHz) ultrasound wave is more attenuated relative to the lower frequency (5 and 2.5 MHz) wave(s) at any given distance (depth).

and choosing the desired probe requires only the toggle of a selector switch. On other machines, the different probes must be physically removed and attached each time. Most US probes have a "central" (i.e. optimal) frequency as well as a range of frequencies on either side of this central frequency, known as the bandwidth. After choosing the appropriate probe, the operator may therefore fine tune the frequency of the US wave emitted from the transducer by actively selecting only the upper, mid, or lower frequencies from each transducer's bandwidth.

Depth

The depth setting must be adjusted so that the structures of interest fall within the field of view (Figure 3.4). The objective is to set the depth to just below the desired target. This serves two purposes: firstly, imaging at a depth greater than necessary results in a smaller

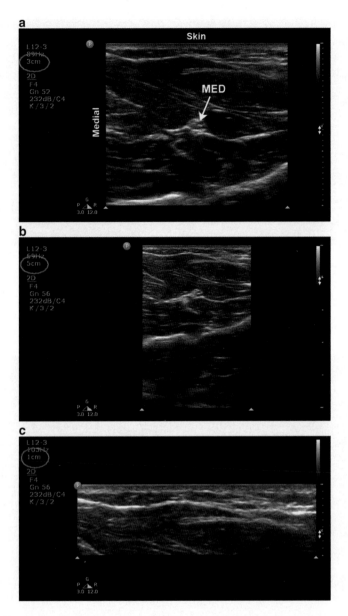

Figure 3.4. Depth. (**a**) Optimal depth setting. The median nerve (MED) and surrounding musculature are apparent. (**b**) Excessive depth setting. The depth setting is too deep such that the relative size of the target structures is diminished. (**c**) Inadequate depth setting. The MED is not visible.

target as the display is a finite size. A smaller target is generally more difficult to visualize and subsequently approach with the needle (Figure 3.4b). Secondly, minimizing the depth optimizes temporal resolution. Temporal resolution may be thought of as the frame rate and refers to the rate at which consecutive unique images are produced (expressed in frames per second) to culminate in continuous real-time imaging. Temporal resolution is dependent upon the rate at which successive US waves are emitted to form a full sector beam (usually in the order of thousands per second). Because US waves are actually emitted in pulses, with the next pulse emitted only when the previous one has returned to the transducer, it follows that for deeper structures this overall emission rate must be slower. Temporal resolution is thus forfeited as depth is increased in yet another trade-off between functions as described above. Modern US machines preserve temporal resolution by reducing the width of the sector beam, which explains the automatic narrowing of the screen image as the depth is increased. Reducing the sector width effectively reduces the number of emitted waves which must return to the transducer, thereby reducing the time before an image is displayed and maintaining frame rate. Unlike during cardiac imaging, when visualizing moving objects is crucial, temporal resolution is of less importance in regional anesthesia and pain management. A low-frame rate, however, could still be significant by creating a blurred image during either needle movement or rapid injection of local anesthetic.

Gain

The gain dial dictates how bright (hyperechoic) or dark (hypoechoic) the image appears. The mechanical energy of the echoes returning to the probe is converted by the US machine into an electrical signal, which in turn is converted into a displayed image. Increasing the gain amplifies the electrical signal produced by all these returning echoes which in turn increases the brightness of the entire image, including background noise (Figure 3.5b).

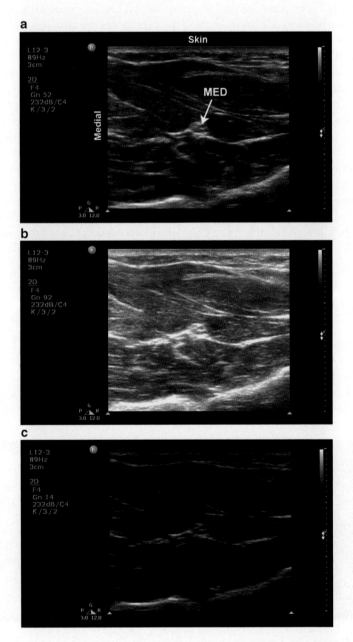

Figure 3.5. Gain. (**a**) Optimal gain setting. The target median nerve (MED) and surrounding musculature in the forearm are apparent. (**b**) The gain is adjusted too high. (**c**) The gain is adjusted too low.

Care must be taken when adjusting the gain dial because, despite the perception by some novices that brighter is better, too much gain can actually create artifactual echoes or obscure existing structures. Similarly, too little gain can result in the operator missing real echo information (Figure 3.5c). Finally, increasing the gain also reduces lateral resolution. Lateral resolution refers to the ability to distinguish objects side by side and is discussed below.

Time Gain Compensation

Similar to the gain dial, the TGC function allows the operator to make adjustments to the brightness. While the gain dial increases the overall brightness, TGC differs by allowing the operator to adjust the brightness independently at specific depths in the field (Figure 3.6). In order to understand the purpose of TGC one must fully appreciate the principle of attenuation. US waves passing through tissues are attenuated, mainly due to absorption but also as a result of reflection and refraction. Attenuation varies depending on both the beam frequency (higher frequency waves are attenuated more, as described above) and the type of tissue through which US travels (represented by the characteristic attenuation coefficient of each tissue type). Attenuation also increases with depth of penetration and so if the machine actually displayed the amplitude of echoes returning to the probe, the image would be progressively darker from superficial to deep. This is because those waves returning from farther away would be more attenuated. While US machines are designed to automatically compensate for attenuation, the machine's automatic correction is not always accurate. In order to create a more uniform image, TGC is most commonly adjusted to increase the brightness of structures in the far field (i.e., deep structures). While some machines have individual controls ("slide pots") for each small segment of the display (Philips, GE) others have more simply "near" and "far" gain (Sonosite). When individual slide pots are present, the optimal configuration is usually to have the gain increasing slightly from superficial to deep to compensate for the attenuation described above.

Focus

The focus button is not present on all machines but when available it may be adjusted to optimize lateral resolution. Lateral resolution refers to the machine's ability to distinguish two objects lying beside one another at the same depth, perpendicular to the US beam (Figure 3.7). Multiple piezoelectric elements arranged in parallel on the face of the transducer emit individual waves which together produce a 3-D US beam. This 3-D US beam

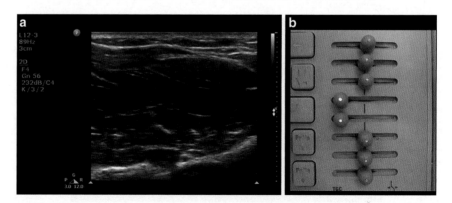

Figure 3.6. Improper time gain compensation setting. (**a**) The median nerve is not visible due to the hypoechoic band in the center of the image. This is caused by inappropriate low setting of the time gain compensation dial (**b**) which creates a band of under gain.

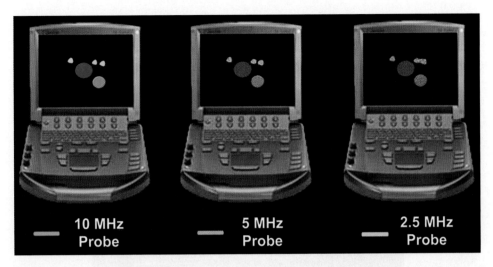

Figure 3.7. Lateral resolution denotes the ability of the ultrasound machine to visually separate two structures lying beside one another in a direction perpendicular to the beam (*x*-axis). As frequency increases, lateral resolution increases but depth of penetration decreases. Low-frequency waves penetrate deeper at the expense of lateral resolution. Note how the ultrasound machine is increasingly unable to resolve each structure distinctly as the frequency decreases.

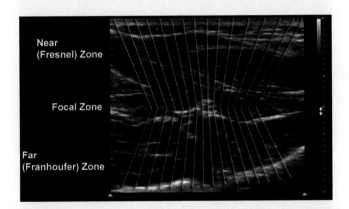

Figure 3.8. Focal zone. The focal zone is the boundary at which convergence of the beams ends and divergence begins. Lateral resolution is best in the focal zone. Lateral resolution denotes the ability of the ultrasound machine to correctly distinguish two structures lying side by side (*x*-axis).

first converges (Fresnel zone) to a point where the beam is narrowest, called the focal zone, and then diverges (Fraunhofer zone) as it propagates through the tissue (Figure 3.8). Conceptually, when the beam diverges, the individual element waves no longer travel in parallel and become increasingly farther apart from one another. Ideally, each individual element wave would strike (and consequently produce a corresponding image) every point in the field, no matter how close two separate structures lie next to one another in the lateral plane. Target objects may be missed by "slipping in between" two individual US waves if these are divergent. Limiting the amount of beam divergence therefore improves lateral resolution and this is optimal at the level of the focal zone. The purpose of the focus dial is to allow the operator to adjust the focal zone to various depths in the field. By positioning the focus at the same level as the target(s) of interest (Figure 3.9), the amount of beam divergence can be limited and lateral resolution maximized accordingly. The focus level is generally represented by a small arrow at the left or right of the image. Some machines actually offer the ability to set multiple focal zones but increasing the number of focal zones simultaneously degrades temporal resolution as the machine spends more time listening for returning echoes and processing each image.

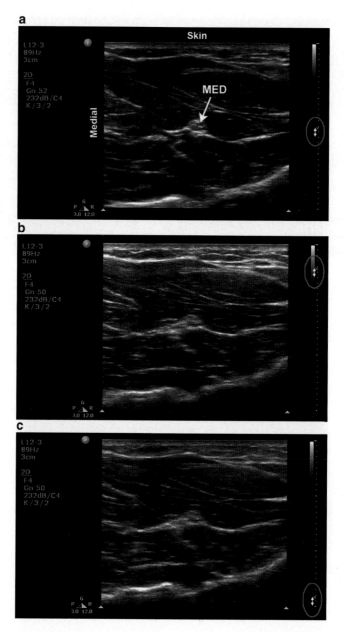

Figure 3.9. Focus. (**a**) Correct focus setting for viewing the median nerve (MED) in the forearm. *Bidirectional arrows* along the *right* border of the image indicate the focus level setting. (**b**) The focus level is set too shallow. (**c**) The focus level is set too deep.

Presets

All machines have presets which use a combination of the settings described above to create an image that is generally optimal for a particular tissue. At a most basic level, this may simply be set for nerves or vessels but other machines may have settings for each particular nerve block. Although these provide a useful starting point, further manual adjustments are generally still required to compensate for patient size and condition.

Color Doppler

Color Doppler technology superimposes Doppler information on the real-time image and facilitates the identification and quantification (velocity, direction) of blood flow. The major benefit, however, of Doppler technology for anesthesiologists performing ultrasound-guided pain procedures is to *confirm the absence* of blood flow in the anticipated trajectory of the needle.

Doppler physics applied to ultrasound relate to the principle that if a sound wave is emitted from a stationary transducer and reflected by a moving object (usually red blood cells), the frequency of that reflected sound wave will change (Figure 3.10). When blood is moving away from the transducer, the reflected wave will return at a lower frequency than the original emitted wave. This is represented by a blue color. Conversely, when blood is moving toward the transducer, the reflected wave returns at a higher frequency than the original emitted wave. This is represented by a red color. Operators should be aware that red is not necessarily associated with arterial blood nor blue with venous blood. The above change in frequency is known as the Doppler shift and it is this principle that can be used in cardiac and vascular applications to calculate both blood flow velocity and blood flow direction. The Doppler equation states that

$$\text{Frequency shift} = \frac{(2vf_t)(\text{cosine}\,\alpha)}{c},$$

where v is the velocity of the moving object, f_t is the transmitted frequency, α is the angle of incidence between the US beam and the direction of blood flow, and c is the speed of US in the blood. It is also important to note that as the beam's angle of incidence

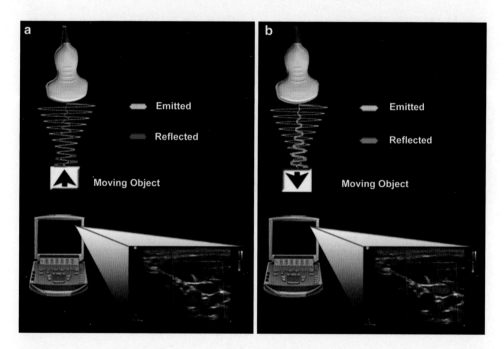

Figure 3.10. Doppler. (a) When a sound wave is emitted from the transducer and reflected from a target object moving toward the transducer, the returning frequency will be higher than the original emitted sound wave. The corresponding image on the ultrasound machine is represented by a *red* color. (b) Conversely, if the target object is moving away from the transducer, the returning frequency will be lower than the original emitted sound wave. The corresponding image on the ultrasound machine is represented by a *blue* color.

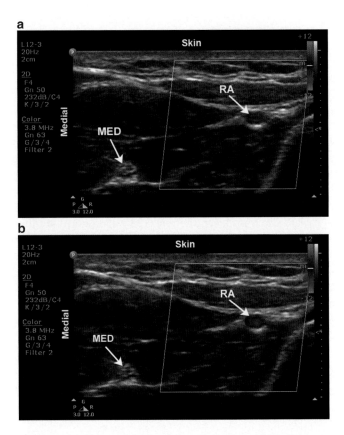

Figure 3.11. Color Doppler. Short axis view of the radial artery. (**a**) No flow is apparent when the beam is perpendicular to the direction in which blood is flowing. (**b**) Adjusting the tilt of the probe alters the angle of insonation, and consequently displays blood flow.

approaches 90°, large errors are introduced into the Doppler equation since the cosine of 90° is 0. In such instances, blood flow in a hypoechoic structure may not be visualized (i.e., false negative – Figure 3.11). Just as overall brightness can be adjusted using the gain function, the amount of Doppler signal displayed can also be adjusted. On some US machines, the Doppler sensitivity is adjusted by turning the gain knob while in Doppler mode. Other machines have a separate Doppler sensitivity knob. It should be noted however that increasing the Doppler sensitivity may result in the production of motion artifacts (i.e., false positive) created by subtle patient movements.

When in Doppler mode, the US machine requires more time to process returning echoes compared to simple B-mode imaging and so temporal resolution may be reduced. This explains why only a small area of the image (usually a rectangle or parallelogram) is monitored for Doppler shift when this function is turned on. The operator may subsequently move this shape over desired targets using either a trackball or touchpad.

Power Doppler

Power Doppler is a newer US technology that is up to 5 times more sensitive in detecting blood flow than color Doppler and can therefore detect vessels that are difficult or impossible to see using standard color Doppler. A further benefit is that, unlike color Doppler, Power Doppler is almost angle independent, reducing the incidence of false negatives described above. Such advantages however come at the expense of more motion artifact with subtle movements such as respiration. One further disadvantage of Power Doppler is that it cannot resolve the direction of flow. Rather than displaying a blue or red color therefore, only one color (usually orange) is used in a range of hues to indicate flow.

Compound Imaging

Compound imaging is one of the more recent technological advances in US. It improves image quality compared with conventional US by reducing speckle and other acoustic artifacts, and improves the definition of tissue planes and needle visibility (Figure 3.12). Conventional US transducers emit sound waves in one direction, perpendicular to the transducer. Modern compound imaging transducers can simultaneously emit and "steer" ultrasound waves at a variety of angles (up to nine), therefore producing images of the same tissue from several different angles of insonation (Figure 3.13). Compound imaging works by electronically combining the reflected echoes from all the different angles to produce a single high-quality image (spatial compound imaging). Frequency compound imaging is similar but uses differing frequencies rather than insonation angles to create a single image.

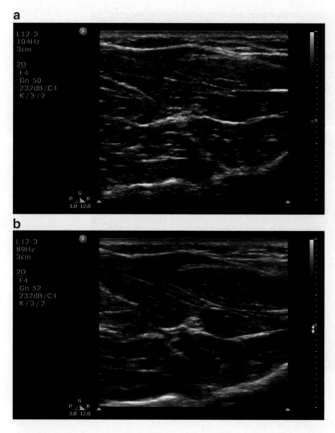

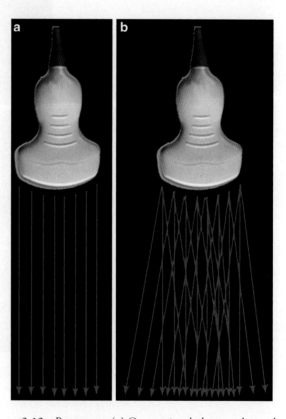

Figure 3.12. (a) Compound imaging in OFF mode. (b) Compound imaging in ON mode. Note the greater speckle artifact and reduction in resolution in (a) compared to (b).

Figure 3.13. Beam steer. (a) Conventional ultrasound transducer emitting sound waves in one direction. (b) Compound imaging transducer emitting sound waves at a variety of angles.

Tissue Harmonic Imaging

THI is another relatively new technology. When sound waves travel through the body tissue, harmonic frequencies are generated (Figure 3.14). These harmonic frequencies are multiples of the original, fundamental frequency. When THI is available, the transducer preferentially captures these higher frequency echoes upon their return to the probe for image processing. Because the harmonic frequencies are higher, there is enhanced axial and lateral resolution with reduced artifact. A further important point is that, unlike conventional US, these higher frequencies are achieved without sacrificing depth of penetration. THI appears to particularly improve visualization of hypoechoic, cystic structures, although it has been reported to worsen needle visibility.

Optimization Button

Many newer machines now implement an automatic image optimization button which serves to instantaneously combine many of the aforementioned features to create the "ideal image." This can be a simple, effective, and quick way to improve the quality of the image though further manual adjustments are sometimes still required.

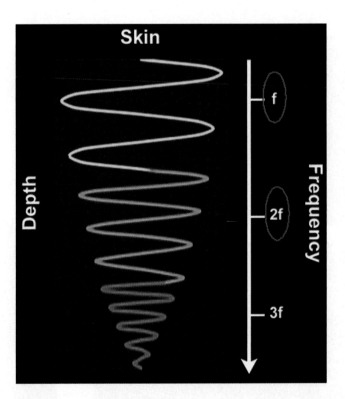

Figure 3.14. Tissue harmonics. As the ultrasound wave travels through tissue, distortion of the wave occurs along the way. The resultant distorted waves are harmonics (multiples) of the fundamental (inputted) frequency (*f*). Higher frequencies, such as 2*f*, 3*f*, etc., result in greater resolution. In tissue harmonic imaging, the ultrasound machine filters out most frequencies, including the fundamental frequency, and preferentially "listens" to one of the harmonics, usually the second harmonic (2*f*), resulting in an image with superior axial and lateral resolution and also fewer artifacts.

Freeze Button and Image Acquisition

US imaging is a dynamic process. The image however is actually made up of a number of "frames" per second (temporal resolution, as described above) that change quickly enough to produce what effectively appears as a real-time display. The freeze button displays the current image on the screen but usually also allows a sequential review of the individual "frames" over a previous short period of time. Such images can then be stored if desired. Image acquisition is important for medicolegal records, teaching, and (less commonly when performing nerve blocks) making measurements. Most machines have the capacity to store still and video images.

REFERENCES

1. Sites BD, Brull R, Chan VW, et al. Artifacts and pitfall errors associated with ultrasound-guided regional anesthesia. Part II: a pictorial approach to understanding and avoidance. *Reg Anesth Pain Med.* 2007;32:419–433.
2. Sites BD, Brull R, Chan VW, et al. Artifacts and pitfall errors associated with ultrasound-guided regional anesthesia. Part I: understanding the basic principles of ultrasound physics and machine operations. *Reg Anesth Pain Med.* 2007;32:412–418.
3. Brull R, Macfaulane AJ, Tse cc. Practical knobology for ultrasound-guided regional anesthesia. *Reg Anesth Pain Med.* 2010:35(2 suppl): S68–73.

4

How to Improve Needle Visibility

Dmitri Souzdalnitski, Imanuel Lerman, and Thomas M. Halaszynski

D. Souzdalnitski (✉)
Department of Anesthesiology, Yale New Haven Hospital, TMP-3, 333 Cedar Street,
New Haven, CT 06510, USA
e-mail: dmitri.souzdalnitski@yale.edu

S.N. Narouze (ed.), *Atlas of Ultrasound-Guided Procedures in Interventional Pain Management*,
DOI 10.1007/978-1-4419-1681-5_4, © Springer Science+Business Media, LLC 2011

Introduction

There are many advantages to the use of ultrasound in interventional pain medicine procedures. Ultrasound technology is currently growing exponentially due to its many advantages of improved and real-time high-resolution ultrasound imaging that results in successful pain management interventions. In addition, use of ultrasound for interventional pain management procedures avoids the many risks associated with radiation exposure to both the patient and practitioner.[1]

With appropriate training and experience, reliable and compulsive tracking of an introduced needle shaft and tip, both critical for effective and safe pain medicine interventions, may be mastered. Failure to visualize the needle, especially the needle tip, during needle advancement is one of the most common errors in ultrasound-guided interventional procedures (UGIP).[2-4]

Manipulation of the needle positioning during a pain management intervention, injection of local anesthetics/steroids or other medications, radiofrequency or cryoablation procedures, and other interventions without adequate needle tip visualization can often result in unintentional vascular, neural, and visceral injury. As an example, the rate of unintentional vascular puncture injuries during peripheral nerve block placement was reduced from 40% in the conventional anatomical landmark techniques to 10% with introduction of real-time visualization of the advancing regional block needle under ultrasound. Trainees can often make repeated errors and exhibit potentially compromising technical and safety behaviors during ultrasound-guided interventional nerve block placement procedures which can be potentially remediated by techniques that can improve needle visualization.[2-7]

A practitioner cannot assume that an interventional/procedural needle will always be clearly identified based on the variable properties and sizes of the several metallic needles. The variety of needle types used will often produce a distinct signal or "echo" under the ultrasound image. Effective visualization of the procedural needle, once introduced under the skin, is challenging for several reasons: variability in echogenicity of needles, varying ultrasound machine image processing technologies by the many ultrasound manufacturers, and transducer probe properties variability. These reasons along with other factors may be manipulated and modified to help improve needle visibility and will be discussed in this chapter.

Training and Phantom Simulation

Training with Adequate Mentorship

An adequate knowledge of human anatomy and ability to produce "typical" cross-sectional anatomical images during sonography are usually not sufficient for adequate needle visualization under all circumstances. The ability to observe, in real time, needle placement and advancement along with several other procedural manipulations under ultrasound guidance can be a challenging task to both the experienced practitioner and novice as it

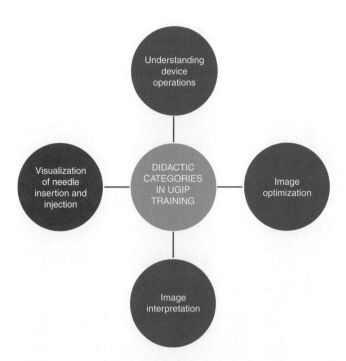

Figure 4.1. Major didactic categories in UGIP training include visualization of needle insertion and injection of local anesthetic solution , understanding device operations, in addition to image optimization and interpretation. *UGIP*-ultrasound guided interventional procedures.

requires a new set of skills. Sites et al has shown that simultaneous needle manipulation along with device operation requires dedicated training[2,3] despite other tendencies to define simple training strategies for ultrasound use by nonradiologists.[8] The American Society of Regional Anesthesia and Pain Medicine and the European Society of Regional Anaesthesia and Pain Therapy Joint Committee suggested that visualization of needle passage along with local anesthetic injection is one of the four important categories of skill required for proficiency in UGIP including understanding device operations, image optimization, and image interpretation[9] (Figure 4.1). In order to become more proficient at these four technical skills, it requires that the practitioner undergo adequate training that includes a continuing medical education regimen under mentorship supervision and instruction. In order to continue to develop the skill set necessary to become more proficient with UGIP, one should also perform ultrasound scanning on self and colleagues, and practice on simulators and phantoms prior to performing UGIP on patients.[9]

Phantoms

Two common errors during UGIP training have been identified and they are (1) failure to visualize the procedural needle during advancement toward its target and (2) ultrasound probe movement without proper needle visualization.[3] An ultrasound *phantom* is a simulation tool that mimics several properties of human tissue including tactile texture and compressibility of human skin, in addition to the typical needle appearance and feel as it is passed under ultrasound. UGIP phantom simulation may also address some important patient safety concerns by improving needle manipulation skills and further develop abilities with needle tip visualization that will alleviate many of the stressors associated with practicing UGIP on patients. Practicing ultrasound-guided needle tip visualization on a phantom simulator will begin to foster development of the necessary skill set for UGIP in a less stressful and low risk setting.[10]

Various modalities have been described to accomplish a "tissue-like" appearance of practice phantoms for ultrasound. Phantoms are typically identified by their "fidelity" that describes how closely the phantom can replicate the accurate texture of anatomical tissue.

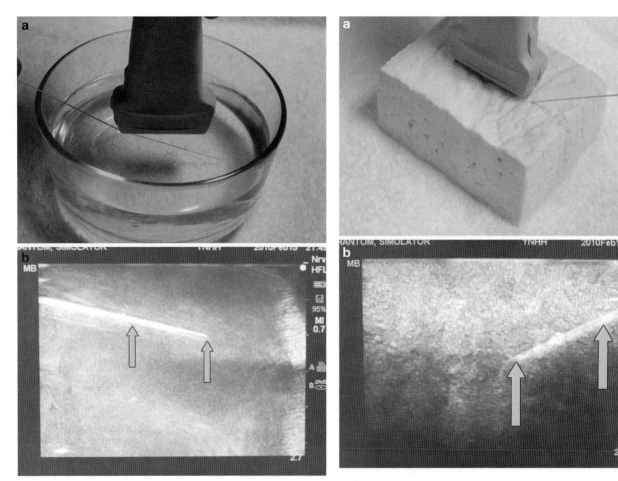

Figure 4.2. Needle appearance in water bath phantom (**a, b**). This is a water bath phantom (**a**), the needle (*arrows*) is easily visualized (**b**).

Figure 4.3. Needle appearance in tofu phantom (**a, b**). Tofu is an inexpensive ultrasound phantom (**a**) where the needle (*arrows*) is easily visualized (**b**).

For example, a high-fidelity phantom would be a cadaver specimen and a low-fidelity phantom would be represented by a water bath.[11] Low-fidelity phantoms have been made from many different materials including water balloons or water baths (Figure 4.2), tofu (Figure 4.3), gelatin or agar, or readily available materials, such as surgical gel pads (Figure 4.4). There have been other simulators described including sponges, cheese, chicken, turkey, porcine phantoms, and other objects.[5,11–14]

The low-fidelity phantoms have limited durability and limitations in sonographic fidelity may also be present. Most recently, phantom simulation technology has improved and phantoms can be made of polymer plastics, polyurethane, and other vinyl materials. As another example, the Blue Phantom (Figure 4.5) (Redmond, WA) and ATS laboratories phantoms (Bridgeport, CT) (Figure 4.6) will appear "tissue-like" under ultrasound imaging and can also include vessels while some others can include phantom nerves, or spine (Figure 4.7).[10,15]

These strategies reflect a growing interest in continued development of newer high-fidelity phantoms technologies.

High-Fidelity Simulation

The ultrasound-guided regional anesthesia simulation phantom (U-GRASP) interactive tool (IT), a newer type of ultrasound simulator has been developed by authors for the trainees mastering their needle visualization technique (Figure 4.8). The U-GRASP IT includes

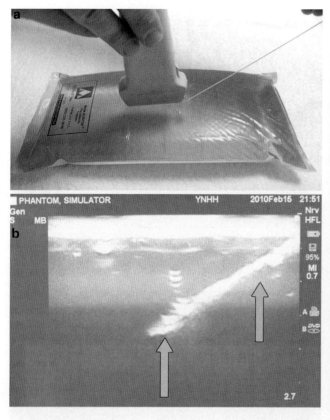

Figure 4.4. Needle appearance in surgical gel pad (**a, b**). This is a surgical gel pad phantom (**a**). Here the needle (*arrows*) is easily visualized (**b**).

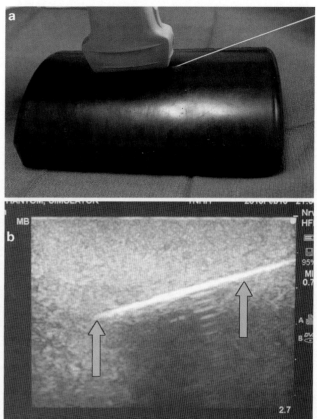

Figure 4.5. Needle appearance in Blue Phantom (**a, b**). Blue Phantom is an ultrasound phantom that includes structures, simulating nerves, and vessels (**a**). Here the needle (*arrows*) is easily visualized (**b**).

a correct phantom that can mimic extremity movement when the ultrasound-guided target is reached and successful neurostimulation is achieved. In addition, the phantom provides feedback in the form of an activating buzzer and an illuminating light emitting diode when a successful block has been performed. The future of simulator phantoms will continue to expand and possibly include error and skill assessment in targeted needle advancement and the data may also be used to score and track UGIP training with an emphasis on improving UGIP outcomes. Recently, there has been development of virtual and 3D/4D UGIP phantoms that are similar to what is being used in surgical training.[16–20]

Some of the ultrasound machines for UGIP provide multimedia tools to facilitate learning of the UGIP. The devices allow the use of the bank of preset images and video of typical procedures, and anatomical cross sections which can be utilized during the procedure of choice to provide a real time on-hand high-quality reference and image interpretation support (Figure 4.9).

Combined Ultrasound and Flouroscopic Phantom Simulators

Many pain practitioners are unfamiliar with UGIP and have no experience or little understanding of ultrasound needle visualization and needle manipulations under ultrasound. These individuals most likely learned and then practiced acquisition of needle tracking skills that are required for the many different types of injections (e.g., cervical and lumbar spine) by simultaneous simulation of x-ray-based techniques and ultrasound simulator. This combination was found to be helpful in the transition from computer tomography-assisted injections for low back pain to the now developing area of UGIP.[21]

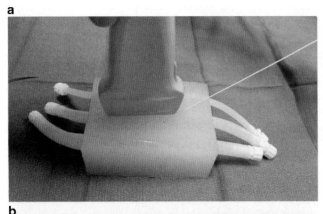

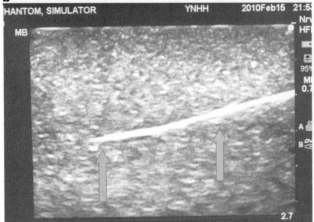

Figure 4.6. Needle appearance in ATS laboratories phantoms (**a**, **b**). The ATS phantom incorporates plastic tubes simulate vessels (**a**). The needle (*arrows*) is easily visualized (**b**).

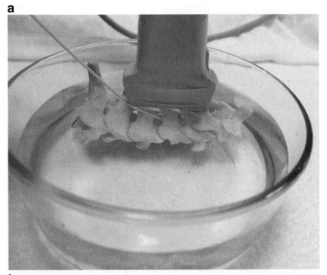

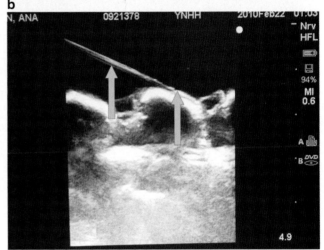

Figure 4.7. Needle appearance in cervical spine water bath phantom simulator (**a**, **b**). A water bath cervical spine and lumbar spine phantom simulate bony structures of the spine. Panel (**a**) shows a cervical spine model in a water bath. Panel (**b**) shows the cervical spine under ultrasound with needle (*arrows*) easily visualized.

However, high-fidelity anatomical and animal lab ultrasound phantoms are currently found most often at university centers or at special conferences and seminars and not widely accessible. A prototype of a combined ultrasound and flouroscopic phantom for cervical transforaminal injections has been developed by authors. It is made from a commercially available cervical spine anatomical model submersed in a polyvinyl medium sonographically simulating human tissue. In addition, this phantom contains anatomical examination and will uptake fluoroscopic dye if mistakenly injected (Figure 4.10). Easy to reproduce, this high-fidelity simulation system may improve trainee proficiency in needle visualization during combined ultrasound-guided and fluoroscopic UGIP.

There is a growing body of evidence along with proven benefit for both technical and "hands-on" skill improvement when simulation of needle localization during UGIP is introduced in surgery, emergency medicine, interventional radiology, and anesthesiology.[2–9,22–24] To establish the utility and cost-effectiveness of technologically advanced simulators, future studies will need to compare high fidelity vs. lower fidelity models.[25] In addition, there are many other medical specialties that have shown the advantage of simu-

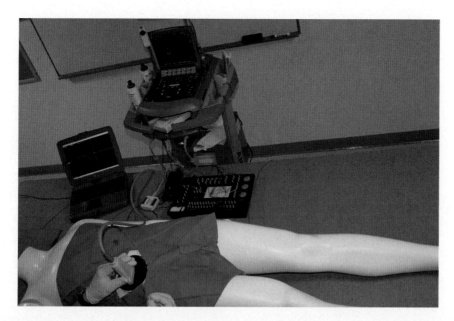

Figure 4.8. Ultrasound-guided regional anesthesia simulation phantom (U-GRASP) interactive tool (IT). This is a high-fidelity ultrasound simulator which allows documentation of trainee performance in the needle positioning during simulated procedures. In addition, it provides the trainee with the immediate feedback through a light and sound indicator which activates as the targeted anatomical structure is approached with the needle tip.

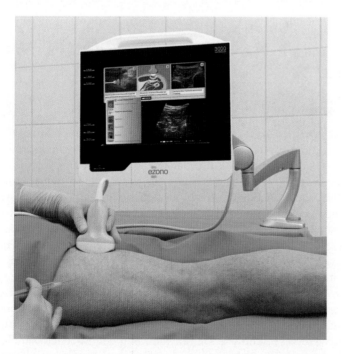

Figure 4.9. Real-time and image interpretation support system (eZONO). The eZONO device allows the operator to use a bank of stored preset images and video, and anatomical cross sections which can be used during the procedure of choice to provide a real time on-hand high quality reference and image interpretation support. Used with permission from eZONO.

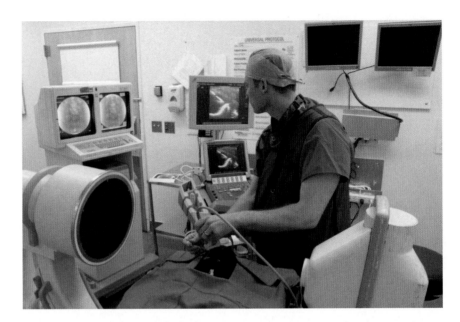

Figure 4.10. Combined ultrasound and fluoroscopic phantom for cervical transforaminal injections. This phantom contains anatomically correct fluid filled vertebral arteries that exhibit pulsed flow under *ultrasound* Doppler examination, and will uptake *fluoroscopic* dye if mistakenly injected through procedural needle. The picture demonstrates the phantom used by a resident physician.

lation on improving manual dexterity which may translate into improved procedural outcomes. The field of pain medicine is rapidly advancing and will surely benefit from incorporating simulation into pain medicine education and training that may also provide a high-yield strategy for overcoming some of the challenges of needle visualization during UGIP.

Procedural Needle-Related Visibility Factors

Basic Sonography and Needle Image Interpretation

One of the important components of an ultrasound machine is the ultrasound transducer (referred to as a probe, or scan-head). This ultrasound probe transmits sound waves, which culminate in an acoustic beam that is generated by an alternating electrical field applied to small piezoelectric crystals located under the ultrasound transducer surface. Typical sound wave frequencies used in UGIP are "ultra" high, within the range of 3–15 MHz, thus the terminology of ultrasound.[26,27] The ultrasound beam is directed away from the transducer footprint and can penetrate through tissue to varying degrees depending upon tissue composition. An acoustic beam can penetrate through muscle, tendon, and other soft tissues to varying degrees depending upon the density of the particular tissue, yet sound waves cannot pass through extremely dense tissue such as bone. The sound waves generated to and through tissue will then be reflected back (to varying degrees) to the ultrasound transducer. Therefore, an ultrasound image results when the transmitted from the ultrasound probe acoustic beam is reflected back to the ultrasound transducer. The ultrasound probe serves not only as the generator of the ultrasound beam, but also serves as the receiver of the "echo," which relays data back to the console and display screen to formulate an image. When a UGIP intervention is performed, the inserted procedure needle being used reflects sound waves back to the ultrasound probe that then deforms the piezoelectric crystals of the transducer to produce an electrical pulse or "echo." The time taken for an ultrasound acoustic beam to return back to the ultrasound probe is proportional to the depth at which the beam is reflected. This relationship is termed the "pulse echo principle" and serves as the basis for real-time visualization of UGIP. Understanding the basic physics principles of sonography will permit the practitioner to continue to improve adequate needle visualization during UGIP and remains crucial for the performance of safe and effective UGIP interventions.[26,27]

Acoustic Impedance as the Basis for Procedure Needle Visualization

Another essential aspect of needle visualization in UGIP is to understand the factors that can change or alter the visibility of ultrasound images such as acoustic impedance. Acoustic impedance of body tissues is dependent on the density of the tissue and the speed at which the ultrasound beam travels through that particular medium. Depending upon the particular body tissue that the ultrasound beam may be traveling through, the speed of sound changes and can range from 1,500 to 1,600 m/s. These small variations in ultrasound beam speed are responsible for variations in signal intensity or brightness. For instance, a part of the procedural needle that has been placed in a fluid-filled vessel will produce a bright hyperechoic signal because there is a large difference between acoustic impedance of each of the structures (needle and fluid). If there are marked differences in acoustic impedance between two different tissue types, for example, between soft body tissues and a metallic needle or bone, the brighter or more hyperechoic the sonographic signal of the needle becomes. This acoustic impedance difference between a needle and soft tissue provides an additional basis for improved needle visualization.

Size (Gauge) of the Procedure Needle and Its Echogenicity

A larger caliber procedure needle is typically more easily visualized under ultrasound than a smaller size diameter needle for two important reasons. First, a large gauge (G) needle has a greater surface area that produces more significant change in acoustic impedance than a smaller G needle and this can translate into a brighter image on the ultrasound screen. Second, the greater surface area of a larger G procedure needle can intercept the ultrasound beam and subsequently there is a higher probability that the ultrasound beam will be reflected back to the transducer, thus producing a brighter signal than smaller G needles (Figure 4.11). As a result, larger gauge needles appropriate for pain management procedures have been recommended for improved needle visibility during UGIP.[28] However, it must be remembered that a larger G procedure needle may be associated with more patient discomfort during needle passage through tissue. Although, during a trial performed by Campos et al to treat chronic inguinal pain, a 14-G needle and cryoablation probe was used and advanced toward the genitofemoral nerve that permitted improved needle visibility under ultrasound, patient discomfort was reduced with local anesthetic skin infiltration prior to needle passage.[29] Appropriate selection of procedure needle G and needle length (discussed later in the chapter) should be chosen based upon the UGIP task and it is important to note that a larger G needle does not necessarily translate into compromised patient safety. As an example, the safety of 21 and 18 G needles was found to be the same in an ultrasound-guided spleen biopsy study.[30]

The Skin Insertion Site Selected and Angle of Procedure Needle Passage

The angle and insertion site selected of a procedure needle for initial skin penetration/insertion plays a critical role in optimizing needle visualization on an ultrasound screen. Poor choice of needle insertion site and needle angle with respect to the ultrasound probe footprint may prevent optimal, clear, and accurate needle visualization on the ultrasound screen. This aspect of behavioral training was one of the five quality-compromising pat-

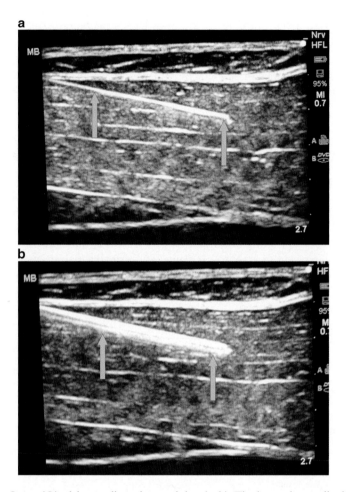

Figure 4.11. Gauge (G) of the needle and its visibility (**a, b**). The larger the needle the greater the ultrasound beam reflection which then improves needle visualization. Panel (**a**) shows 21 G needle (*arrows*), while an 18-G needle (*arrows*) is shown in panel (**b**). Even small increase in needle size makes it better visible. Porcine phantom.

terns identified by Sites et al during UGIP trainee behavior.[3] If the angle of the procedure needle insertion is too steep or acute in relation to the ultrasound probe footprint surface, then a smaller or shorter portion of the ultrasound beam will be reflected back from the needle to the transducer resulting in decreased needle visibility (Figure 4.12).[28] A simple approach suggested to overcome this obstacle is to introduce the procedure needle at as much of a perpendicular angle of insertion to the ultrasound probe footprint surface/ultrasound beam direction as possible. To obtain the most optimal sonographic image of a procedure needle, the ultrasound beam should approach the needle and be reflected back to the ultrasound probe at a perpendicular (90°) angle. When the ultrasound probe acoustic beam and procedure needle are at a 90° angle to one another, the transducer maximizes the reception of the reflected ultrasound beam from the needle. An alternative way to position the procedure needle and ultrasound probe as close to 90° to one another as possible is to press or tilt the opposite end of the ultrasound transducer using the "heel in" maneuver[31] (Figure 4.13).

Many regional anesthesia and UGIP procedures are performed with a linear array ultrasound probe. However, the linear array probe may produce additional patient discomfort during the tilting or heel in maneuver used to obtain optimal procedure needle to ultrasound probe orientation. This increased sensitivity to heel in manipulations may be especially true for certain chronic pain patients and a potential solution to this patient discomfort concern is the use of a curvilinear ultrasound probe. The curvilinear probe will

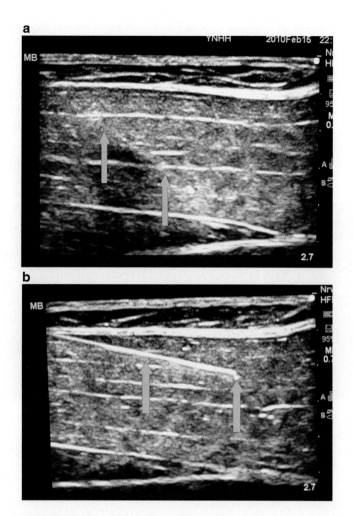

Figure 4.12. Angle of needle insertion and its visibility (**a, b**), At a steeper angle of needle insertion (acute angle of incidence), less of the ultrasound beam is reflected back to the transducer (*arrows*), which worsens needle visibility (**a**). A solution to this obstacle is to introduce the needle at a greater angle of incidence (**b**) (*arrows*).

permit a relatively painless heel in maneuver for almost all patients while obtaining an excellent procedure needle and ultrasound probe orientation and maximizing both tissue and procedure needle visualization[32] (Figure 4.14). However, it must be remembered that the curvilinear ultrasound probe (more ideal for deeper structures) does not provide an optimal scanning image for more superficial targets as does a linear array ultrasound transducer.

The most optimal angle for a procedure needle to the skin surface interface is performance of a needle insertion angle range between 30° and 45°.[32] In various clinical situations, it may not be feasible to gain this optimal angle interface for needle insertion, so echogenic needles have been designed to overcome some of these situations (not being able to obtain more adequate angles for needle insertion). These echogenic needles can be visualized at small or steep angles of insertion to the skin in a range as low as 15–30° due to special echogenic properties of the procedural needles.[33]

Echogenic Procedure Needles

When imaged properly, almost any procedure needle will generate an ultrasound image or return an echo under ultrasound scanning. However, needles have been designed and engineered with special properties to be used in conjunction with ultrasound that will

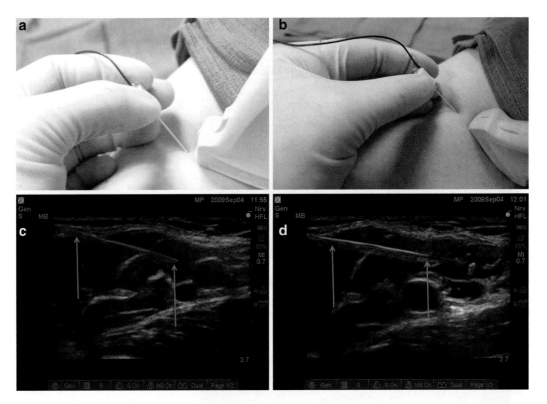

Figure 4.13. Probe heel in to change the angle (**a, b**). The heel in maneuver increases the angle of incidence from probe to needle improving reflection of the needle and improved visualization. Panel (**a**) demonstrates an in-plane linear probe approach. Panel (**b**) demonstrates an in-plane heel in maneuver. Panel (**c**) demonstrates the needle (*arrows*) appearance with the in-plane linear probe approach. Panel (**d**) demonstrates the needle appearance (*arrows*) with the in-plane heel in maneuver.

enhance and optimize their ultrasound image quality and have been termed echogenic procedure needles. Many recent advances have provided additional properties in needle technology that will improve needle echogenicity. Small angled indentations or notches have been created in the needle shaft resulting in an irregular surface of the procedure needle that will increase scatter of ultrasound waves. Theoretically, the irregular or notched surface of the procedure needle will provide a brighter signal and clearer ultrasound image at variable angles of needle insertion to the skin (Figure 4.15). The greater number of indentations or notches created in the shaft of a procedure needle will possibly translate into improved needle visualization on the ultrasound image screen.[34] However, as the number of indentations increases, there is a simultaneous increase in degree of roughness of the procedure needle shaft, which may be associated with greater friction at the needle–tissue interface. The friction at the needle–tissue interface can be disruptive to the process of smooth needle movements that are necessary during a nerve block procedure and may prove to be disadvantageous and/or create additional patient discomfort.[35]

The polymer encased procedure needle is another technological advancement which improves needle echogenicity.[36] A special polymeric needle coating, treated with a bubbling agent, creates microbubbles on the needle shaft surface during needle insertion and passage. Therefore, as the procedure needle is advanced into and through tissues, an increase in acoustic impedance is created between the tissue–needle interface and this measure may improve needle echogenicity and ultrasound image quality (Figure 4.16). In addition, when polymeric-coated needles are used during nerve stimulation and targeted nerve localization procedures, the applied polymer coat to the procedure needle shaft serves as an insulator for electrical stimulation and minimizes stimulation to tissues around the shaft of the procedure needle. The combination of the above described technological advances in procedure needle design (indentations and polymeric coating) has created a basis for development of the modern echogenic needles currently available on the market

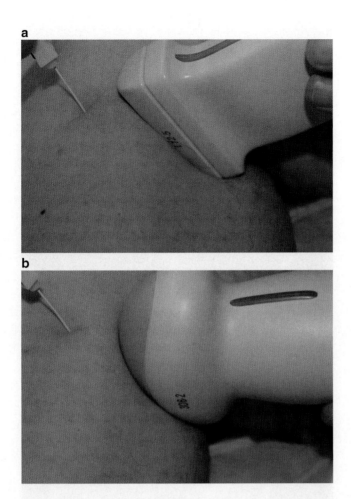

Figure 4.14. Curved vs. linear probe (**a, b**). The heel in maneuver is ergonomically improved with a curved ultrasound probe and has the added advantage of causing less patient discomfort. Panel (**a**) shows the heel in maneuver with a linear probe. Panel (**b**) shows the heel in maneuver with a curved probe.

(Figure 4.17). There are other engineering innovations currently under development toward improving upon procedure needle visibility for UGIP. One of these newer approaches consists of installation of a low-frequency generator at the end of the procedure needle, opposite to the procedure needle tip.[35] This generator creates large amplitude vibrations along the needle shaft making the procedure needle more visible under ultrasound imaging. The effectiveness of this and some other promising needle design developments are currently under investigation.

A study by Phelan et al comparing echogenic needles to standard nonechogenic needles did not provide any measurable objective performance improvement for UGIP during the short axis approach for interventional procedures.[23] One potential disadvantage of a bright echogenic needle is the potential for an increase in unwanted shadowing from the procedure needle on the ultrasound image as well as some other artifacts.[31] To reduce artifact created from the procedure needle shaft and to further improve upon needle tip visualization during UGIP, new technologies are focusing on developments to improve needle tip visibility rather than the entire needle shaft.

Procedure Needle Tip

Precise visualization of the UGIP needle tip is of primary importance and critical in order to minimize or avoid unintentional vascular injury or injections and other complications

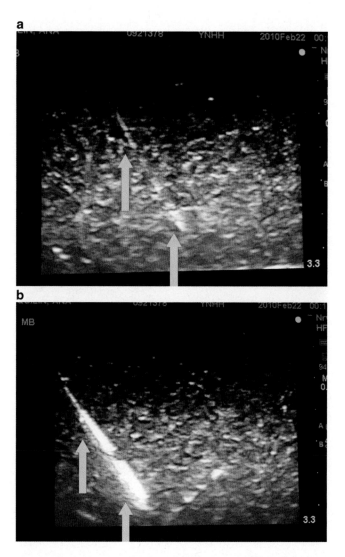

Figure 4.15. Indentation improves reflection of ultrasound (**a, b**). This echogenic needle has indentation on the needle shaft that improves ultrasound beam reflection at more variable angles of insertion. Panel (**a**) shows generic nonechogenic needle (*arrows*) at an acute angle of incidence. Panel (**b**) shows a grooved echogenic needle (*arrows*) at an acute angle of incidence with improved visibility (Pajunk, USA). Blue Phantom.

related to nerve and tissue damage created by procedure needles. Sites et al have recently showed that the most common error of trainees during UGIP occurred while residents were advancing the needle and not maintaining needle tip visualization on the ultrasound screen. The additional commonly performed errors were inadequate needle visualization and identification of the needle tip during intramuscular injections, which have been identified as one of the five quality-compromising patterns of resident behaviors during UGIP techniques.[3]

The procedure needle tip bevel will usually scatter the ultrasound beam because of irregularity of the needle tip surface compared to the needle shaft and also because of the less steep angle of the needle tip compared to the proximal needle shaft. It was secondary to the realization that the procedure needle bevel up position improved needle tip visualization of the ultrasound image that introduced the development of grooved shaft echogenic needles (Figure 4.18). Other additional technological advances have been developed toward improving upon procedure needle tip visibility and ultrasound image quality. A special transducer-receiver placed at the tip of the needle has significantly improved needle tip visualization in one study.[37] The sensor placed on the needle tip was made of a

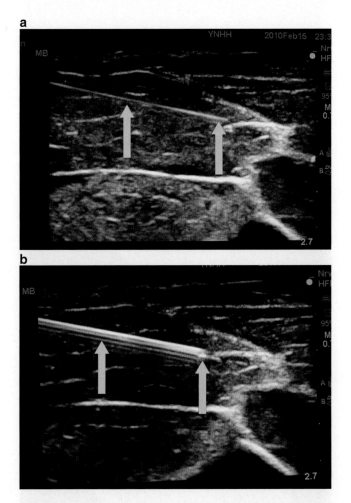

Figure 4.16. Polymer coated vs. nonechogenic needle (**a, b**). A polymer coated echogenic needle compared to a nonechogenic needle. Panel (**a**) shows a 21-G nonechogenic needle (*arrows*). Panel (**b**) shows a 21-G polymer coated echogenic needle (*arrows*). Porcine phantom.

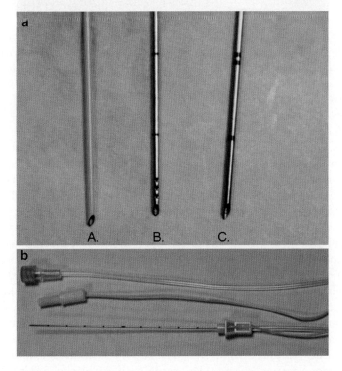

Figure 4.17. Needle with indentations, covered with polymer (**a, b**). These are samples of neurostimulation needles with combined polymeric coating and indentations in the shaft which further improve needle echogenicity, and subsequent visualization. Panel (**a**) A Braun, *B* Havels, *C* Pajunk needles. Panel (**b**), a sample of echogenic needle with neurostimulation properties (B Braun).

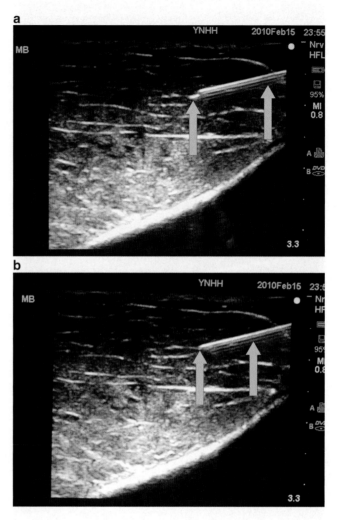

Figure 4.18. Bevel up vs. bevel down or bevel at the side (**a, b**). The bevel up position provides improved visualization of the needle tip because the ultrasound beam is maximally reflected in this position. Panel (**a**) shows a bright needle tip when the needle is in bevel up position (*arrow*). Panel (**b**) shows the exact same needle rotated to bevel down position, and demonstrates worsened visualization of the needle tip (*arrow*).

piezoelectric polymer that detected ultrasound waves and converted them into an electrical signal that was transferred back to the ultrasound probe receiver to aid the image quality of procedure needle tip positioning. Unfortunately, this transducer-receiver needle tip design device malfunctioned in 4 of 16 patients and has not been widely used. However, there are other new prototypes of advanced piezoelectric needle designs that have been developed. Placement of a piezoelectric actuator on a customized 18 G insulated Tuohy needle has permitted better distal needle tip visualization in one recent study.[38]

There has also been a marked and increased echogenicity achieved by creating dents or larger irregularities in only the needle tip and sparing of the procedure needle shaft. The placement or incorporation of these notches in procedure needle tips are created in a fashion similar to that of the design for increased texture needle technology described above. These notched tip procedure needles act to highlight the needle tip echogenicity from the remainder of the needle shaft and as a result, the needle tip is more visible under ultrasound imaging (Figure 4.19).

Superior needle tip image quality design and needle shaft image visibility are the factors to be considered for an ideal procedure needle for nerve blocks and UGIP techniques. Another factor that is paramount for an ideal UGIP needle would be its versatility. The UGIP needle should be useable for all types of tissue, easily visualized at any angle, main-

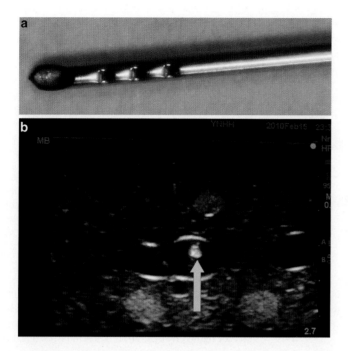

Figure 4.19. Echogenic tip. This Havels echogenic tip needle utilizes grooves in the needle tip to improve needle tip echogenicity. Panel (**a**) shows the Havels needle with grooves in the distal needle tip. Panel (**b**) shows the highly echogenic needle tip within an ultrasound phantom (*arrow*). Blue Phantom.

tain a sharp depiction of the needle rim, produce low artifact formation without shadowing, and contain qualities that maintain good detection and differentiation from the surrounding tissues and structures.[39] Many of the currently used echogenic needles tested are still far from an ideal echogenic design. However, recent technological advances are rapidly closing the gap between the current echogenic needle design and the ideal echogenic needle to be used during regional anesthesia and UGIP procedures.[40]

The Ultrasound Device and Procedure Needle Visibility

Ultrasound Imaging Artifacts and Procedure Needle Visibility

Ultrasound imaging of needle visibility depends not only upon the properties of the procedure needle used, but also upon the technology and capabilities of both ultrasound transducer and ultrasound machine. The ultrasound probe image resolution that results during an ultrasound examination is dependent on the piezoelectric crystal density of the scan-head, its crystal type, and the transducer's receiver properties. Ultrasound image resolution is also dependent upon the power of the ultrasound machine image processor.[31,41] Advances in both ultrasound transducers and ultrasound image processor technologies continue to assist the practitioner in procedure needle visualization; however, it is imperative that the practitioner gains knowledge of potential artifacts from needle imaging and experience in its interpretation.

Sonographic artifacts related to acquiring and processing of the image by an ultrasound machine may impair both tissue structures and procedure needle visibility in various ways. In some cases, a hyperechoic target may appear hypoechoic or anechoic when the returning ultrasound sound waves are degraded, which can be an effect of acoustic beam misalignment and is termed *anisotropy*. Anisotropy can be secondary to aberrant reflection

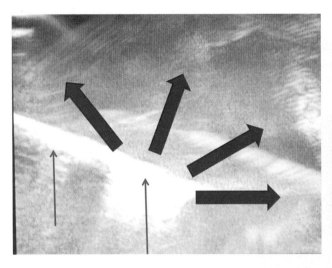 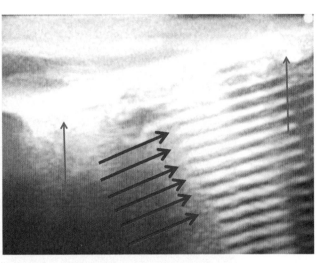

Figure 4.20. Scattering decreases needle visibility. Needle scatter can decrease the visualization of needle. The *red arrows* represent ultrasound beam scatter, which can cause artifact and worsen needle (*blue arrows*) visualization. Here the needle is inserted in a water bath.

Figure 4.21. Reverberation decreases needle visibility. Reverberation can cause reflection of the needle off the structures below and can impair needle visualization. Here the needle (*blue arrows*) is placed in a surgical gel pad phantom and there is clear artifact termed reverberation (*red arrows*). Surgical gel phantom.

and/or refraction (described below) and remains independent of operator acoustic beam misalignment. Reflection from a smooth surface, such as a procedure needle, is termed *specular reflection*. Reflection from an irregular surface can cause dispersion of the ultrasound beam with subsequent degradation of the received ultrasound signal, which is termed *scattering* (Figure 4.20). Scattering can cause image degradation and artifact; however, scattering may be used to an advantage with the newer developed echogenic procedure needles. When multiple surfaces reflect an ultrasound acoustic beam between each other and the ultrasound transducer, it is termed *reverberation* (Figure 4.21). If ultrasound sound waves are deviated from its path of incident and then reflected from a deeper structure, it is termed *refraction*. *Attenuation* is another factor that can cause ultrasound acoustic beam degradation. Attenuation is described as a decrease in ultrasound signal strength or amplitude as it passes through certain tissue types and can be caused by many of the above listed factors including reflection, refraction, and scattering. The additive or distorting effects of attenuation, aberrant reflections, and less so with refraction can distort the displayed ultrasound image and may lead to an inability to correctly identify both the procedure needle and surrounding anatomical structures as well as needle proximity to other tissue structures.

Impact of Various Sonographic Modes on Procedure Needle Visibility

Compound Spatial and Frequency Image Reconstruction Following Acoustic Beam Steering and Variable Frequency

A commonly used solution to overcome the problem of deflection created by an ultrasound signal reflected from a procedure needle is to use a *beam steering* sonographic system that enables the production of *compound spatial imaging*. Beam steering ultrasound systems essentially steer the acoustic beam reflected away from the procedure needle back to the ultrasound probe by altering the internal ultrasound beam angle of incidence (Figure 4.22). Older ultrasound probes are limited to mechanical steering, but the newer modern sonographic machines, with broad bandwidth transducers, have specific functions that can change the transmit focus. Broad bandwidth transducers permit the ultrasound probe to produce and accept ultrasound signals at different angles in automatic mode that can produce an improved sonographic image.[42]

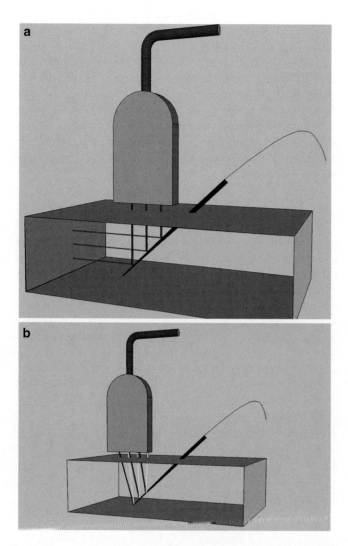

Figure 4.22. Beam steering may improve needle visibility. Beam steering improves needle visualization by increasing the angle of incidence between probe and needle and therefore increasing needle visibility. On panel (**a**) the beam is not steered toward the needle and fewer of the ultrasound beams in *blue* are reflected, in *red*, back to the transducer. On panel (**b**) the ultrasound beams in *blue* are steered toward the needle and reflected back in *yellow*.

Compound spatial imaging is achieved by computational process. This is performed by mechanical beam steering that then combines three of more frames from different steering angles into a single frame. Compound spatial imaging allows greater clarity, resolution, and better procedure needle contour definition.[43]

Frequency compound sonography obtains scans from several different frequencies, producing variable speckle artifact patterns in each frame. The frames produced are then averaged, which reduces the speckle and grainy appearance observed in conventional sonography. This result is an improved anatomical ultrasound image of tissue structures, but not a procedure needle imaging quality enhancement.[44]

Frequency of the Ultrasound Probe (AKA Depth) Acoustic Power and Gain

The ultrasound probe most commonly used during UGIP is a 5–10-MHz frequency transducer. This particular ultrasound scan-head frequency is known to provide good spatial resolution for nerves and nerve plexus at 1–5 cm depth.[45] A lower frequency, 2–5 MHz, ultrasound probe is often used to visualize deeper nerve and nerve plexus structures. However, resolution of both anatomical structures and the procedure needle becomes less definitive at increasing depth and use of lower frequency ultrasound transducers. The higher frequency ultrasound probe, transducer frequencies up to 18 MHz, is most often used for interventions on the most superficial structures such as nerves of the hand and forearm.[46] Ultrasound device controls that can adjust depth, acoustic power, and gain will permit an option(s) to focus the ultrasound beam to an optimal level and provide an improved ultrasound image. However, this adjustment potential of the ultrasound machine may have only a limited impact on procedure needle visibility outside of its regular optimization of the sonographic image.

Time Gain Compensation and Harmonic Imaging

Time gain compensation control options on an ultrasound machine will permit adjusting image brightness at variable depths. In addition, changes and adjustments made in gain compensation may minimize many of the sonographic artifacts produced when the ultrasound acoustic beam travels through the skin and other superficial layers. The time gain compensation control option may not only reduce noise produced by tissue artifacts, but can also reduce artifact from the paramount signal of the procedure needle.

Another function of the more modern ultrasound devices is harmonic imaging. This function provides the ability to suppress reverberation and several other types of noise artifact produced by skin and body wall structures. Harmonic imaging technology is based on an understanding that body tissues produces a weak, but a usable harmonic signal that can be detected and amplified by the sonographic unit. Harmonic imaging capability then uses these detected harmonic signals and applies low frequency-high amplitude noise that can be used to improve an ultrasound image.[47] The reports resulting from harmonic imaging of procedure needle visualization are mixed and vary from superior ultrasound imaging to procedure needle images that are considered inferior when compared with a conventional ultrasound device without harmonic imaging capability.[44,48] The impact of the new type of harmonic imaging, broadband techniques, is to be explored.

Brightness, Motion, and Doppler Modes

Conventional B-mode (B stands for brightness) serves as the currently used gray scale sonographic device modality, typically used when performing UGIP. M-mode (M stands of motion) ultrasound machines are used to evaluate the movement of structures within the body. Typically, modern ultrasound machines display the M-mode image adjacent to a smaller version of the original B-mode image on the display screen. When using 2D ultrasound devices, M-mode is focused on the targeted structure and will display its movement over time in the form of an undulating line that is altered according to the moving tissue structures. M-mode has limited use during UGIP and it does not affect or improve upon procedure needle visibility.

A third imaging modality equipped in modern ultrasound machines is the Doppler mode, comprised of Doppler sensitivity and power Doppler. Doppler mode capability can differentiate blood flow in blood vessels from other similar looking tissue structures, and can be utilized to theoretically prevent unintentional vessel penetration or trauma by a procedure needle since the blood vessel can be identified (Figure 4.23). Doppler capabilities may also be used to enhance procedure needle imaging quality and clarity in conjunction with other methods and tools described in the "enhancement" section.

3D and 4D Ultrasound Imaging

Typical 2D ultrasound imaging captures and displays a flat ultrasound image in two planes and is analogous or similar to current fluoroscopy. 3D ultrasound technology captures images in multiple planes and at different angles. The resulting 3D ultrasound image can

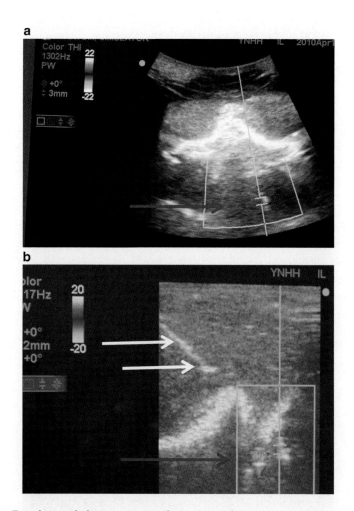

Figure 4.23. Doppler may help to prevent inadvertent vessel penetration or intravascular injection (**a**, **b**). Using Doppler can assist in the visualization of vessels to be avoided when undergoing ultrasound-guided procedures. Panel (**a**) shows the detection of blood flow with Doppler in the vertebral artery (*red arrow*) at the level of cervical spine C7 in a prone position. Panel (**b**) shows a needle (*white arrows*) avoiding the prior identified vessel (*red arrow*) on Doppler ultrasound in a lateral position. Combined ultrasound and fluoroscopic phantom for cervical transforaminal injections.

then be displayed in a 3D representation or schema of scanned structures. Advantages of static 3D imaging are described by Clendenen et al when comparing differences between plain radiographic imaging (analogous to 2D sonography) and conventional computer tomography (analogous to static 3D ultrasound imaging).[49] 3D ultrasound imaging in real time (dynamic 3D and sometimes termed as 4D imaging) adds time as a fourth axis to traditional X, Y, and Z dimensions. Dynamic 3D imaging (4D) allows for real-time tracking of an intervention that is comparable to real-time CT or MRI technologies, but with levels of simplicity, safety, and cost which are difficult to compare. Current 4D ultrasound technology has limitations related to scanning and visibility of superficial interventions that is based on the same current limitations that are associated with 3D ultrasound probe frequency.[49] However, we have recently witnessed significant improvements in ultrasound technology and anticipate that such technology will continue to rapidly improve.

Initially, 3D ultrasound imaging was produced by a freehand move of the regular 2D ultrasound probe over the skin. This maneuver was then followed by a reconstruction procedure that is similar to one used in computed tomography, but is cumbersome and time intensive.[50] Despite the introduction of special 2D transducers fitted with a rotating receiver inside the ultrasound probe and providing excellent biplane and multiplane 3D images, the image reproduction is static and not imaged in real time. With 4D ultrasound imaging, there is a small but noticeable lag in the real-time 3D image of the procedure needle. In addition, there have been no obvious benefits reported in terms of better procedure needle visualization with the special 2D ultrasound transducers[31] and these transducers are cumbersome for UGIP purposes.

Current technological limitations of 3D ultrasound transducers are derived from the difficulty in producing small and maneuverable ultrasound probes that are capable of housing the necessary and advanced scanning mechanical machinery (Figure 4.24). However, real-time tracking of procedure needles with these types of ultrasound transducers could be potentially superior to images produced by current sonographic technologies, especially in experienced hands (Figure 4.25).

Another recent advance in 3D ultrasound technology is the matrix array transducer. Creation of 3D and 4D ultrasound images have been developed independent of the mechanically steered array ultrasound probe with the use of a matrix array transducer. These probes are smaller and lighter and have better ergonomic profiles. The development of matrix array ultrasound transducers has resulted in smaller transducers while also

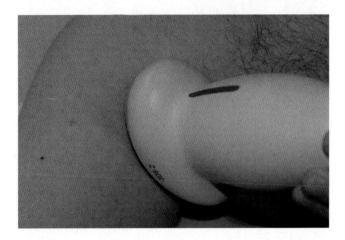

Figure 4.24. 3D needle ultrasound and needle visibility. This is a 3D ultrasound probe. Currently 3D ultrasound probes are larger than their 2D counterparts. However, newer, smaller 3D ultrasound probes are in development.

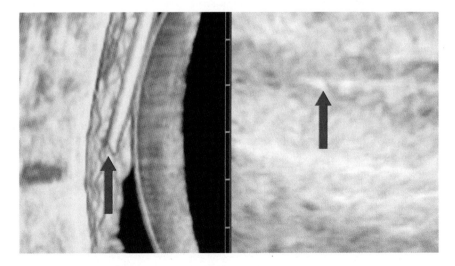

Figure 4.25. 3D image of the needle in the phantom. Here, a needle is visualized within an ultrasound phantom under 3D ultrasound in real time, also termed 4D ultrasound. The needle is clearly visualized in 3D on the left (*left red arrow*) and is less visible under conventional ultrasound on the right (*right red arrow*).

increasing speed of data acquisition and processing by roughly 3 times faster than a conventional mechanically steered array ultrasound transducer. This translates into a true 4D experience and could lead to improved transducer maneuverability and procedure needle visualization.[49,51]

Recent Advances in Ultrasound Imaging and Procedure Needle Visibility

Complex signal processing, broadband transducers, increased scanner bandwidth, upgradable software, and other recent technological developments have made investigational improvements in ultrasound image quality.[52–54] Increasing ultrasound beam frequency of sonographic systems up to 50 MHz could lead to improved image quality, especially when the UGIP target structures are superficial or during UGIP in the pediatric patient population.[55] Combining ultrasound with other imaging technologies including fluoroscopy, computer tomography, and magnetic resonance imaging[56,57] may represent a high yield strategy for better localization of procedure needles during an UGIP intervention. One of the newest dual imaging systems currently being developed is a photoacoustic and ultrasound imaging combination.[58] These advances along with other technologies in sonographic imaging are in transition from research to possible clinical implementation and the impact of these technologies on procedure needle visibility is yet to be determined.

To obtain optimal procedure needle sonographic image visibility, it is first important to acquire manual dexterity, apply the advanced ultrasound technologies, and maintain experienced needle/ultrasound transducer manipulations. Additional measures to assist in providing improved procedural needle visualization are automatic optimization technologies of the ultrasound image that have been developed and are available on modern ultrasound machines. These automatic optimization technologies permit the practitioner to choose between preset modes optimized to visualize certain tissues and structures such as vascular, muscular, breast, and others.[59] Recent advances in sonographic border detection has resulted in technology that can identify and assume automatic color marking of nerves (yellow), muscles (brown), arteries (red), and veins (blue) and will possibly be available in the near future.[60,61]

Incorporation of UGIP systems into the Internet network may provide specific clinical benefits by permitting real-time online consultations by pain management specialists, target structure imaging enhancement suggestions, procedure needle visualization assistance, and confirmation provided by experienced ultrasound practitioners.[62] However, image optimization of sonographic target structures does not automatically provide adequate procedure needle visibility. Even despite the many advances made toward ultrasound imaging technological improvements, it has not always translated into better procedure needle visualization.[31] One probable explanation for the dissociation between targeted structure ultrasound imaging optimization and advances toward procedure needle visualization improvement is that traditional application of ultrasound in medicine is typically focused on imaging and diagnosis. Although there continues to be some efforts achieved and attempts made to improve upon sonographic systems so that they may be adjusted to permit interventional instruments and procedure needles to produce more optimal visibility under ultrasound imaging. Unfortunately, such systems have usually been limited toward improving upon sonographic visualization of surgical instruments or computer-assisted imaging units and development of robotic systems for UGIP.[63–66] The advancements in ultrasound technology and improvement in development of procedure needles for UGIP seem to be somewhat disconnected, possibly due to the narrow specialization of procedure needles and ultrasound machine manufacturers. However, this gap has recently been reduced due to the fact that there are a growing number of improved procedure needles and UGIP being developed across several different fields of medicine. There have been advances in developing technology that can diminish sonographic artifacts produced by the gas of radiofrequency ablation and those created during interventions associated with cryoablation that remain pertinent to pain medicine.[29,67]

There are reasons to believe that a concerted coordination of effort toward procedure needle and sonographic equipment manufacturers to improve upon needle visibility for UGIP interventions is underway. Such development efforts will likely translate into an association with sonographic technology designed specifically for the growing field of interventional pain medicine and may represent a promising, practical, scientific, and business niche for the specialty. The current important issue that remains a crucial variable is the need to develop further technology that will improve upon consistently securing appropriate alignment of the procedure needle with the ultrasound transducer. This continues as one of the important aspects of UGIP and interventional pain medicine that if mastered, will in the end produce a successful interventional procedure for the patient.[31]

Needle-Probe Alignment

Need for Procedure Needle and Ultrasound Probe Alignment

A typical ultrasound beam width that is emitted from an ultrasound probe is only about 1 mm (Figure 4.26). Therefore, imaging a procedure needle can often be complicated as a result of misalignment of the ultrasound beam and the needle during an "in-plane" technique of regional anesthesia and UGIP procedures. It remains relatively easy for the procedure needle to deviate from under the narrow ultrasound beam, so diligence remains necessary as even small movements of the ultrasound probe or needle will result in the loss of the procedure needle image on the ultrasound screen. As a result of an inability to maintain the ultrasound image of a procedure needle, both regional anesthesia and UGIP techniques may lead to prolonged procedure times or result in an increased complication rate due to unintentional tissue and structural damage. Therefore, successful ultrasound procedure needle visualization remains important and careful needle positioning, advancement, and manipulation in relation to the ultrasound probe are of critical importance.[4,31]

"In-Plane" and "Out-of-Plane" Needle Approach: Classical Probe-Needle Interpositions

Several strategies have been suggested for procedure needle ultrasound visualization and imaging, yet two classical techniques known as the "in-plane" (IP) approach and the "out-of-plane" approach (OOP) continue to be advocated. For the IP approach, the procedure needle is inserted midline, parallel, and under the long axis of the ultrasound probe footprint with a concept of procedure needle visualization as a hyperechoic bright line. The OOP approach is achieved by inserting the needle under, midline, (usually) and perpendicular to the ultrasound probe footprint in a short axis to the ultrasound beam where the needle tip/shaft appears as a bright hyperechoic dot (Figure 4.27).

An identified disadvantage of the IP approach that is often cited is that the procedure needle can more easily deviate away from the narrow ultrasound beam and result in or cause potential complications and lengthen block procedure time if the needle cannot be imaged throughout the selected pain management intervention. Another potential disadvantage of the IP approach is the associated reverberation created from the long axis of the needle shaft that may impair detection of structures below the imaged procedure needle shaft. A disadvantage of the OOP approach is associated with an inability or increased difficulty to accurately follow the procedure needle to the selected target. Another complication associated with the OOP technique is lack of assurance or inability to confirm whether the hyperechoic dot seen on the ultrasound image is an approximation of the procedure needle tip or an approximation of the needle shaft. An important consideration when comparing or selecting between the two techniques (IP or OOP) is that the IP approach requires 2–3 times more needle length insertion to reach the desired target when

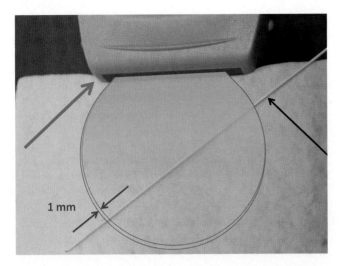

Figure 4.26. The need for alignment. The ultrasound probe (*blue arrow*) emits a very narrow beam (*rounded shape*) close to 1 mm width (*red arrows*) which widens with distance from the probe. This small area can make it difficult to visualize the needle (*black arrow*) if it is misaligned. Tofu phantom.

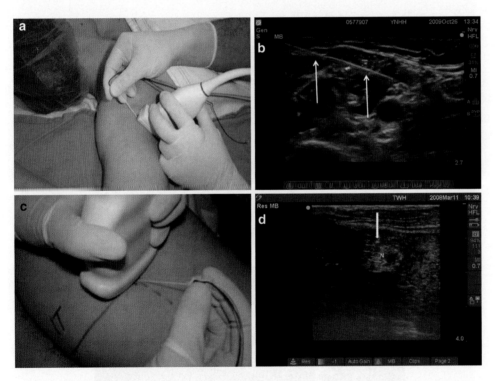

Figure 4.27. In-plane (IP) and out-of-plane (OOP) techniques. This is the in-plane technique. The needle is held inserted parallel to the probe (**a**) and is seen (*white arrows*) in the long axis on ultrasound (**b**). The out-of-plane technique is demonstrated in panel (**c**). The out-of-plane approach is achieved by inserting the needle in the short axis of the beam and therefore the needle tip (*white arrow*) appears as a bright hyperechoic dot (**d**). N sciatic nerve above popliteal fossa.

compared to the OOP approach along with the associated potential to create additional patient discomfort. It remains clear that there are some drawbacks to both IP and OOP procedure needle approaches when performing regional anesthesia and UGIP. Therefore, gaining experience with both approaches is necessary in order to select the most appropriate technique for each particular procedure. As an additional alternative, the oblique plane approach is yet another technique that may be considered when selecting ultrasound-guided pain management in a search to minimize or eliminate some of the drawbacks from either an IP or OOP approach for procedure needle visualization.[68]

Oblique Plane Needle Approach for Ultrasound-Guided Pain Management

The oblique plane approach is achieved by viewing the target anatomical structures (including nerves and vessels) in the short axis and places the procedure needle in long axis to the ultrasound probe. This approach permits the operator to obtain an optimal view of the underlying target and surrounding structures while maintaining continuous visualization of procedure needle and needle shaft during movement and manipulation[68,69] (Figure 4.28). The oblique plane approach has been found to be useful in certain procedures where the target nerve may be traditionally difficult to visualize. As an example of such a situation, the femoral nerve (lateral and inferior to the femoral artery) typically has a fattened shape as it is wedged between the iliacus muscle and hyperechoic fascia that may lead to some degree of obstruction of an optimal sonographic view. The oblique approach often retains the advantages of the OOP technique while enabling a clearer view of the procedure needle shaft and tip during advancement.[68]

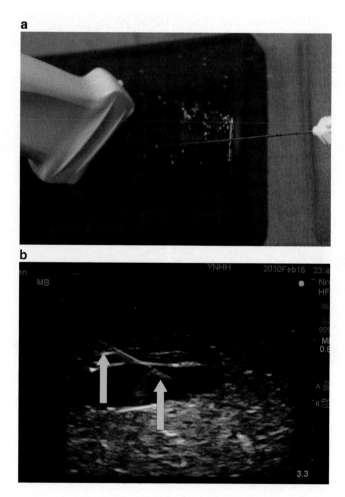

Figure 4.28. The oblique plane technique (**a, b**). The oblique plane approach is achieved by viewing the short axis view to visualize the target anatomical structures including nerves and vessels, but places the needle in long axis to the probe. Panel (**a**) shows the needle and probe positioning for the oblique view. Panel (**b**) shows the image of the needle (*arrows*) on ultrasound in the oblique view. Blue Phantom.

Biplane Needle Imaging Approach for Ultrasound-Guided Pain Management

Some of the 2D ultrasound units and machines with 3D capabilities permit combining images in different planes (in "real-time") on the same ultrasound screen. This allows the practitioner to observe both anatomical structures and the needle in two or more planes simultaneously. For example, a vessel could be viewed in either long axis or a transverse axis at the same time on a split ultrasound screen display. A biplane transducer is used for 2D ultrasound and 3D ultrasound probes produce multiplane images. Both bi- and multiplane imaging techniques may have great potential for improving needle visualization and UGIP procedures, but as the technology is still relatively new its utility has yet to be established. However, the biplane imaging capabilities are unlikely to replace the cornerstone techniques of basic procedure needle and transducer alignment, which greatly improve needle tip and shaft visibility. [26]

Mechanical and Optical Procedure Needle Guides

The importance of procedure needle alignment with the ultrasound probe beam has prompted the consideration and development of various types of guides for needle stabilization and for needle path direction. These procedure needle guides are intended for alignment and synchronization of the needle with the ultrasound transducer probe position, and essentially keep the needle path under the ultrasound beam. Several types of procedure needle guides have been described such as the mechanical needle guide that is a device attached directly to the ultrasound probe and used for aligning the procedure needle so its trajectory remains under the ultrasound beam. Such procedure needle guide devices are designed to match with specific types of ultrasound probes and with the intent that as the procedure needle is being advanced, it will be directed in a path under the ultrasound beam (Figure 4.29). Initially, these types of guide devices were introduced into clinical practice for the performance of biopsies and the guide devices helped to facilitate procedures performed by less experienced practitioners.[70] The developed ultrasound guide procedure needle devices are routinely mentioned in the literature as it describes techniques for optimizing needle visualization under ultrasound for regional anesthesia.[26]

Mechanical needle guidance has shown to significantly (2×) reduce the time necessary to safely perform UGIP procedures. Use of such devices has also demonstrated superior needle visualization when tested by inexperienced residents performing simulated UGIP procedures on porcine phantoms. Needle visibility proved to be approximately 30% better with the use of mechanical procedure needle guide devices and trainees ranked their satisfaction with needle guidance devices significantly better than "free-hand" techniques.[13,71] However, the routine performance of UGIP typically requires frequent adjustments in needle path direction(s) that could be a potential drawback of a rigid mechanical guide device. It may not be easy to achieve optimal visualization of surrounding tissue, nerve target structures, and procedure needle direction with use of a rigid mechanical needle guide device since it is often necessary and required that dynamic needle adjustments are performed during UGIP.[31] Therefore, the role of rigid mechanical needle guide devices for facilitation of procedure needle visualization during pain management interventions and procedures is still yet undetermined.[31]

Adjustable mechanical needle guide devices have been developed and trialed in order to overcome the drawbacks of rigid mechanical devices.[72] Various types of mechanical devices to guide procedure needles have created a basis and prompted the production of robotic-guided UGIP systems. Although, practical applications of robot guided approaches for UGIP currently appear to be limited. A potential solution for the shortcomings of the various needle guide devices was developed and described by Tsui by means of a laser system-based device. The laser guide device is designed to facilitate UGIP needle and ultrasound probe alignment.[73] This optical procedure needle guide is comprised of a laser beam allowing easy adjustment of the procedure needle position as needed (Figure 4.30). It has

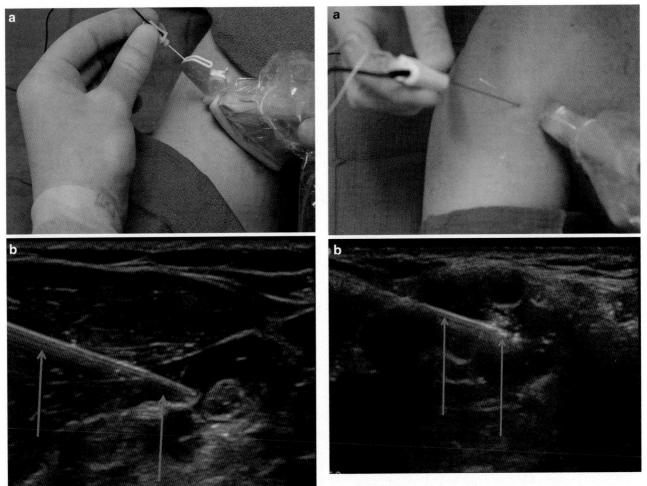

Figure 4.29. Mechanical needle guides (**a, b**). Mechanical needle guides can improve needle visibility significantly by stabilizing both transducer and needle. Panel (**a**) shows the CIVCO mechanical needle guide. Panel (**b**) shows the needle (*arrows*) under mechanical guidance.

Figure 4.30. Optical needle guide (**a, b**). The Tsui device enhances needle visualization by improving alignment. Panel (**a**) shows the Tsui device clearly demarcating the angle of entry and the needles relation to the probe with the light beam (*red*). Panel (**b**) shows the needle (*arrows*) insertion under the optic guide guidance.

been determined that this optical needle guide provides an unambiguous visual trace of accurate needle-beam alignment, and may therefore be useful in teaching and developing bimanual coordination for trainees. Longer procedure needles are typically necessary when using this laser device since a larger portion of the procedure needle shaft should protrude from the skin during the UGIP procedure so as to permit alignment of the needle and laser beam.[31]

Advanced Procedure Needle Positioning Systems

Most experienced practitioners who use ultrasound prefer to perform UGIP using "freehand" techniques in which the operator can freely manipulate the ultrasound transducer with one hand and procedure needle with the other hand. The freehand technique affords flexibility in positioning the procedure needle during its placement and advancement toward the targeted structure(s).[31] Even for an experienced practitioner, it can sometimes be difficult to maintain both the needle and target in view while avoiding various tissue structures, blood vessels, and other nerve structures.[2–4,74]

One potential solution toward improving a practitioner's guide of predicting a procedure needle trajectory is an advanced positioning system that uses optical or electromagnetic tracking systems.[75-78] This particular tracking system uses a sensor attached to an ultrasound probe and another sensor attached to the procedure needle's hub. This device uses an electromagnetic tracking system and performs calculations that can predict procedure needle trajectory that is then extrapolated and displayed (on the screen) as an estimation of a procedure needle anticipated path.

The initial developments for the electromagnetic tracking system were described as separate units that were designed to acquire ultrasound images from conventional ultrasound machines that have an output port.[79] This kind of positioning system would recreate sonographic images obtained from the ultrasound machine and combine this actual image with predicted needle path on the separate screen. The latest technology permits incorporating advanced positioning systems into current ultrasound machines (Figure 4.31). Most sonographic

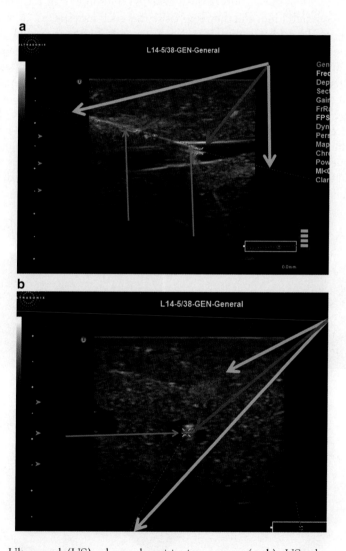

Figure 4.31. Ultrasound (US) advanced positioning systems (**a, b**). US advance positioning systems use optical or electromagnetic tracking technologies that calculate the needle projection which is then displayed as a prediction of needles future path on the screen. Panel (**a**) shows the needle in an in oblique plane approach (*blue arrow + green arrow*) and extrapolates the direction of the needle shown by the *dotted green line*. The tip of the needle is marked by device *red arrow*. Panel (**b**) shows the needle in an out-of-plane approach and again extrapolates the direction of the needle (*blue arrow*) shown by a *dotted green line* (*green arrow*). Again, the needle tip is marked by device (*red arrow*). Ultrasound GPS, used with permission of Ultrasonix. Blue Phantom.

equipment manufacturers are actively developing this particular type of technology for advanced positioning procedures that are to be used in UGIP for 2D, 3D, and 4D systems. Combined ultrasound and cat-scan or ultrasound and MRI radiofrequency ablations along with other pain medicine interventions may employ advanced interventional tool positioning systems in the near future.[66,77]

The "ART" of Scanning for Better Procedure Needle Visualization

Advances in needle positioning systems that permit UGIP to become more efficient, interactive, safe, and objective such that it will likely compensate for some of the current difficulties and shortcomings in learning UGIP will continue to develop. However, it is unlikely that such a positioning system will replace currently practiced needle–transducer alignment skills as they will remain an integral part of UGIP performance. Marhofer and Chan described various movements of the ultrasound transducer that can improve procedure needle tip visualization, and they emphasize that such movements of the transducer and needle should be deliberate and slow. Marhofer and Chan further emphasize that the practitioner move or manipulate only one part of the system at a time (i.e., only move the ultrasound transducer or the needle to optimize procedure needle tip visualization). These slow and deliberate movements should be kept separate or independent from one another (move either needle or probe) in order to minimize repositioning steps or maneuvers (probe sliding, tilting, rotating) that may prolong UGIP performance. The chapter continues to describe the "ART" of ultrasound scanning techniques as a useful tool for effective ultrasound transducer movements where (1) sliding is referred to as alignment (A), either in plane or out of plane as the transducer slides on the skin surface, (2) rotation (R) refers to clockwise and counter clockwise movement of the ultrasound transducer, and (3) tilting (T) refers to angling the transducer to maximize the ultrasound beam signal to maintain as best as possible an angle of incidence at 90° (Figure 4.32).

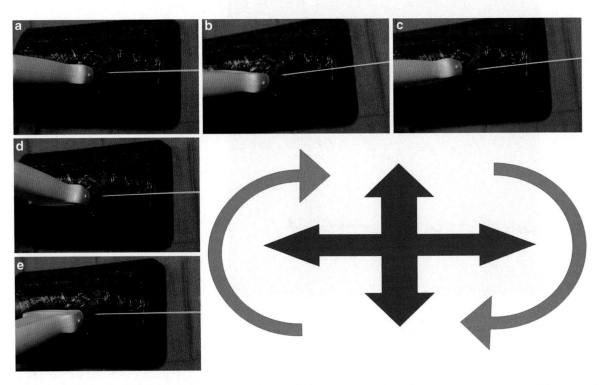

Figure 4.32. Probe and needle alignment by rotation, sliding, and tilting. Probe and needle alignment by rotation, sliding, and tilting are all important factors in successful needle visualization. Panel (**a**) shows the probe and needle aligned in the in-plane technique. Panels (**b**) and (**c**) rotate the probe clockwise and counterclockwise. Panels (**d**) and (**e**) tilt the probe forward and back. Blue Phantom.

Ergonomics for Better Procedure Needle Visibility

Unintentional or nondeliberate ultrasound probe movement was found to be the second most common error performed by trainees during regional anesthesia and UGIP procedures.[3] A satisfactory ultrasound image of target structures (e.g., nerve) and procedure needle could be easily and quickly lost with even minor or small manipulations (sliding) of the ultrasound probe that has been prepared (placed in ultrasound gel) for regional anesthesia and UGIP. These seemingly minor or small ultrasound probe movements, caused commonly during attempts to reach for supplies or poor ergonomics, for example, are errors that must be considered to avoid prolonging UGIP procedure performance. Sites et al demonstrated that novice practitioners created errors (approximately 10%) that comprised of poor ergonomics and operator fatigue.[3] Operator fatigue during UGIP typically presented as the need to switch hands holding the ultrasound probe during the performance of a procedure, the need for use of both hands on the ultrasound probe, and hand tremors or shaking. These fatigue issues and small or minor ultrasound probe movements may potentially further compromise procedure needle visualization as well as UGIP efficiency and success.

In order to overcome some issues compromising UGIP success, the ultrasound probe should be manipulated and measures should be taken to properly stabilize ultrasound probe positioning while also taking steps to minimize operator fatigue. To improve ultrasound probe stabilization techniques, the operator should use freehand techniques during UGIP procedures. Freehand techniques are performed by having the operator's ultrasound transducer hand function as both ultrasound transducer stabilizer and for localizing and maintaining the target structure on the ultrasound image screen. The practitioner may also consider using the resting fingers of the hand used to hold the ultrasound probe to apply pressure downwards which may minimize probe movement and reduce operator fatigue (Figure 4.33). The freehand technique may also lessen slipping of the ultrasound probe on the gel covered skin surface.

When performing UGIP procedures, it is always useful to do a preprocedural ultrasound scan of targeted structures and surrounding tissue area and then mark or identify (on the patients skin) optimal probe position outlining the ultrasound probe footprint positioned where the most ideal target image is best visualized. This quick, easy, and beneficial

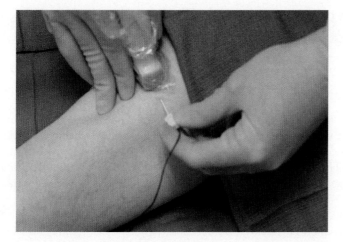

Figure 4.33. Freehand technique. Freehand techniques are performed by having the operator's ultrasound transducer hand function as both ultrasound transducer stabilizer and for localizing and maintaining the target structure on the ultrasound image screen. The practitioner may also consider using the resting fingers of the hand used to hold the ultrasound probe to apply pressure downward which may minimize probe movement and reduce operator fatigue. The technique may also lessen slipping of the ultrasound probe on the gel covered skin surface.

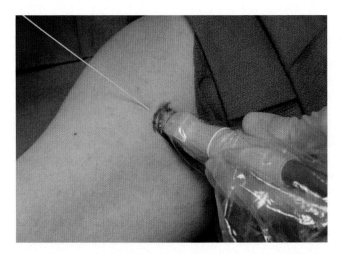

Figure 4.34. Marking of the skin. Marking of the patient skin site affords the operator improved alignment. This is especially true in cases of patient movement or loss of prior probe needle alignment.

measure may minimize or avoid excessive ultrasound probe and needle movements during UGIP intervention that could translate into inefficient and time-consuming UGIP procedures as well as possible unintentional structural damage (Figure 4.34). To further optimize procedure needle ultrasound visualization and decrease operator fatigue, simple measures should be taken to improve practitioner ergonomics. Some simple measures to improve operator ergonomics are to prepare all the necessary supplies before the ultrasound probe is prepared and placed in a sterile sheath as well as raising the patient's bed height to maintain proper operator posture. To further improve procedure needle and ultrasound probe alignment, in addition to decreasing operator fatigue, there are special carts designed for UGIP, ultrasound adhesive gels, and stabilizing mechanical arms to minimize ultrasound transducer movements.[60,81–83]

Enhancement and Techniques to Improve Procedure Needle Localization

Basic Sonographic Effect of Enhancement

Enhancement is the description of what occurs and what is seen on an ultrasound image when tissues with low acoustic impedance, such as blood within a vascular structure, enhances its containing vessel wall as an ultrasound signal which makes it appear hyperechoic. Similarly, the concept of enhancement may also improve the visualization of a procedure needle within a vascular structure or certain tissues (e.g., fat) that have lower acoustic impedance when compared to the needle (Figure 4.35).

An understanding and application of the enhancement concept could provide value in situations in which procedure needle localization and tracking may prove to be difficult during UGIP procedures. Despite the use of echogenic procedure needles and use of advanced sonographic technology along with skilled and experienced needle and ultrasound probe manipulation, performing UGIP in all situations may not be enough to be successful with the proposed intervention.[4,26,31,84] Application of the useful strategy of enhancement and other techniques described below may prove beneficial toward highlighting procedure needle localization under ultrasound.

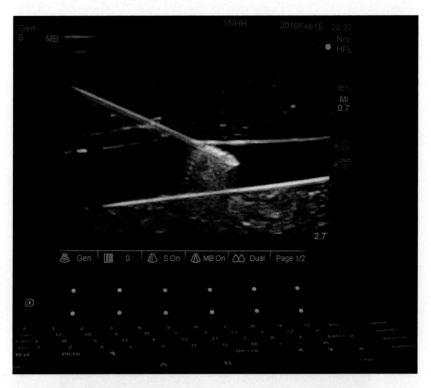

Figure 4.35. Needle enhancement. Needle enhancement within the vessel wall occurs because of an increased difference in acoustic impedance between needle and vessel fluid. The needle shaft at the site of entry into the vessel wall does not enhance as brightly as the tip within the vessel wall.

Enhancement with Priming, Insertion of Stylet or Guide Wire, and Vibration

There are instances in which the procedure needle may prove difficult to visualize despite correct procedure needle and ultrasound transducer alignment and positioning. In some of these difficult to maintain needle visualization situations, a procedure needle could be localized, simply by moving the entire needle (or a stylet/guide wire that has been placed in the lumen of the needle). Chapman et al describes movement of the inserted procedure needle in short "side to side" and "in and out" motions that deflect adjacent tissues and may improve the visualization of the needle path and trajectory.[26] However, movement of the entire procedure needle may cause additional patient discomfort and it could result in unintentional tissue structural damage if the needle tip is not visualized.[31]

When continuous ultrasound scanning of procedure needle insertion and passage toward a target structure is not successful the needle tip may be localized by inserting a small guide wire or stylet through the needle to the needle tip. Chapman et al describes priming a procedure needle by submersion of the needle in sterile water can cause enhancement of the needle during ultrasound scanning.[26] Another technique that can be used is with the Doppler function of the ultrasound machine to detect procedure needle vibrations.[85] With the color flow Doppler function of the ultrasound device activated, a slightly bent stylet is inserted into the procedure needle and then rotated causing lateral vibration of the needle. This vibration of the needle is detected and visualized by color flow Doppler and may assist in improving procedure needle visibility on the real-time ultrasound screen (Figure 4.36). Devices are now commercially available that utilize this principle of vibrating the procedure needle to improve needle visibility. Such technology is used by attaching a small device onto the procedure needle shaft that when activated can produce small vibrations at the needle tip (maximum amplitude 15 µm that are imperceptible to touch) that then generate a signal with color flow Doppler.[31]

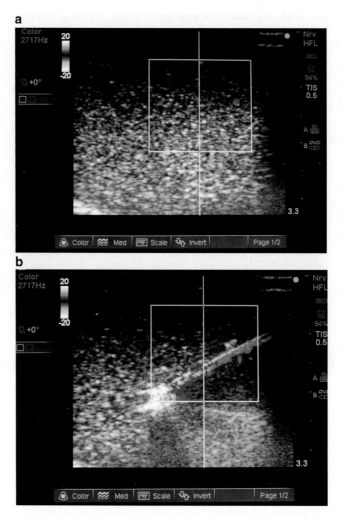

Figure 4.36. Improved procedural needle visualization under Doppler ultrasound (**a, b**). Applying vibration to the needle with a stylet inserted and moved will cause slight needle movement and improve visualization under Doppler ultrasound. Panel (**a**) shows the needle under ultrasound without vibration. Panel (**b**) shows color Doppler signal with movement of the needle stylet.

Another approach that may improve procedure needle visualization (while using Doppler) has been accomplished by applying vibratory actions to the tissue around the target structure rather than to the needle. By activating the color flow Doppler option, the ultrasound probe or transducer is being activated to vibrate at various frequencies. Then the amount of tissue vibration that is caused by the ultrasound probe at each of the frequencies is measured by using a quantitative power Doppler algorithm built into the scanner.[86] This advanced ultrasound imaging technique could help to produce better procedure needle localization and may have potential for use in many pain management procedures and interventions.

Hydrolocalization of the Procedure Needle

There are several studies that describe injection of a small amount of fluid (0.5–1 ml) through the needle in order to assist in confirming procedure needle tip location or position. This maneuver is usually performed by first moving the inserted procedure needle and observing the movement of the surrounding tissue and then by fluid injection while

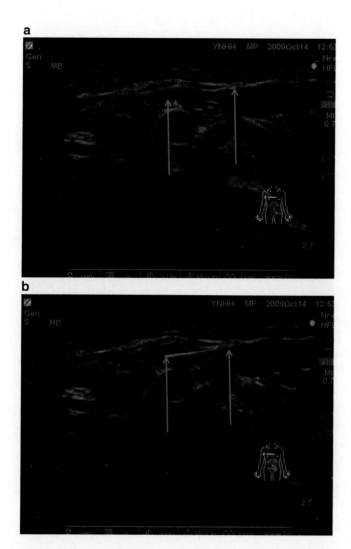

Figure 4.37. Hydrolocalization technique (**a**, **b**). Hydrolocalization is carried out by injecting the fluid that can improve needle tip visualization by first forming an anechoic pocket which then enhances the needle tip. Panel (**a**) demonstrated that the procedural needle (*right arrow*) tip (*left arrow*) is difficult to visualize. Injection of fluid, shown in panel (**b**), made the tip (*left arrow*) of the procedural needle (*right arrow*) to be easily localized.

looking for the appearance of a small hypoechoic or anechoic pocket at the site of the needle tip created by the injected fluid.[5,6,87,88] Hydrolocalization is the term or name given to this maneuver by Bloc et al.[88] It can be carried out with sterile water, normal saline, an injection of local anesthetic, or 5% dextrose (Figure 4.37). Use of a 5% dextrose solution, in order to preserve motor function and response, is most optimal for combined ultrasound-guided and nerve stimulation techniques during the performance of peripheral nerve blocks.[83,89,90]

Procedure Needle Visibility by Agitated Solutions or with Ultrasound Contrast Agents

Similar to hydrolocalization described above, injection of microbubbles uses a small bolus of agitated saline placed through the procedure needle. This technique may assist in ultrasound-guided needle tip visibility and could further improve visualization and localization

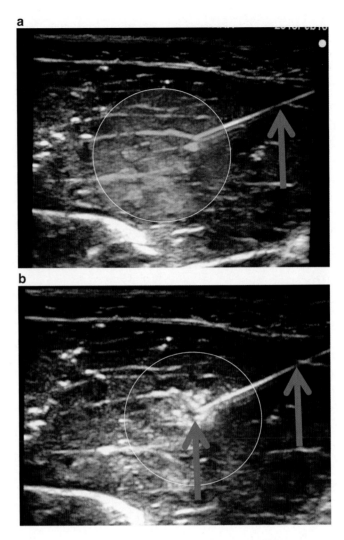

Figure 4.38. Microbubble injection technique (**a, b**). The microbubble injection technique uses a small bolus of agitated saline which is injected through the needle tip and can further improve visualization and localization of the needle. Panel (**a**) shows the needle prior to injection. Panel (**b**) shows the needle tip and surrounding area after injection of the microbubbles. Microbubbles can disrupt the visualization of structure deep to the microbubbles seen in panel (**b**). porcine phantom.

of both the procedure needle or threaded catheter[91,92] (Figure 4.38). Microbubbles may produce needle enhancement by taking advantage of the acoustic impedance mismatch between injected microbubbles and the surrounding tissues.[93] However, the microbubbles injection technique has received some criticism when practicing UGIP as it has the potential disadvantage of creating an acoustic shadow and potentially obscuring the image of target structures.[31]

The microbubbles represent one of the varieties of ultrasound contrast media. The pre-made ultrasound contrast agents are available on the market and they typically employ encapsulated lipid-based nanoparticles or polymeric micelles.[93] These injectable contrast agents can significantly increase the amount of ultrasound backscatter imaging and this may improve procedure needle visibility under conventional ultrasound or color flow Doppler. The disadvantages of injecting contrast agents are the costs associated with the agents as they are expensive and they require an additional intravenous injection. There are no studies performed describing the use of these contrast agents for improved needle visualization in regional anesthesia or pain medicine, but they may be potentially useful if employed for UGIP procedures. There is an understanding that if ultrasound contrast technology is developed, this technique could become a useful adjunct or tool for improving upon procedure needle tip visualization.

Localization of the Procedure Needle Tip with the Aid of Nerve Stimulation

It is known that it can sometimes be difficult to determine the proximity of the procedure needle tip in relation to targeted nerve structures on the ultrasound screen. Tsui et al reported that nerve stimulation can be used to aid in the UGIP training settings and to assist in verifying position of the needle tip in relation to nerve structures.[89,90] Chantzi et al has confirmed that the combined technique using both ultrasound and percutaneous nerve stimulation may serve as a reliable method for procedure needle tip location verification.[94] Combined ultrasound and nerve stimulation techniques by anesthesia residents and practitioners who are not skilled at ultrasound-guided procedures or with little ultrasound experience may be able to improve their skills when attempting to identify nerve structures in situations of difficulty in needle tip localization. UGIP combined with nerve stimulation has been shown to increase the success rate of pain management interventions.[95,96]

In addition, because procedure needles used during nerve stimulation techniques are polymer coated, they are by definition echogenic, and remain attractive for use with UGIP procedures (Figure 4.17). One of the drawbacks for this technique is that by combining UGIP and nerve stimulation, it requires the availability of both an ultrasound machine and necessary equipment for neurostimulation that must all be made available in the sterile field. Another potential disadvantage of the combined technique is that nerve stimulation controls and the ultrasound image screen are located on two separate display panels (ultrasound and neurostimulator) that could cause difficulty with visualization and simultaneous calibration on two individual devices. The processes required in setting and changing of device adjustment controls could possibly lead to unintentional procedure needle or ultrasound probe movement. A potential solution for this problem would be an ultrasound machine that also has the ability of incorporating the mechanics of a nerve stimulator.[97] Therefore, when stimulating procedure needles and perineural catheters to confirm anatomical locations and proximity to target sites during nerve block techniques, there would be added benefits of both adjunctive ultrasonography and nerve stimulation that could be controlled simultaneously.[98] In addition, when both, the needle and target, are adequately imaged, the nerve stimulation as an adjunct to ultrasound guidance may have a limited role because a positive motor response to nerve stimulation does not increase the success rate of the block. In addition nerve stimulation when combined with UG does have a and high false-negative rate that suggests these blocks are usually effective, even in the absence of a motor response.[99,100] Potential problems with adequate neurostimulation when used in conjunction with UGIP could be related to the ultrasound gel. When 5% dextrose was used, as a nonconducting medium, it did not affect electrical conduction during electrical stimulation. Thus, it is important to avoid using saline or gel as a sound medium because it may hinder any subsequent attempts to electrically stimulate the nerve.[90]

Summary

In order to unmistakably visualize the procedural needle under the ultrasound and manipulate the needle effectively, a new set of skills is to be acquired. These skills are the critical assets which unlikely will ever be substituted by advanced ultrasound technology and enhanced procedural needles. The techniques discussed in this chapter intend to help to improve needle visualization during UGIP. They should be used in combination, depending on the nature and localization of the procedure.

REFERENCES

1. Peng PW, Narouze S. Ultrasound-guided interventional procedures in pain medicine: a review of anatomy, sonoanatomy, and procedures: part I: nonaxial structures. *Reg Anesth Pain Med.* 2009;34(5):458–474.
2. Sites BD, Gallagher JD, Cravero J, Lundberg J, Blike G. The learning curve associated with a simulated ultrasound-guided interventional task by inexperienced anesthesia residents. *Reg Anesth Pain Med.* 2004;29(6):544–548.
3. Sites BD, Spence BC, Gallagher JD, Wiley CW, Bertrand ML, Blike GT. Characterizing novice behavior associated with learning ultrasound-guided peripheral regional anesthesia. *Reg Anesth Pain Med.* 2007;32(2):107–115.
4. Sites BD, Brull R, Chan VW, et al. Artifacts and pitfall errors associated with ultrasound-guided regional anesthesia. Part II: a pictorial approach to understanding and avoidance. *Reg Anesth Pain Med.* 2007;32(5):419–433.
5. Dessieux T, Estebe JP, Bloc S, Mercadal L, Ecoffey C. Evaluation of the learning curve of residents in localizing a phantom target with ultrasonography. *Ann Fr Anesth Reanim.* 2008;27(10):797–801.
6. Bloc S, Mercadal L, Dessieux T, et al. The learning process of the hydrolocalization technique performed during ultrasound-guided regional anesthesia. *Acta Anaesthesiol Scand.* 2010;54(4):421–425.
7. Ivani G, Ferrante FM. The American Society of Regional Anesthesia and Pain Medicine and the European Society of Regional Anaesthesia and Pain Therapy Joint Committee recommendations for education and training in ultrasound guided regional anesthesia: why do we need these guidelines? *Reg Anesth Pain Med.* 2009;34(1):8–9.
8. Bennett S. Training guidelines for ultrasound: worldwide trends. *Best Pract Res Clin Anaesthesiol.* 2009;23(3):363–373.
9. Sites BD, Chan VW, Neal JM, et al. The American Society of Regional Anesthesia and Pain Medicine and the European Society of Regional Anaesthesia and Pain Therapy Joint Committee recommendations for education and training in ultrasound-guided regional anesthesia. *Reg Anesth Pain Med.* 2009;34(1):40–46.
10. Pollard BA. New model for learning ultrasound-guided needle to target localization. *Reg Anesth Pain Med.* 2008;33(4):360–362.
11. Tsui B, Dillane D, Pillay J, Walji A. Ultrasound imaging in cadavers: training in imaging for regional blockade at the trunk. *Can J Anaesth.* 2008;55(2):105–111.
12. Xu D, Abbas S, Chan VW. Ultrasound phantom for hands-on practice. *Reg Anesth Pain Med.* 2005;30(6):593–594.
13. van Geffen GJ, Mulder J, Gielen M, van Egmond J, Scheffer GJ, Bruhn J. A needle guidance device compared to free hand technique in an ultrasound-guided interventional task using a phantom. *Anaesthesia.* 2008;63(9):986–990.
14. Bruyn GA, Schmidt WA. How to perform ultrasound-guided injections. *Best Pract Res Clin Rheumatol.* 2009;23(2):269–279.
15. Keegan B. Anthropomorphic phantoms and method. US Patent Application 2005/0202381. 2005.
16. Zhu Y, Magee D, Ratnalingam R, Kessel D. A training system for ultrasound-guided needle insertion procedures. *Med Image Comput Comput Assist Interv.* 2007;10(pt 1):566–574.
17. Magee D, Zhu Y, Ratnalingam R, Gardner P, Kessel D. An augmented reality simulator for ultrasound guided needle placement training. *Med Biol Eng Comput.* 2007;45(10):957–967.
18. Gurusamy KS, Aggarwal R, Palanivelu L, Davidson BR. Virtual reality training for surgical trainees in laparoscopic surgery. *Cochrane Database Syst Rev.* 2009;(1):CD006575.
19. Grottke O, Ntouba A, Ullrich S, et al. Virtual reality-based simulator for training in regional anaesthesia. *Br J Anaesth.* 2009;103(4):594–600.
20. Ullrich S, Grottke O, Fried E, et al. An intersubject variable regional anesthesia simulator with a virtual patient architecture. *Int J Comput Assist Radiol Surg.* 2009;4(6):561–570.
21. Galiano K, Obwegeser AA, Bale R, et al. Ultrasound-guided and CT-navigation-assisted periradicular and facet joint injections in the lumbar and cervical spine: a new teaching tool to recognize the sonoanatomic pattern. *Reg Anesth Pain Med.* 2007;32(3):254–257.
22. Matveevskii AS, Gravenstein N. Role of simulators, educational programs, and nontechnical skills in anesthesia resident selection, education, and competency assessment. *J Crit Care.* 2008;23(2):167–172.

23. Phelan MP, Emerman C, Peacock WF, Karafa M, Colburn N, Buchanan K. Do echo-enhanced needles improve time to cannulate in a model of short-axis ultrasound-guided vascular access for a group of mostly inexperienced ultrasound users? *Int J Emerg Med.* 2009;2(3):167–170.

24. Steadman RH. The American Society of Anesthesiologists' national endorsement program for simulation centers. *J Crit Care.* 2008;23(2):203–206.

25. Friedman Z, Siddiqui N, Katznelson R, Devito I, Bould MD, Naik V. Clinical impact of epidural anesthesia simulation on short- and long-term learning curve: high- versus low-fidelity model training. *Reg Anesth Pain Med.* 2009;34(3):229–232.

26. Chapman GA, Johnson D, Bodenham AR. Visualisation of needle position using ultrasonography. *Anaesthesia.* 2006;61(2):148–158.

27. Sites BD, Brull R, Chan VW, et al. Artifacts and pitfall errors associated with ultrasound-guided regional anesthesia. Part I: understanding the basic principles of ultrasound physics and machine operations. *Reg Anesth Pain Med.* 2007;32(5):412–418.

28. Schafhalter-Zoppoth I, McCulloch CE, Gray AT. Ultrasound visibility of needles used for regional nerve block: an in vitro study. *Reg Anesth Pain Med.* 2004;29(5):480–488.

29. Campos NA, Chiles JH, Plunkett AR. Ultrasound-guided cryoablation of genitofemoral nerve for chronic inguinal pain. *Pain Physician.* 2009;12(6):997–1000.

30. Liang P, Gao Y, Wang Y, Yu X, Yu D, Dong B. US-guided percutaneous needle biopsy of the spleen using 18-gauge versus 21-gauge needles. *J Clin Ultrasound.* 2007;35(9):477–482.

31. Chin KJ, Perlas A, Chan VW, Brull R. Needle visualization in ultrasound-guided regional anesthesia: challenges and solutions. *Reg Anesth Pain Med.* 2008;33(6):532–544.

32. Tsui BC, Doyle K, Chu K, Pillay J, Dillane D. Case series: ultrasound-guided supraclavicular block using a curvilinear probe in 104 day-case hand surgery patients. *Can J Anaesth.* 2009;56(1):46–51.

33. Nichols K, Wright LB, Spencer T, Culp WC. Changes in ultrasonographic echogenicity and visibility of needles with changes in angles of insonation. *J Vasc Interv Radiol.* 2003;14(12):1553–1557.

34. Deam RK, Kluger R, Barrington MJ, McCutcheon CA. Investigation of a new echogenic needle for use with ultrasound peripheral nerve blocks. *Anaesth Intensive Care.* 2007;35(4):582–586.

35. Simonetti F. A guided wave technique for needle biopsy under ultrasound guidance. *Proc SPIE.* 2009;7261:726118.

36. Culp WC, McCowan TC, Goertzen TC, et al. Relative ultrasonographic echogenicity of standard, dimpled, and polymeric-coated needles. *J Vasc Interv Radiol.* 2000;11(3):351–358.

37. Perrella RR, Kimme-Smith C, Tessler FN, Ragavendra N, Grant EG. A new electronically enhanced biopsy system: value in improving needle-tip visibility during sonographically guided interventional procedures. *AJR Am J Roentgenol.* 1992;158(1):195–198.

38. Klein SM, Fronheiser MP, Reach J, Nielsen KC, Smith SW. Piezoelectric vibrating needle and catheter for enhancing ultrasound-guided peripheral nerve blocks. *Anesth Analg.* 2007;105(6):1858–1860. table of contents.

39. Maecken T, Zenz M, Grau T. Ultrasound characteristics of needles for regional anesthesia. *Reg Anesth Pain Med.* 2007;32(5):440–447.

40. Takayama W, Yasumura R, Kaneko T, et al. Novel echogenic needle for ultrasound-guided peripheral nerve block "Hakko type CCR". *Masui.* 2009;58(4):503–507.

41. Daoud MI, Lacefield JC. Distributed three-dimensional simulation of B-mode ultrasound imaging using a first-order k-space method. *Phys Med Biol.* 2009;54(17):5173–5192.

42. Bertolotto M, Perrone R, Bucci S, Zappetti R, Coss M. Comparison of conventional ultrasound and real-time spatial compound imaging in evaluation of patients with severe Peyronie's disease. *Acta Radiol.* 2008;49(5):596–601.

43. Cheung S, Rohling R. Enhancement of needle visibility in ultrasound-guided percutaneous procedures. *Ultrasound Med Biol.* 2004;30(5):617–624.

44. Mesurolle B, Bining HJ, El Khoury M, Barhdadi A, Kao E. Contribution of tissue harmonic imaging and frequency compound imaging in interventional breast sonography. *J Ultrasound Med.* 2006;25(7):845–855.

45. Brull R, Perlas A, Chan VW. Ultrasound-guided peripheral nerve blockade. *Curr Pain Headache Rep.* 2007;11(1):25–32.

46. Ricci S, Moro L, Antonel liIncalzi R. Ultrasound imaging of the sural nerve: ultrasound anatomy and rationale for investigation. *Eur J Vasc Endovasc Surg.* 2010;39(5):636–641.

47. Yen CL, Jeng CM, Yang SS. The benefits of comparing conventional sonography, real-time spatial compound sonography, tissue harmonic sonography, and tissue harmonic compound sonography of hepatic lesions. *Clin Imaging.* 2008;32(1):11–15.

48. Cohnen M, Saleh A, Luthen R, Bode J, Modder U. Improvement of sonographic needle visibility in cirrhotic livers during transjugular intrahepatic portosystemic stent-shunt procedures with use of real-time compound imaging. *J Vasc Interv Radiol.* 2003;14(1):103–106.

49. Clendenen SR, Riutort KT, Feinglass NG, Greengrass RA, Brull SJ. Real-time three-dimensional ultrasound for continuous interscalene brachial plexus blockade. *J Anesth.* 2009;23(3): 466–468.

50. Kwak J, Andrawes M, Garvin S, D'Ambra MN. 3D transesophageal echocardiography: a review of recent literature 2007–2009. *Curr Opin Anaesthesiol.* 2010;23(1):80–88.

51. French JL, Raine-Fenning NJ, Hardman JG, Bedforth NM. Pitfalls of ultrasound guided vascular access: the use of three/four-dimensional ultrasound. *Anaesthesia.* 2008;63(8):806–813.

52. Hansen R, Masoy SE, Johansen TF, Angelsen BA. Utilizing dual frequency band transmit pulse complexes in medical ultrasound imaging. *J Acoust Soc Am.* 2010;127(1):579–587.

53. Huijssen J, Verweij MD. An iterative method for the computation of nonlinear, wide-angle, pulsed acoustic fields of medical diagnostic transducers. *J Acoust Soc Am.* 2010;127(1):33–44.

54. Martinez-Graullera O, Martin CJ, Godoy G, Ullate LG. 2D array design based on Fermat spiral for ultrasound imaging. *Ultrasonics.* 2010;50(2):280–289.

55. Foster FS, Mehi J, Lukacs M, et al. A new 15–50 MHz array-based micro-ultrasound scanner for preclinical imaging. *Ultrasound Med Biol.* 2009;35(10):1700–1708.

56. Gebauer B, Teichgraber UM, Werk M, Beck A, Wagner HJ. Sonographically guided venous puncture and fluoroscopically guided placement of tunneled, large-bore central venous catheters for bone marrow transplantation-high success rates and low complication rates. *Support Care Cancer.* 2008;16(8):897–904.

57. Phee SJ, Yang K. Interventional navigation systems for treatment of unresectable liver tumor. *Med Biol Eng Comput.* 2010;48(2):103–111.

58. Vaithilingam S, Ma TJ, Furukawa Y, et al. Three-dimensional photoacoustic imaging using a two-dimensional CMUT array. *IEEE Trans Ultrason Ferroelectr Freq Control.* 2009;56(11): 2411–2419.

59. Nelson BP, Melnick ER, Li J. Portable ultrasound for remote environments, part I: feasibility of field deployment. *J Emerg Med.* 2010 (In press).

60. Sites BD, Spence BC, Gallagher J, et al. Regional anesthesia meets ultrasound: a specialty in transition. *Acta Anaesthesiol Scand.* 2008;52(4):456–466.

61. Palmeri ML, Dahl JJ, MacLeod DB, Grant SA, Nightingale KR. On the feasibility of imaging peripheral nerves using acoustic radiation force impulse imaging. *Ultrason Imaging.* 2009;31(3): 172–182.

62. Meir A, Rubinsky B. Distributed network, wireless and cloud computing enabled 3-D ultrasound: a new medical technology paradigm. *PLoS One.* 2009;4(11):e7974.

63. Linguraru MG, Vasilyev NV, Del Nido PJ, Howe RD. Statistical segmentation of surgical instruments in 3-D ultrasound images. *Ultrasound Med Biol.* 2007;33(9):1428–1437.

64. Boctor EM, Choti MA, Burdette EC, Webster Iii RJ. Three-dimensional ultrasound-guided robotic needle placement: an experimental evaluation. *Int J Med Robot.* 2008;4(2):180–191.

65. Freschi C, Troia E, Ferrari V, Megali G, Pietrabissa A, Mosca F. Ultrasound guided robotic biopsy using augmented reality and human-robot cooperative control. *Conf Proc IEEE Eng Med Biol Soc.* 2009;1:5110–5113.

66. Wood BJ, Locklin JK, Viswanathan A, et al. Technologies for guidance of radiofrequency ablation in the multimodality interventional suite of the future. *J Vasc Interv Radiol.* 2007;18(1 pt 1):9–24.

67. Hiraoka A, Hirooka M, Koizumi Y, et al. Modified technique for determining therapeutic response to radiofrequency ablation therapy for hepatocellular carcinoma using US-volume system. *Oncol Rep.* 2010;23(2):493–497.

68. Fredrickson M. "Oblique" needle-probe alignment to facilitate ultrasound-guided femoral catheter placement. *Reg Anesth Pain Med.* 2008;33(4):383–384.

69. Phelan M, Hagerty D. The oblique view: an alternative approach for ultrasound-guided central line placement. *J Emerg Med.* 2009;37(4):403–408.

70. Phal PM, Brooks DM, Wolfe R. Sonographically guided biopsy of focal lesions: a comparison of freehand and probe-guided techniques using a phantom. *AJR Am J Roentgenol.* 2005;184(5): 1652–1656.

71. Wang AZ, Zhang WX, Jiang W. A needle guide can facilitate visualization of needle passage in ultrasound-guided nerve blocks. *J Clin Anesth.* 2009;21(3):230–232.

72. Buonocore E, Skipper GJ. Steerable real-time sonographically guided needle biopsy. *AJR Am J Roentgenol.* 1981;136(2):387–392.

73. Tsui BC. Facilitating needle alignment in-plane to an ultrasound beam using a portable laser unit. *Reg Anesth Pain Med.* 2007;32(1):84–88.

74. Sites BD, Brull R. Ultrasound guidance in peripheral regional anesthesia: philosophy, evidence-based medicine, and techniques. *Curr Opin Anaesthesiol.* 2006;19(6):630–639.

75. Wood BJ, Zhang H, Durrani A, et al. Navigation with electromagnetic tracking for interventional radiology procedures: a feasibility study. *J Vasc Interv Radiol.* 2005;16(4):493–505.

76. Levy EB, Tang J, Lindisch D, Glossop N, Banovac F, Cleary K. Implementation of an electromagnetic tracking system for accurate intrahepatic puncture needle guidance: accuracy results in an in vitro model. *Acad Radiol.* 2007;14(3):344–354.

77. Krucker J, Xu S, Glossop N, et al. Electromagnetic tracking for thermal ablation and biopsy guidance: clinical evaluation of spatial accuracy. *J Vasc Interv Radiol.* 2007;18(9):1141–1150.

78. Glossop ND. Advantages of optical compared with electromagnetic tracking. *J Bone Joint Surg Am.* 2009;91(suppl 1):23–28.

79. Paltieli Y, Degani S, Zrayek A, et al. A new guidance system for freehand, obstetric ultrasound-guided procedures. *Ultrasound Obstet Gynecol.* 2002;19(3):269–273.

80. Marhofer P, Chan VW. Ultrasound-guided regional anesthesia: current concepts and future trends. *Anesth Analg.* 2007;104(5):1265–1269.

81. Molnar J. Regional anesthesia system and cart. US Patent 2009275892. 2009.

82. Hickey K, Parashar A, Sites B, Spence BC. Biomedical positioning and stabilization system. US Patent 2007129634. 2007.

83. Tsui BC. Dextrose 5% in water as an alternative medium to gel for performing ultrasound-guided peripheral nerve blocks. *Reg Anesth Pain Med.* 2009;34(5):525–527.

84. Sites BD, Spence BC, Gallagher JD, Beach ML. On the edge of the ultrasound screen: regional anesthesiologists diagnosing nonneural pathology. *Reg Anesth Pain Med.* 2006;31(6):555–562.

85. Faust AM, Fournier R. Color Doppler as a surrogate marker of needle-tip location in ultrasound-guided regional anesthesia. *Reg Anesth Pain Med.* 2009;34(5):525.

86. Greenleaf JF, Urban MW, Chen S. Measurement of tissue mechanical properties with shear wave dispersion ultrasound vibrometry (SDUV). *Conf Proc IEEE Eng Med Biol Soc.* 2009;1:4411–4414.

87. Chung HH, Cha SH, Lee KY, Kim TK, Kim JH. Fluid infusion technique for ultrasound-guided percutaneous nephrostomy. *Cardiovasc Intervent Radiol.* 2005;28(1):77–79.

88. Bloc S, Ecoffey C, Dhonneur G. Controlling needle tip progression during ultrasound-guided regional anesthesia using the hydrolocalization technique. *Reg Anesth Pain Med.* 2008;33(4):382–383.

89. Tsui BC, Kropelin B. The electrophysiological effect of dextrose 5% in water on single-shot peripheral nerve stimulation. *Anesth Analg.* 2005;100(6):1837–1839.

90. Tsui BC, Kropelin B, Ganapathy S, Finucane B. Dextrose 5% in water: fluid medium for maintaining electrical stimulation of peripheral nerves during stimulating catheter placement. *Acta Anaesthesiol Scand.* 2005;49(10):1562–1565.

91. Dhir S, Ganapathy S. Use of ultrasound guidance and contrast enhancement: a study of continuous infraclavicular brachial plexus approach. *Acta Anaesthesiol Scand.* 2008;52(3):338–342.

92. Swenson JD, Davis JJ, DeCou JA. A novel approach for assessing catheter position after ultrasound-guided placement of continuous interscalene block. *Anesth Analg.* 2008;106(3):1015–1016.

93. Kang E, Min HS, Lee J, et al. Nanobubbles from gas-generating polymeric nanoparticles: ultrasound imaging of living subjects. *Angew Chem Int Ed Engl.* 2010;49(3):524–528.

94. Chantzi C, Saranteas T, Paraskeuopoulos T, Dimitriou V. Ultrasound and transcutaneous neurostimulator combined technique as a training method for nerve identification in anesthesia residents. *Reg Anesth Pain Med.* 2007;32(4):365–366.

95. Dingemans E, Williams SR, Arcand G, et al. Neurostimulation in ultrasound-guided infraclavicular block: a prospective randomized trial. *Anesth Analg.* 2007;104(5):1275–1280.

96. Dufour E, Quennesson P, Van Robais AL, et al. Combined ultrasound and neurostimulation guidance for popliteal sciatic nerve block: a prospective, randomized comparison with neurostimulation alone. *Anesth Analg.* 2008;106(5):1553–1558.

97. Urbano J, Cannon M, Engle l. Integrated nerve stimulator and ultrasound imaging device. US Patent 2008119737. 2008.

98. de Tran QH, Munoz L, Russo G, Finlayson RJ. Ultrasonography and stimulating perineural catheters for nerve blocks: a review of the evidence. *Can J Anaesth.* 2008;55(7):447–457.

99. Beach ML, Sites BD, Gallagher JD. Use of a nerve stimulator does not improve the efficacy of ultrasound-guided supraclavicular nerve blocks. *J Clin Anesth.* 2006;18(8):580–584.

100. Chan VW, Perlas A, McCartney CJ, Brull R, Xu D, Abbas S. Ultrasound guidance improves success rate of axillary brachial plexus block. *Can J Anaesth.* 2007;54(3):176–182.

II

Spine Sonoanatomy and Ultrasound-Guided Spine Injections

5

Spine Anatomy and Sonoanatomy for Pain Physicians

Bernhard Moriggl

B. Moriggl (✉)
Department of Anatomy, Histology and Embryology, Division of Clinical and Functional Anatomy,
Innsbruck Medical University, Muellerstrasse 59, Innsbruck A-6020, Austria
e-mail: bernhard.moriggl@i-med.ac.at

S.N. Narouze (ed.), *Atlas of Ultrasound-Guided Procedures in Interventional Pain Management*,
DOI 10.1007/978-1-4419-1681-5_5, © Springer Science+Business Media, LLC 2011

Introduction

First and far most *recognition of limits* in performing ultrasound (US) imaging of the spine, associated spaces and joints is imperative before feasibilities may be fully appreciated. It is thus not surprising that some of the descriptions on approaches within parts of the spine (and pelvis) by means of sonography were published that can simply not withstand critical analysis. In addition, more than elsewhere in applying US in pain medicine one has to be familiar with the usage of the right transducer (frequency) in the right area at individual patients and different settings. That way, all available transducers, technologies and possible frequencies play a practical role in proper spine imaging! Finally, influence of positioning, movements and alterations of the spine (and thus age!) are tremendous and may either be challenging or make manoeuvres impossible.

Accordingly, this chapter will *first* include a briefing on *relevant anatomical peculiarities* and *variability* of the spine from skull to coccyx *absolutely basic* to understand possibilities/limits in performing blocks and injections, respectively. Throughout the *second* part on *relevant US images*, emphasis will be laid on differentiation between "superficial," meaning bony contours (mainly posterolateral) or synovial joint capsules/entrances and "deep," that means articular cavities of zygapophysial (ZJ) and sacroiliac joints (SIJ), the vertebral canal, epidural space (EDS), paravertebral space, intervertebral foramina and nerve roots, sacral foramina and the vertebral artery.

As a rule, deep structures or spaces in the above-mentioned sense may only be reliably visualised ultrasonographically if "acoustic windows" are present (or created!) and used properly.

That way and generally speaking, there is no US access to vertebral bodies or intervertebral discs and intervertebral foramina (thus nerve roots) of the thoracic spine (TS) and sacrum (S). Addressed structures are partly accessible in the lumbar spine (LS) but reliable visualisation is closely associated with BMI and/or individually highly different tissue properties that markedly influence echogenicity. So, with the important exception of the cervical part, direct visualisation of the sympathetic trunk is impossible. In the cervical spine (CS), a wider approach to the anterior aspect – including discs – is possible but partly limited by both, air ways and mandible.

Despite named difficulties it will be shown that spine imaging using US, spine *sonoanatomy*, is as challenging as it is fascinating if one is familiar with and aware of intrinsic limitations!

Basic Spine Anatomy (Figures 5.1–5.13)

Cervical Spine

While all transverse processes (TP) of cervical vertebrae, C1–C7, possess foramina transversaria – hosting the vertebral artery (VA) and sympathetic plexuses from C6 upwards. Only C3–C6 constantly show an anterior (usually the bigger) and posterior tubercle with the groove for the spinal nerve between them. Regularly, the posterior tubercles C3 through C5 are situated lower and lateral to the anterior ones. In clear contrast to the rest of the spine, the TP lie beside the vertebral bodies and are slightly directed downwards and anteriorly (Figures 5.1 and 5.2). As TP are crucial landmarks for orientation it is important to add that:

Apart from the atlas (C1) and C7, all other TP are relatively short (Figure 5.1b).

The TP of C1 projects more laterally than all others (Figure 5.1b).

The TP of C2 is often rudimentary as an anterior tubercle is not clearly developed (Figures 5.1a and 5.2a, b).

The anterior tubercle of TP C6, usually referred to as the biggest ("carotid tubercle," tubercle of Chassaignac), may vary considerable in size (!), even between both sides of the same individual (Figure 5.1a). The TP of C7 has no anterior tubercle (Figures 5.1a, 5.2a, b, 5.23c and 5.24b!) all TP may vary according to size and length.

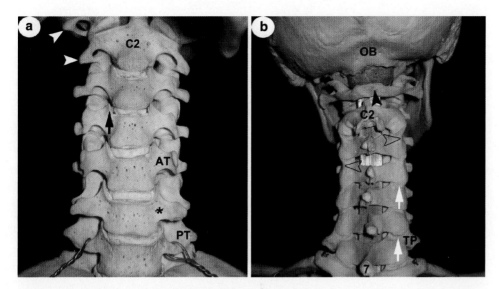

Figure 5.1. (a) CS anterior view. C2 axis; *white arrowheads* pointing at transverse processes of atlas and axis with their foramina transversaria; *black asterisk* indicates groove at the base of transverse process C6; AT left anterior tubercle of C5. Note: in this individual, the C5 AT is bigger than that of C6, especially the right one! C7 has only a posterior tubercle, PT; from C5 to C3 all PT are lateral and lower to the AT; *black arrow* points at uncinate process; (b) CS posterior view. OB occipital bone; seven spinous process, SP, of vertebra prominens; C2 axis with bifid tip of SP; *black arrowhead* points at rudimentary posterior tubercle of the atlas' slim posterior arch. *Open arrowheads* point at the waist of articular pillars, *white arrows* at posterior entrance into cervical zygapophysial joints. Note asymmetry of length of TP in segments C2–C6! See text for more details.

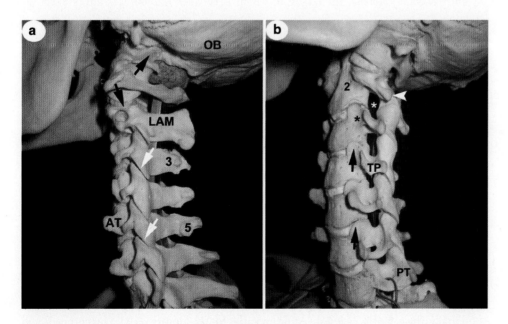

Figure 5.2. (a) CS lateral view. OB occipital bone; LAM lamina of axis; three and five asymmetry of tubercles at spinous processes; AT anterior tubercle C5 of considerable size; *white arrows* point at cervical zygapophysial joints, *black* ones indicate joint gaps of atlanto-occipital and atlanto-axial joints, respectively. Note their different orientation and width of gaps. (b) CS antero-lateral view. PT posterior tubercle of C7; TP transverse process C4; *black arrows* point at uncinate processes; *black asterisk* indicates groove at base of transverse process C3, *white* one in intervertebral foramen C2/3. Two body of axis; *white arrowhead* on rudimentary TP of axis; Note that foramina are only fully appreciated when CS is viewed from antero-lateral and slightly inferior (the ones of C5/6 and 6/7 therefore incompletely seen); compare with view in (a)! See text for more details.

Figure 5.3. Bilateral cervical ribs (with ligamentous extensions). The smaller with ankylosis to transverse process, TP, of C7. Note asymmetry of transverse processes from C6 upwards, especially comparing anterior tubercles!

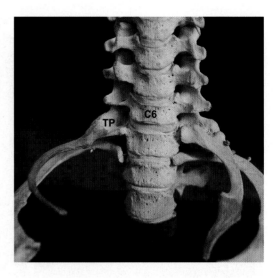

Another noteworthy and constant morphological feature true for C3–C6(7) is the marked but unnamed groove at the base of TP. Above this groove the upper surfaces of corpses C3–C7 raise lip-like to form the *uncinate processes*. They reach as far cranial as the lower contour of the next body; so they completely cover (and protect) the whole lateral aspect of the intervertebral disc! (Figures 5.1 and 5.2b).

Cervical ribs (Figure 5.3) of various length and massiveness may occur if the rib anlagen of the TP remains independent; most commonly seen bilateral (more frequent on left side if unilateral). Such an entity should be thought of if sensory disturbances occur related to the brachial plexus.

Intervertebral foramina, the largest of which is between C2 and C3, are not seen in lateral views (Figure 5.2a, b).

In contrast to C7, the tips of spinous processes (SP) appear bifurcated in most individuals, but very often asymmetrical, unequal in size and not infrequently poorly developed or just indicated at C5 and C6. Moreover, SP often deviate either to right or left (Figure 5.1b).

Cervical zygapophysial joints (CZJ), also named "facet joints," are plain joints with their inferior articular surfaces facing forwards and downwards, in conformity the superior ones backwards and upwards. In general, the narrow joint gaps are best appreciated in a lateral view! Only that between C2 and C3 differs as the two surfaces of C3 are at an angle of 142° to each other (Figures 5.1b, 5.2a and 5.4a, b). Viewed from posterior, superior and inferior *articular processes* (AP) of each vertebra ("articular pillars") with their marked waist between them, creates a wavy appearance of the lateral borders of the CS from C2–C7 (Figure 5.1b).

Due to the lack of both, a vertebral body and a SP, the *atlas* is unique among vertebrae. It has two arches, anterior and posterior. The latter is usually very slim, its height approximately only half the size of a regular lamina (LAM), and its "median" posterior tubercle often rudimentary or absent. As a result, the atlanto-occipital and atlanto-axial gaps (acoustic windows) are considerably wider compared to those between LAM and SP of C2–C7 (Figures 5.1b and 5.2a). The distance from skin to the posterior arch differs significantly, not least influenced by the individual shape of the neurocranium.

Finally, the atlanto-occipital (AOJ) and atlanto-axial joints (AAJ), "upperhead" and "lowerhead joints" are also unique among CS diarthroses: the former is an ellipsoid joint, the latter part of a (functionally) rotary one with a considerable wide joint gap. Importantly, the AAJ is bordered by the C2 dorsal root ganglion (DRG; dorsomedial), and the vertebral artery (VA; lateral); consecutively the VA regularly runs inferior and medial to the AOJ (Figures 5.2a and 5.4a, b). In case of elongation, the VA may also cross both joints dorsally (Figure 5.17a bottom)!

In summary, all mentioned features of CS-anatomy should remind US users that there is (a) *no symmetry* within one individual and (b) practically *relevant interindividual variabil-*

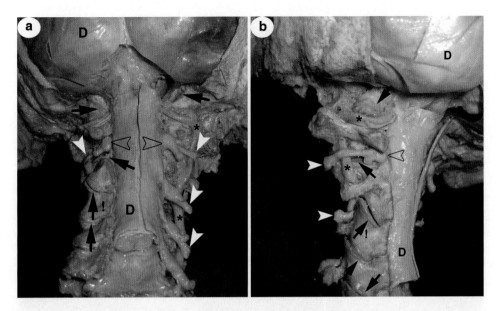

Figure 5.4. (a) Atlanto-occipital, atlanto-axial and cervical zygapophysial joints, AO, AA, CZJ, posterior view. Posterior arch of atlas, SP and LAM C2–C5 as well as occipital bone removed. D dura mater; *black arrows* indicate AOJ, AAJ and CZJ of C3/4 and C2/3! *White arrowheads* show ventral rami of spinal cervical nerves; *open arrowheads* show second dorsal root ganglia. Note the course of the vertebral artery (*black asterisks*) relative to AO and AAJ as well as to nerve roots. (b) Postero-lateral view of specimen in (a). Symbols for labelling as in (a). Note width of AAJ-gap. See text for more details.

ity (Sir William Osler: "… and as no to faces are the same, so no two bodies are alike …"). Special attention has to be paid to *atlas and axis* with their respective joints!

Thoracic Spine

The second through the tenth thoracic vertebrae, T2–T10, may be viewed as "typical." In contrast to the situation at the CS, the sturdy transverse processes (TP) lie lateral and a little posterior to the articular processes and are directed upwards (except T10) and posteriorly. They articulate with the tubercles of their respective ribs, the neck of which lies anterior (thus hidden) to the transverse processes until T4. From there to T9, the ribs' neck progressively projects the TP (Figure 5.5a); important for paravertebral blocks (narrow acoustic windows). There is little variability as far as the size and length of these TPs. In contrast, TP of T11 and T12 are often rudimentary, and as occurs in the LS, show accessory and mamillary processes in various degrees and shapes. In addition, T12 often develops an indicated (rudimentary) costal process (CP) (Figure 5.5b).

The spinous processes (SP) of the second through ninth thoracic vertebrae are arranged like roof tiles. This is most accentuated from T5 to T9, creating an osseous barrier (no acoustic window!). As a consequence, a transverse section through both TP of a given vertebra will show the SP of the next higher segment (Figure 5.5a)! Quite similar to the situation in the CS, the SP of a (perfectly regular) TS often deviate, meaning their tips are paramedian, sometimes even by turns of each segment in certain parts (Figure 5.5a, b). Orientation of the SP of T10 varies; most commonly it only slightly descends, while those of T11 and 12 extend directly dorsally, giving space (=allowing better access) between them (Figure 5.5b).

A typical feature of T1–T10 is the width of their lamina (LAM) which exceeds over that of their bodies (Figure 5.6a). Together with the SP, both LAM of a single vertebra form a bow. Not so with T11 and T12 (due to their similarity with lumbar vertebrae, see also below): their LAM is sturdy and narrow, essentially facing posteriorly (Figure 5.5b).

The thoracic zygapophysial joints (TZJ) are plain joints as those in the CS (with similar narrow cavity), but position of the joint surfaces represents segments of a cylinder (except the one between T11 and T12): they face back and slightly outwards at the superior, forward and inwards at the inferior AP. As in the CS, the inferior AP almost com-

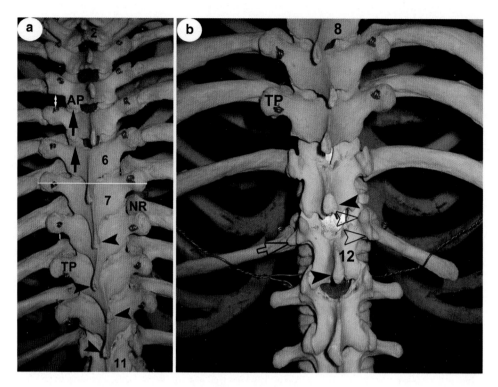

Figure 5.5. (a) Posterior view of TS from T2 to T11. 2, 6, 7 and 11 lamina of respective thoracic vertebra; AP inferior articular process of T4; *black arrows* point at posterior entrance into thoracic zygapophysial joints. Note differences in upper and lower part of TS. TP transverse process of T9; NR neck of eighth rib; *white double arrows* indicate examples of different "acoustic windows" in different thoracic levels; *black arrowheads* indicate tips of spinous processes, SP, T8–T11; the *white line* through both TP of T7 hits the SP of T6! (b) 8, 12 lamina, LAM, of respective thoracic vertebra; TP transverse process of T10; TP of T11 and 12 are rudimentary but clearly show mamillary as well as accessory processes (*open arrowheads*); *open arrow* points at an equivalent of a lumbar costal process in T12! *Black arrowheads* indicate tips of SP T11 and 12. Note width between LAM and SP at T11/12 level compared to segments above! See text for more details.

pletely covers the superior AP of the next vertebra (not so at T12/L1). This arrangement impedes access to most of the joint entrances in contrast to the more exposed *costotransverse joints* (Figure 5.6b). Synovial capsules of all costotransverse articulations are surrounded by a rather strong ligamentous apparatus! There are no such joints at T11 and T12 (rudimentary transverse processes and lack of costal tubercles at ribs 11 and 12).

Due to peculiarities of *anatomy* mentioned, the TS is a *difficult part for US exploration* and one has to consider *uppermost, lowermost* and *middle part* differently.

Lumbar Spine

With the exception of the fifth lumbar vertebra, L1–L4 show similar features and are therefore representative. Their costal processes (CP) or "transverse processes" (TP) (see below) are regularly slim and long, pointing lateral in essence. The dorsal surface of CP face strictly posterior. Apparently different to the TS, CP are situated anterior (!) to the AP. This is because they constitute the homologue of a rib (and therefore CP is the more accurate terminology). In case of non-fusion with the vertebra, a *lumbar rib* occurs in approximately 8% of individuals. Apart from this entity, there is noteworthy variability concerning length, width/height and "massiveness" of CP. This includes marked differences in different levels as well as on both sides of a single spine. Especially, a rudimentary (very short and slender) CP is of practical relevance, most frequently seen at L4 (Figures 5.7 and 5.9b). Uninfluenced by such variability, at the root of each CP a small but rough *acces-*

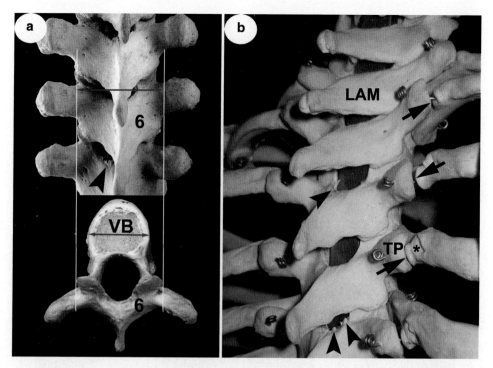

Figure 5.6. (a) Posterior view of middle part of TS with insert of a typical thoracic vertebra. Six lamina, LAM, of T6; *double arrows* compare width of LAM with that of body, VB; *black arrowhead* points at a typical bony spur from upper margin of T7 LAM (partly ossification of yellow ligament!). (b) Postero-lateral view of upper thoracic spine. LAM lamina of T1; *asterisk* tubercle of fourth rib, TP transverse process of T4; *black arrows* indicate costotransverse diarthroses, *black arrowheads* beginning ossification of yellow ligaments. Note that windows between LAM are relatively wide in this part of TS (compare with Figure 5.5a, b). See text for more details.

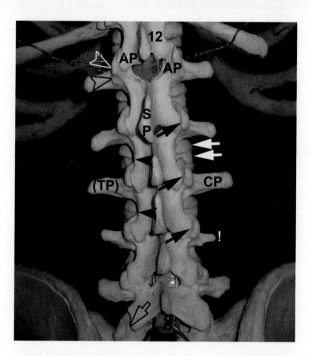

Figure 5.7. Posterior view of LS. Twelve lamina, LAM, of T12; AP facing articular processes of T12 (inferior AP) and L1 (superior AP); *open arrowheads* indicate mamillary process at superior AP and accessory processes at root of costal process, CP ("transverse," TP); SP spinous process of L1; *black arrows* point at lumbar zygapophysial joints, LZJ, *white* ones indicate vertebral body of L2 and intervertebral disc, respectively; *black arrowheads* at waists of LAM L2 and L3. Note (!) rudimentary CP of L4 and different "shapes" of CP throughout LS. *Open arrow* points at the LSJ that differs from LZJ above. See text for more details.

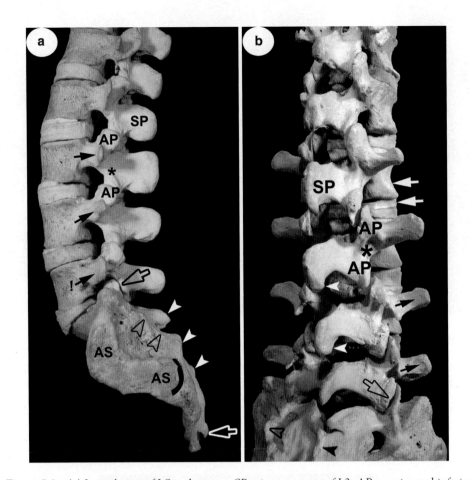

Figure 5.8. (a) Lateral view of LS and sacrum. SP spinous process of L2; AP superior and inferior articular process of L3 with "interarticular portion" (*asterisk*) in between; *black arrows* indicate costal processes L3–L5, the latter more massive than all others (!). *Black open arrow* points at joint gap of LSJ (those of LZJ not visible!). AS articular surface, *arched line marks* posterior end (compare with Figure 5.11b); the median sacral crest (*white arrowheads*) and lateral sacral crest (*open arrowheads*) are labelled; *white open arrow* points to (left) sacral horn. Note the huge distance and area between lateral sacral crest and AS, the sacral tuberosity! See text for more details. (b) Postero-lateral view of LS (and sacrum). Interspinous and interlaminar spaces widened by abolition of lordosis compared to (a). *White arrowheads* indicate caudal extension of SP, *white arrows* vertebral body of L2 and intervertebral disc, respectively; *open arrowhead* lateral sacral crest, *black arrowhead* median sacral crest. L3 and L5 with particularly prominent accessory processes at root of CP (compare with Figure 5.7). Note shape and orientation of lamina L5, considerably different from others! Sacrum: note incomplete fusion at the upper part of median sacral crest. See text for more details.

sory process is present in most cases. Together with another protrusion, *mamillary process*, at the dorsal margin of the superior AP, they are remnants of true transverse processes, which are only seen in the TS (Figures 5.5b, 5.7 and 5.8b). Very often both are distinguishable by means of sonography. One of the outstanding signs of L5 is the massiveness of its CP (Figures 5.8a and 5.9b). Moreover, its dorsal surface looks slightly upwards.

The *spinous processes* are massive (L5 the least substantial in contrast to its CP), rectangular and sagittally orientated. Their upper margin is approximately in line with the lower margins of both CP; the lower margin reaches at least to the level of the intervertebral disc (in projection). The dorsal border is thickened, often revealing an extension at its caudal end (Figures 5.8a, b and 5.9b).

Opposed to the TS, the width of the high but sturdy L1–L4 laminae (LAM) is much less than that of their bodies. Therefore, a considerable part of vertebral bodies and dorsal aspects of intervertebral discs are seen in a dorsal view. Showing a clear waist, all LAM are narrowest between superior and inferior AP, at the so-called interarticular part (Figure 5.7).

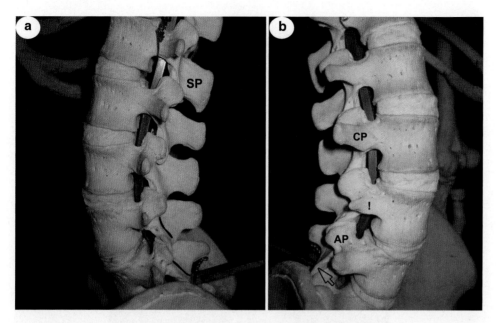

Figure 5.9. (a) Lateral view of LS. SP spinous process of L1; compare with Figure 5.8a (similar grade of lordosis) for interindividual differences, especially concerning shape, massiveness, etc. as well as orientation of SP L1–L5. They are responsible for different interspinous space. Note orientation of laminae (outlined) of L4 and L5. (b) Antero-lateral view of LS (L2–L5). AP superior articular process of L5; CP costal process L3; compare with (a) and Figure 5.7 (same individual) for side differences, especially concerning shape, massiveness and orientation of CP L2–L5. *Open arrow* points at articular surface of inferior AP of L5 (orientation!). See text for more details.

At the same time, this waist indicates the level and position of lumbar dorsal root ganglia, DRG. The LAM faces posteriorly from L1 to L3, posteriorly and slightly upwards in L4 while the extensively broad but low L5 LAM looks more upwards than posterior (Figures 5.8b and 5.9a).

The articular facets of the lumbar zygapophysial joints (LZJ) are principally convex (at the inferior AP) and concave (at the superior AP), in essence facing laterally and medially, respectively. This is why joint gaps are best seen in a posterior view (Figure 5.7). However, the position of the facets is highly variable, not infrequently asymmetrical and showing angulations. Restriction of movements is realised by a very strong ligamentous apparatus, especially by transversely oriented dorsal capsular ligaments (Figure 5.10). At the lumbo-sacral joint (LSJ) the "ZJ" between the inferior AP of L5 and superior AP of sacrum, variability concerning facets is even higher (asymmetry in 60%!), but joint surfaces at the inferior AP of L5 look principally anterolateral (Figures 5.7, 5.8a, b and 5.9b). The articulation is additionally protected from overloading by the strong iliolumbar ligament.

LS-anatomy reveals that this part of the spine is *more* "open" to *US examination* as compared to the thoracic part, not least by augmentation of acoustic windows through motion. However, structures of interest lie deeper and in addition, a solid knowledge of *variability* is crucial.

Sacrum

The curved sacrum is formed by fusion of five sacral vertebrae with their respective inter-vertebral discs and ligaments. It explains why after fusion is completed we no longer see lateral processes (neither TP nor CP) but what is called lateral part at the pelvic surface and *lateral sacral crest* at the convex dorsal surface (Figures 5.8a and 5.11a, b), which is obviously more important for US. While the aforementioned crest, representing remnants of the transverse processes, is always clearly seen (and thus a good landmark in US images), the intermediate sacral crest is often poorly developed (representing union of articular

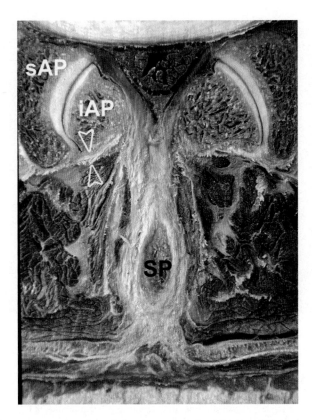

Figure 5.10. Transverse section through lumbar zygapophysial joint, LZJ, between L3 and L4. SP and iAP spinous process and inferior articular process of L3; sAP superior articular process of L4. Note hooked shape of LZJ on left side compared to right as well as thickness of capsular ligament (*open arrowheads*)!

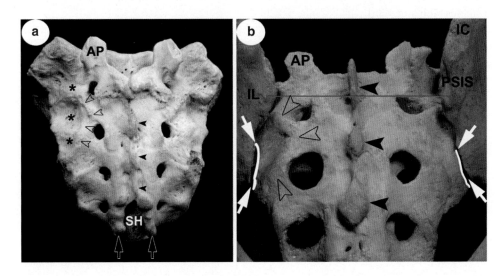

Figure 5.11. (a) Isolated sacrum, dorsal surface. Compare with Figure 5.8a. AP superior articular process; SH sacral hiatus; *open arrowheads* indicate lateral sacral crest, *black arrowheads* median sacral crest; *white open arrows* point at sacral horns; *asterisks* mark the sacral tuberosity. Note the relatively small posterior sacral foramina in this specimen as compared to (b). Sacrum in situ, dorsal view. IL ilium with iliac crest, IC, and posterior superior iliac spine, PSIS; *white arrows* delineate entrance into posterior most (=directly accessible) part of sacroiliac joint cavity, SIJ; *curved lines* mark posterior rim of sacral articular surfaces as in Figure 5.8a (see there for comparison!). Note that the gap seen above does not lead to or correspond with SIJ! The transverse line through both PSIS indicates level of cross section in Figure 5.13a. See there and text for more details. Other symbols of labelling as in (a).

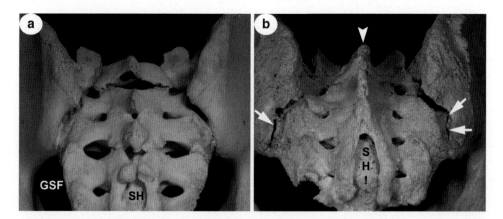

Figure 5.12. (a) Sacrum in situ, dorsal view. SH sacral hiatus; GSF greater sciatic foramen. Note incomplete ossification with partly open sacral canal and non-fusion of S1 segment. (b) Sacrum in situ, dorsal view. Note prominent but shortened median sacral crest (*white arrowhead*) due to non-fusion of laminae of S4 that results in an extraordinary high SH! Entrance into SIJ (*white arrows*) partly obscured by ossification. Compare both (a) and (b) with Figure 5.11a, b! See text for more details.

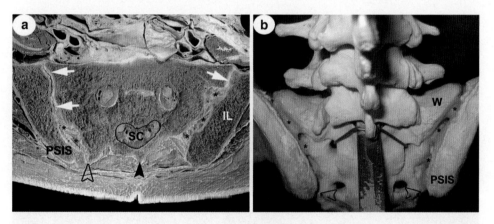

Figure 5.13. (a) Cross section through pelvis at the level of PSIS. SC sacral canal; *black arrowhead* points at median sacral crest, open one at (very prominent) lateral sacral crest. Note that at this level the joint cavity of the sacroiliac articulation (*white arrows*) is in far distance from the dorsal body surface. The space from joint cavity to lateral sacral crest is filled with interosseous ligaments (*asterisks*) attached to facing iliac and sacral tuberosities. The latter is almost completely covered by the wing of ilium, IL! Compare with (b). Sacrum in situ viewed from above. *PSIS* posterior superior iliac spine; *W* wing of sacrum; *open arrows* point at lateral sacral crests; a mass (*asterisks*) simulates interosseous ligaments.

processes). The *median sacral crest* is formed by fusion of the spinous processes (SP) of S1–S4, thus the most prominent of all longitudinal ridges. Not infrequently, this fusion includes only three SP or is incomplete throughout the midline (Figure 5.12a, b)! Incomplete fusion is seen in 10% of adults aged 50, in which cases the sacral canal appears partly opened (comparable to the vertebral canal at the LS)! Regularly, however, both laminae of the fifth sacral segment fail to fuse in the midline to leave the *sacral hiatus* that leads into the sacral canal. The height and shape of the hiatus depend on the number and mode of fused SP (see above!) but is in its caudal part always laterally bordered by the *sacral cornu*, the most important of all palpable landmarks (Figure 5.11a). Interestingly, complete synostosis of all sacral parts and elements happens as late as with 25–35 years of age, in some individuals never, which explains all forms of variants so frequently encountered and thus practically important (Figures 5.11a and 5.12b).

Concerning above-mentioned variability, the *posterior* or *dorsal sacral foramina* differ from small to huge as well as their number (Figures 5.11a, b and 5.12a). The latter occurs as frequent as in one third of the population, either due to *sacralisation* of a lumbar vertebra or a coccygeal element (both with five foramina on either side). This is seen more often in males. Sacral foramina, anterior or posterior, should not be misinterpreted as equivalents to the intervertebral foramina of the rest of the spine! In the sacrum, they lie within the sacral canal as lateral openings.

It is of utmost importance to realise that a considerable area of the dorsal surface of the sacrum, roughly corresponding to the sacral tuberosity, is overlaid by the wing of ilium. As the tuberosity lies mainly above the auricular surface, most of the SIJ cavity is also completely and deeply hidden (Figure 5.13a, b). As a consequence, only the most posterior part of the joint cavity (gap) is visible from posterior! (Figure 5.11b), and this is important for US approach.

Although most of the *dorsal* surface of the sacrum is *easily accessible* by US, the *anatomy of the sacrum is tremendously influenced by its most variable progress of ossification (fusion) and non-ossification.*

Sonoanatomy of the Cervical Spine

Superficial (Figures 5.14–5.21)

While there is no chance to image atlas (C1) and axis (C2) from ventrally, the posterior arch of C2 with its typical features mentioned in the anatomy part (see above), and articular pillar, lamina as well as the bifurcated (two tubercles) spinous process of C2 are easily seen and may serve as ideal landmarks. As for C2, the same is true down to C6 (Figure 5.14a–c). In addition, the *occipital bone* is well appreciated with US with appropri-

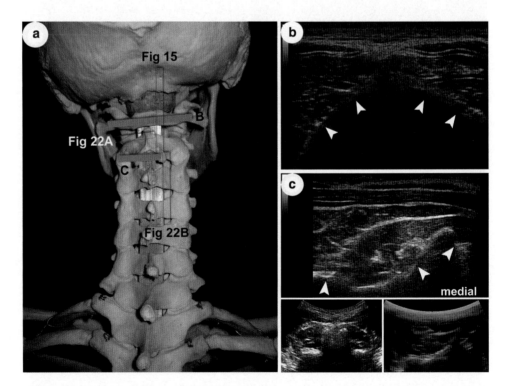

Figure 5.14. (a) Scanning planes for US images (b), (c), and for Figure 5.15 as well as Figure 5.22 relative to skull and upper CS; posterior view. (b) Dorsal surface of posterior arch of atlas (*arrowheads*). Note that the quality of image is not least depending on highly variable degree of bone curvature! (c) Bony outlines of axis, C2. *Arrowheads* indicate from medial to lateral: bifid spinous process, SP, lamina, and inferior articular process. To get a better overview of vertebrae, usage of curvilinear probes is recommendable; see inserts *bottom right* (paramedian) and *left* (median position of transducer). See text for more details.

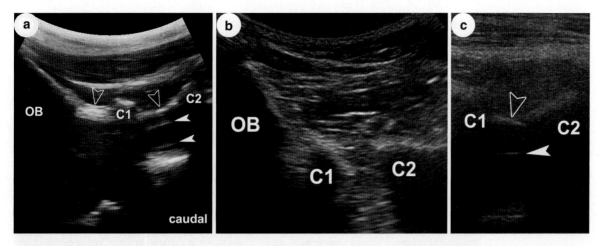

Figure 5.15. (a) See Figure 5.14a for scanning plane! All labelling also applies for (b) and (c). OB occipital bone; C1 posterior arch of atlas; C2 lamina of axis; *open arrowheads* point at atlanto-occipital and atlanto-axial membrane, respectively; *white arrowheads* indicate dura mater (see legend of Figure 5.22 for details). Note narrow interosseous gaps in (b) due to retro-flexion! See text for more details.

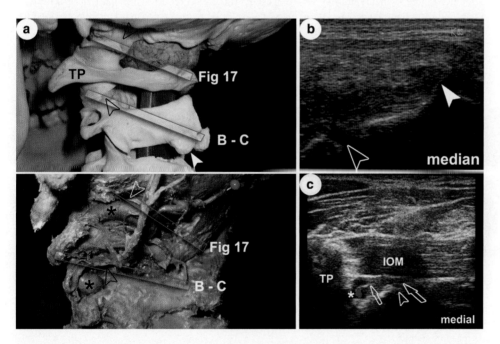

Figure 5.16. (a) Scanning planes for US images (b), (c) and for Figure 5.17 relative to skeleton (upper) and special preparation (lower) of uppermost CS and skull base. *Open arrowheads* mark AA and AOJ; *white arrowhead* indicates left tubercle of C2 spinous process, SP; *asterisks* show vertebral artery, VA. Note that the VA shows elongation, so part of the AOJ is hidden; *TP* transverse process of atlas; all labelling also applies for (b) and (c). (b) Demonstration of AAJ gap. (c) *IOM* inferior oblique muscle. Note that this scan is more horizontal and reaches more lateral (no SP seen) compared to (b) to show TP, VA as well as 2nd dorsal root ganglion and ventral ramus (*open arrows*). See also Figure 5.4b! (basic anatomy) and text for more details.

ate transducers and thus atlanto-occipital as well as atlanto-axial windows are easily detectable (Figure 5.15a, b). To give practical examples, these bony surfaces may be used as landmarks for approaching both AAJ and AOJ as well as the greater occipital nerve (GON) more centrally (Figures 5.16a–c, 5.17a, b and 5.18a–c). The above-mentioned

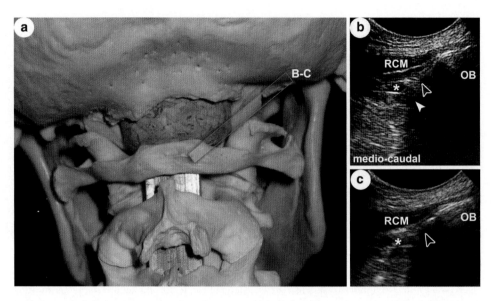

Figure 5.17. (a) Scanning plane for US images (b) and (c) relative to occipital bone (OB), and uppermost CS; see Figure 5.16a for comparison. (b) and (c) different appearance of AOJ-gap (*open arrowhead*); note regular relation of vertebral artery (*asterisk*) infero-medial to joint; *white arrowhead* in (b) indicates bone shadow by lateral mass of atlas; *RCM* rectus capitis major muscle. See text for more details.

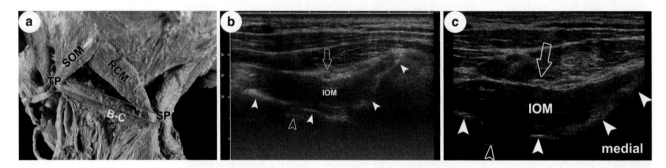

Figure 5.18. (a) Scanning plane for US images (b) and (c) in an anatomic specimen of short muscles of neck; *open bar* on inferior oblique muscle; SOM superior oblique muscle; RCM rectus capitis major muscle; OB occipital bone, TP transverse process of atlas, SP spinous process of axis; postero-lateral view. (b) and (c) *white arrowheads* indicate from medial to lateral: SP, lamina and superior articular process of axis and lateral mass of atlas, respectively. The GON (*open arrow*) lies "on top" of IOM. Note that in both images the AAJ (*open arrowhead*) is also seen. See text for more details.

joints lie relatively deep compared to the CZJ and are bordered by the vertebral artery (VA). CZJ can be located either from lateral or posterior and capsular ligaments may be detectable where stronger. Lying directly on bone, the third occipital nerve, TON and "medial branches" C3 and C4 are visible (Figure 5.19a–c). The outlines of transverse processes from C3 to C6 including anterior and posterior tubercles are accessible from lateral and thus most valuable landmarks, e.g. for nerve root location and general orientation (Figure 5.20a–c and 5.24a).

Anterior longitudinal scans reveal the typical shape of *vertebral bodies* (and anterior aspects of discs in between) covered by the *anterior longitudinal ligament*, in transverse views the anterior tubercles of TP C3–C6 and the marked groove at the base of each TP are appreciated. As C7 lacks an anterior tubercle, its TP appears completely different and

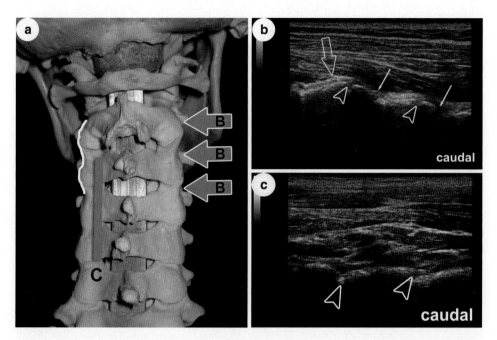

Figure 5.19. (a) Scanning planes for US images (b) and (c) relative to CS; posterior view. Note wavy lateral outline of CS by typical shape of articular pillars (*white line*). (b) Visibility of (entrance into) joint gaps (*open arrowheads*) depends on obliquity of lateral scan; *arrows* indicate medial branches C3 and C4; *open arrowhead* points to TON. This image was done with an 18-MHz probe! (c) Scan on dorsal surface of articular processes. Note that gaps are only indicated (compared to **b**) by "steps" (*open arrowheads*). See text for more details.

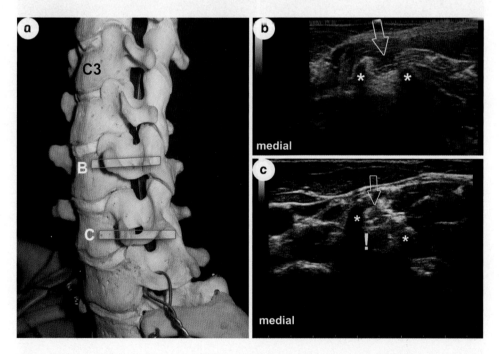

Figure 5.20. (a) Scanning planes for US images (b) and (c) relative to CS; antero-lateral view. (b) and (c) TP transverse processes of C5 and C6 (hit at their lateral end); *asterisks* mark anterior and posterior tubercles; *open arrows* point at ventral rami. Note the mirror artefact (!) in (c) that may be misinterpreted as the true nerve! See also Figure 5.24 and text for more details.

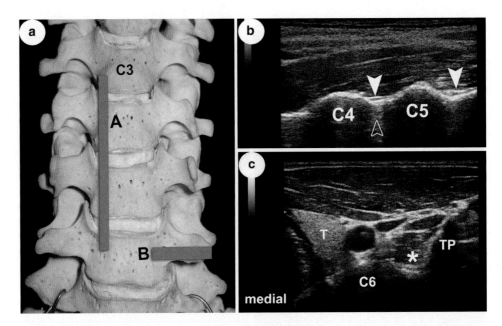

Figure 5.21. (a) Scanning planes for US images (b) and (c) relative to CS; anterior view. (b) C4 and C5 vertebral bodies of respective vertebrae; *arrowheads* indicate anterior longitudinal ligament; *open arrowhead* indicates intervertebral disc. (c) TP transverse process; *asterisk* in longus colli muscle indicates groove at base of TP; *T* thyroid gland. See text for more details.

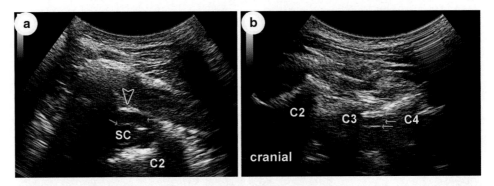

Figure 5.22. (a) Transverse scan through atlanto-axial space into vertebral canal with spinal cord, SC; *arrows* point at dura and epidural space, EDS, respectively. The latter ends dorsally at the atlanto-axial membrane (*open arrowhead*); C2 bone shadows by body and superior articular process of atlas. (b) Demonstration of vertebral canal with SC in a paramedian longitudinal scan. C2 right tubercle of spinous process of axis; C3 and C4 laminae of respective vertebrae; *arrows* point – from superficial to deep – at: yellow ligament (double contour!), EDS and dorsal surface of dural sac. See Figure 5.14a for scanning planes, Figure 5.15 for comparison (!) and text for more details.

the VA has no bony covering at that segment (Figure 5.21a–c; C6 and Figures 5.23c and 5.24b).

Deep (Figures 5.22–5.25)

Demonstrating EDS, dura mater (D), and *spinal cord* is done from posterior and preferably paramedian, the biggest acoustic window to be found between atlas and axis and atlas and occiput. With maximum ante-flexion, however, the other interlaminar gaps allow sufficient access as well (Figure 5.22a, b and compare with Figure 5.15a, b). The VA runs

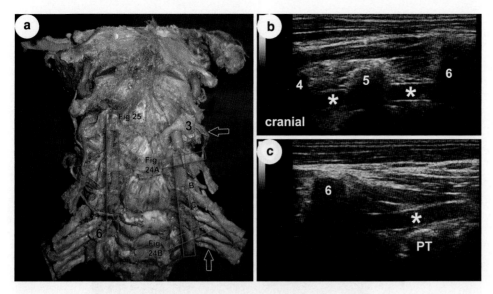

Figure 5.23. (a) Scanning planes of US images (a) and (b) and for Figures 5.24 and 5.25 in an anatomic preparation of CS with injected (*red latex*) vertebral artery, VA, and ventral rami of spinal nerves C3–T1 (*open arrows*); anterior view. Three and six anterior tubercles of transverse processes of respective vertebrae. (b) and (c) lower cervical and prevertebral part of VA (*asterisks*); PT posterior tubercle of transverse process of seventh cervical vertebra. See text for more details.

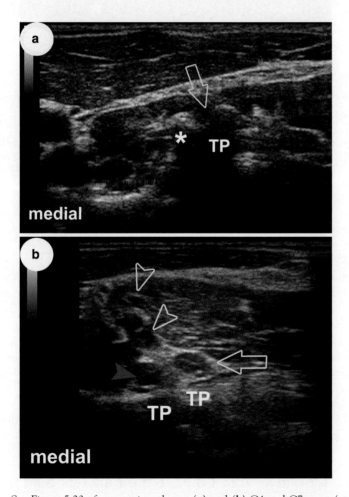

Figure 5.24. See Figure 5.23a for scanning planes. (a) and (b) C4 and C7 roots (*open arrows*) at transverse processes, TP. Note different appearance of TP of vertebra prominens relative to that of fourth, its length and lack of an anterior tubercle (*asterisk*). This is why the VA (*arrowhead*) is freely accessible at that level in transverse views. Note the relation to nerve root and do not mix both with other "*black balls*" also seen (C5 and C6 roots, *open arrowheads*). See text for more details.

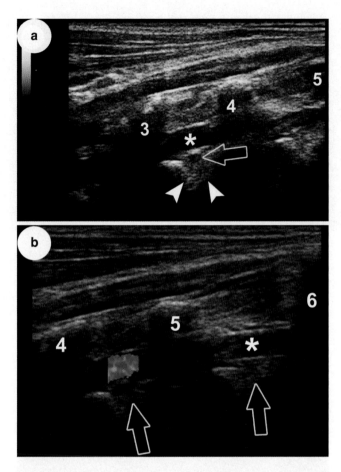

Figure 5.25. See Figure 5.23a for scanning plane (**a**) and (**b**) cervical part of VA (*asterisks* and *blue colour*) through and between transverse processes from third to sixth vertebra. Note that nerve roots lie dorsal to artery, in (**a**) outlines of the intervertebral foramen is seen too. See text for more details.

through the foramina transversaria, its "free" part, obviously limited, easily detectable with an anterior longitudinal approach (Figure 5.23a–c). Although more challenging, showing the VA in relation to the AOJ and AAJ is also feasible in most cases (Figures 5.16c and 5.17b, c). *Ventral rami* of *spinal nerves* can be traced at least till their position within the respective sulcus from C3 to C7 (Figure 5.24a, b: US C3 und C7). Moreover, it is often possible to reliably demonstrate their relationship with the VA in mentioned segments; the nerves lie dorsal to it and can be followed right to their exit from the intervertebral foramina (Figure 5.25a, b)! At least from C3/4 downwards, anterior aspects of the *intervertebral discs* can be visualised (Figure 5.21b). This is not possible for their antero-lateral circumference due to the bony covering by uncinate processes as mentioned above.

Sonoanatomy of the Thoracic Spine

Superficial (Figures 5.26 and 5.27)

All of the dorsal surface of the thoracic vertebrae can be appreciated with US. Especially the contour of the transverse and articular processes together with the *necks of ribs*, are ideal

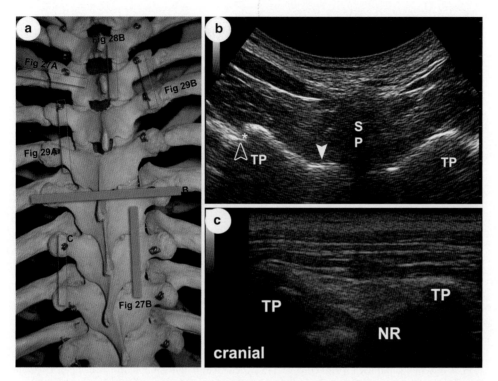

Figure 5.26. (a) Scanning planes of US images (a) and (b) relative to TS; posterior view. (b) TP dorsal surface of transverse processes T7; SP shadow by spinous process of T6! *White arrowhead* on lamina of T7; *open arrowhead* marks tubercle of seventh rib. Note gap between TP and tubercle (entrance into costo-vertebral joint; *asterisk*). (c) TP transverse processes of T8 and T9; NR neck of ninth rib. See text for more details.

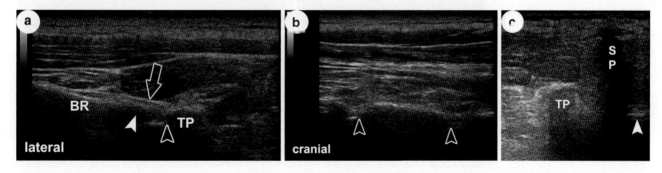

Figure 5.27. See Figure 5.26a for scanning planes in (a) and (b), Figure 5.28a for plane of US image shown in (c). (a) TP transverse process of T4; BR body of rib; *arrowhead* marks tubercle of rib; *open arrowhead* points at costotransverse joint (gap); *open arrow* indicates lateral costotransverse ligament. (a) Scan on dorsal surface of articular processes. Note that gaps are only indicated (compared to b) by "steps" (*open arrowheads*). (c) TP rudimentary transverse process of T11; SP bone shadow by spinous process of T10; *arrowhead* points at right lamina. See text for more details.

landmarks to find acoustic windows for entering the paravertebral space. The ribs within the "intertransverse window" are ultrasonographically seen in longitudinal scans from level T4 or T5 downwards as they project the transverse processes, (Figure 5.26a–c). Likewise, entrance into the *costotransverse joints* is often possible and the *lateral* costotransverse *ligament* is clearly detectable; not so with the TZJ (Figure 5.27a, b). Due to their small dimensions, *TP* of vertebra *T11* and *T12* may cause difficulties in identification and/ or orientation in that lower most part of the TS (Figure 5.27c).

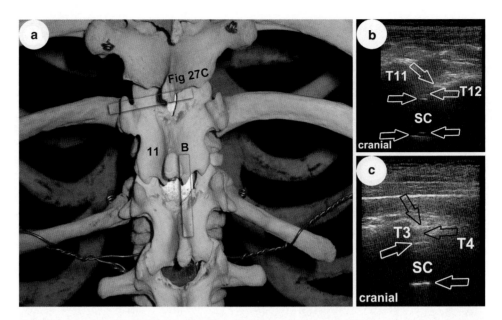

Figure 5.28. (a) Scanning plane of US image in (b) relative to lower part of TS; posterior view. Eleven marks lamina of thoracic vertebra T11. See Figure 5.26a for scanning plane of US image (c). In (b) and (c) T11 and T12 as well as T3 and T4 mark laminae of respective vertebrae; demonstration of vertebral canal with spinal cord, SC, in paramedian longitudinal scans; *arrows* point – from superficial to deep – at: yellow ligament (double contour!), epidural space (EDS), dorsal (and ventral) surface of dural sac, posterior longitudinal ligament. See text for more details.

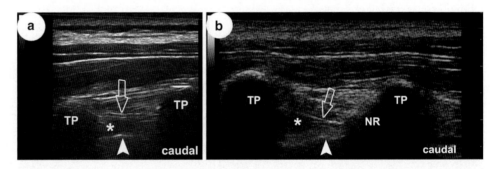

Figure 5.29. See Figure 5.26a for scanning planes in (a) and (b). (a) and (b) Longitudinal scans between transverse processes, TP, of vertebrae T4/T5 and T5/T6, respectively. *Open arrows* point at superior costotransverse ligament. Note that in (a) the neck of the rib, NR, is not seen! *Arrowheads* indicate pleura; *asterisks* in thoracic paravertebral space. See text for more details.

Deep (Figures 5.28 and 5.29)

Throughout this part of spine, with the exception of spaces between T11/12 and T12/L1, visualising the *vertebral canal* and its content by a median scan is usually impossible. Limited visualisation may be feasible paramedian from T1 to T4 as well as from T10 to T12 (Figure 5.28a–c). Nevertheless, considering the fact that there is often additional narrowing by deformities or ossification (e.g. often the yellow ligaments, see anatomy Figure 5.6b) makes US application challenging to often impossible. Quite in contrary, using US for paravertebral blocks is really promising (see "superficial") and because one may image the superior *costotransverse ligament* as well as the *pleura!*, although we have to admit limitations in following needle tip ore placing catheters (Figure 5.29 a, b).

Sonoanatomy of the Lumbar Spine

Superficial (Figures 5.30–5.33)

All of the *dorsal surface* of the lumbar vertebrae can be appreciated with US. Orientation may be achieved in starting in the midline, spinous processes (SP), and walk off laterally over articular processes (AP) until costal processes (CP) are reached (Figures 5.30b, c and 5.31b). Proper orientation is of particular value when performing medial branch blocks for facet joint pain. The lumbar medial branches lie in tiny little osseofibrous tunnels (roofed by the mamillo-accessory ligament) between mamillary and accessory process of a vertebra (Figure 5.30a). This anatomical detail is relevant, as it is one of the reasons why block may fail when done too caudally, especially true when ligament is ossified. Despite the fact that the medial branches themselves are invisible, accuracy of an ultrasound-guided block comes near to fluoroscopy. Often disregarded, however, and apart from the necessity to scan in longitudinal and transverse planes for a meaningful algorithm and optimal orientation, slightly oblique scanning is sometimes helpful, not least due to individually different orientation of CP (Figures 5.30a and 5.31b). It is also noteworthy that, although sometimes proposed, no linear array transducers should be used. This is inappropriate due to both, ultrasound physics and given anatomy of the LS and one of the common mistakes made. In contrast, losing orientation in case of very slim and/or short (=rudimentary) TP as normal variant is a typical pitfall (Figure 5.7).

LZJ can be located. It is crucial to understand that these articulations are (1) relatively tight diarthroses with tense ligamentous restriction and that (2) shape as well as

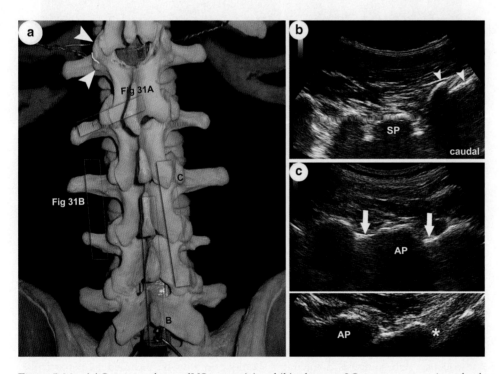

Figure 5.30. (a) Scanning planes of US images (a) and (b) relative to LS; posterior view. *Arrowheads* point at mamillary and accessory processes, *yellow line* indicates course of lumbar medial branch in between them, *circle* indicates target point for medial branch block; see Figure 5.31. (b) Median longitudinal scan to show (and count) lumbar spinous processes (SP spinous process L5) starting from the median sacral crest (*arrowheads*). (c) Upper and lower part demonstrate typical, nevertheless different appearances of scans over articular processes, AP, depending on individual anatomy of the LS as well as transducer orientation. Note that white outline of laminae (*arrows*) in lower image are not continuous throughout (*asterisk*) due to their waists; compare to upper image. See text on LS anatomy for more details.

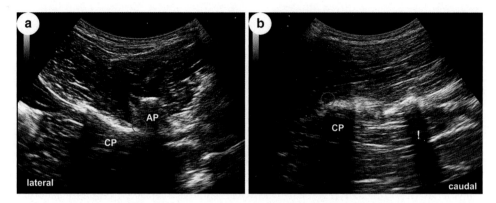

Figure 5.31. See Figure 5.30a for scanning planes of (**a**) and (**b**). (**a**) Slightly oblique scan to show AP articular processes L1 and L2, CP costal process L2. (**b**) Lateral longitudinal scan shows typical acoustic shadowing of different width (!) by costal processes, CP (of L3). *Circle* indicates target point of medial branch block.

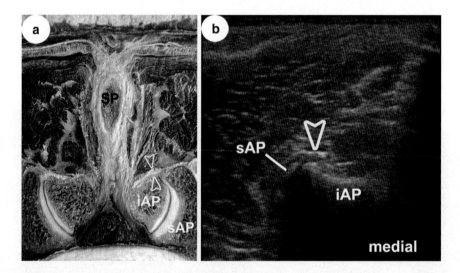

Figure 5.32. (**a**) Transverse section through lumbar zygapophysial joint, LZJ, between L3 and L4. Spinous process (SP) and inferior articular process (iAP) of L3; superior articular process (sAP) of L4. Note hooked shape of LZJ on left side compared to right as well as thickness of capsular ligament (*open arrowheads*)! (**b**) Transverse US image corresponding to anatomical cross section in (**a**) with similar labelling. Note that anechoic gap between bony contours does not represent the true anatomic joint space. See text for more details.

orientation of the articular facets is extremely variable in different people as well as on both sides of a single individual (Figure 5.32a and text on LS anatomy). The practical consequence: US-guided LZJ injection should primarily be regarded as periarticular. The hypo- to anechoic gap interrupting the surface outline of articular processes (AP) represents the distance between the posterior most, bony parts of articulating medial facet and lateral facet of two joining vertebrae. That way, it indicates the dorsal entrance point into a LZJ (Figure 5.32b). Under ideal conditions, the covering ligaments (joint capsule) may be visible as hyperechoic structures (Figures 5.32b and 5.33a). The extension of the joint space itself, both radiologic (between bone) and true anatomic (between cartilage) cannot be appreciated with US. In summary: LZJs can be reliably located with US but not imaged to the deep. Apart from that and finally, in case of pathologically altered LZJ, trying to look for a gap with US may be frustrating if simply absent (Figure 5.33b).

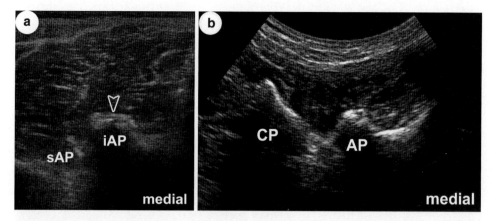

Figure 5.33. (a, b) Examples of LZJ entrances in different individuals and conditions. (b) Scanned from lateral and oblique (CP seen) and with curvilinear probe. For labelling, see Figure 5.32. Note narrow gap in (a) compared to Figure 5.32b. In (b) no gap is seen, but bony surface of AP irregular due to pathologic protuberances. See text for more details.

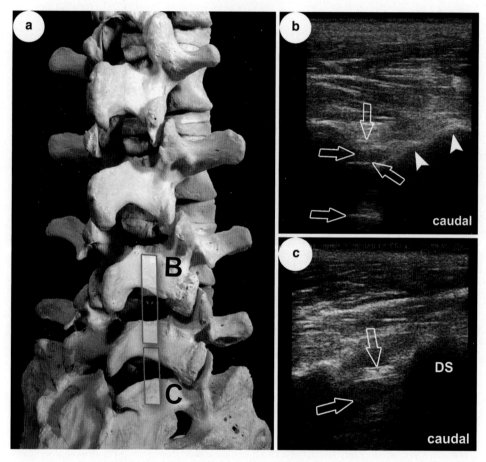

Figure 5.34. (a) Scanning planes for US images (a) and (b) relative to lower part of LS; postero-lateral view. Note non-fusion of S1-laminae! (b) and (c) Demonstration of vertebral canal in the segments between laminae L4/L5 and L5/sacrum, respectively. DS dorsal surface of sacrum; note orientation of L5 lamina (*arrowheads*)! *Arrows point* – from superficial to deep – at: yellow ligament (double contour!), epidural space, EDS, (dorsal and ventral) surface of dural sac. Note the thickness of yellow ligament in the lower segment! See text for more details.

Deep (Figures 5.34–5.36)

To see and interpret structures within the *vertebral canal* it is best to use a paramedian longitudinal plane, with spine flexed to widen the acoustic window! Thus, even an approach between laminae of L5 and sacrum is possible (Figure 5.34a–c). Moreover in the

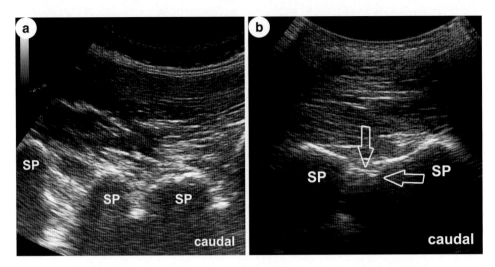

Figure 5.35. (a, b) Median longitudinal scans at lower lumbar spine showing influence of maximum flexion (b) in visualisation of the spinal canal. *SP* spinous processes. Only in (b) structures may be visualised under good conditions, but quality is poor (compared to Figure 5.34b). At least yellow ligament and epidurals space can be identified (*arrows*). See text for more details.

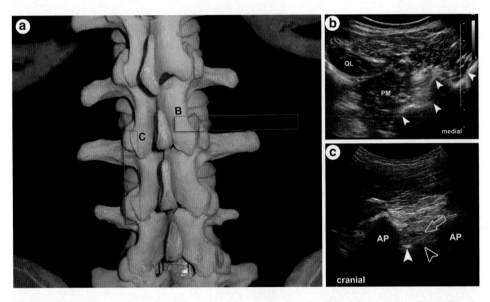

Figure 5.36. (a) Scanning planes of US images (a) and (b) relative to LS; posterior view. (b) Transverse image obtained with transducer positioned "paravertebral" and scanning direction to antero-medial. *Arrowheads* indicate from deep to superficial: antero-lateral circumference of vertebral body, lateral margin of interarticular portion, articular process and lamina; QL quadratus lumborum muscle; PM psoas major muscle. (c) Longitudinal scan between two articular processes, AP, immediately adjacent to lamina. *Open arrow* points at lumbar root L3 exiting intervertebral foramen; *arrowhead* indicates dorsal surface of vertebral body, *open arrowhead* indicates intervertebral disc. See text for more details.

lumbar spine, calcified yellow ligaments are less frequent. However, ossification occurs and may hinder US exploration and approach. It is then advisable to look for a median acoustic window between TP, accepting that image quality may decrease significantly (Figure 5.35a, b).

As windows between CP are relatively wide and laminae very slim, US exploration may reach rather deep, especially when the US probe is positioned "paravertebral" and scan is directed in antero-medial direction. That way, considerable parts of the *vertebral bodies (and discs)* can be seen (Figure 5.36a–c). It is necessary to mention, however, that all of what is said here concerning "deep" is often not feasible in marked obesity.

Sonoanatomy of the Sacrum and Sacroiliac Joint

Superficial (Figures 5.37–5.40)

Excellent images of the *dorsal surface* of the sacrum are the rule. The dorsal sacral foramina and their ligamentous covering are beautifully seen with US and serve as ideal landmarks for orientation. The same is true for the more prominent sacral crests (Figures 5.37a–5.40c). Clinically we need to identify all of these structures as they guide us to the deeper ones (e.g. trans-sacral block, caudal epidurals or sacroiliac joint (SIJ) injections). Apart from that, by counting these foramina one may detect sacral elongations that mean incorporation of either lumbar or coccygeal elements. Finally anomalies are readily seen by US (e.g. bifid spine) and all forms of variations and incomplete ossifications may be detected.

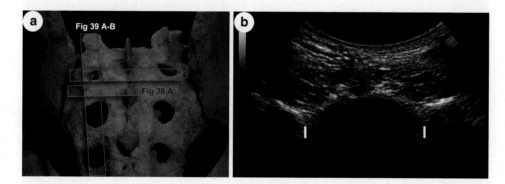

Figure 5.37. (a) Scanning levels of US image in (b), for image Figures 5.38a and 5.39a, b. (b) Overview of dorsal surface in a transverse US scan at level of posterior sacral foramen I. Note indentation instead of a crest! See text for more details.

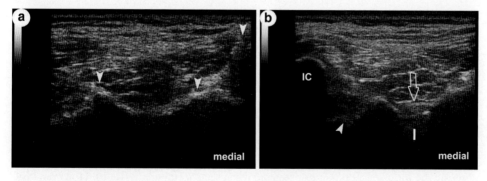

Figure 5.38. (a) US visualisation of sacral crests. From median to lateral, *arrowheads* indicate median, intermediate and lateral sacral crest. Note marked elevation of lateral crest! See text for more details. (b) See Figure 5.42a for scanning plane. Slightly oblique scan over iliac, IC, and lateral sacral crest at the level of dorsal sacral foramen I. *Open arrow* shows covering ligaments of foramen; *arrowhead* points at sacral tuberosity. See text for more details.

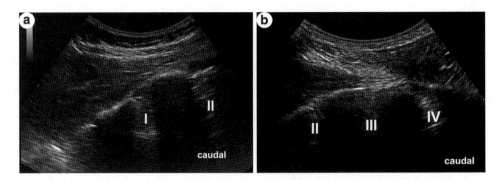

Figure 5.39. Both images (**a**) and (**b**) show dorsal sacral foramina from one to four, I–IV. Note their different dimensions and the overall convexity of dorsal sacral surface. See text for more details.

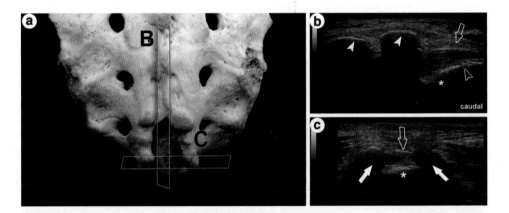

Figure 5.40. Scanning planes of US images in (**a**) and (**b**); posterior view of lower third of sacrum with sacral hiatus. (**b**) US over end of median sacral crest (*arrowheads*) and sacral hiatus; the latter is closed in the living by the sacro-coccygeal ligament (*open arrow*) *asterisk* marks bony floor of hiatus; *open arrowhead* indicates sacro-coccygeal gap. (**c**) Transverse scan over sacral horns (*white arrows*). See text for more details.

Deep (Figures 5.41 and 5.42)

There is often a misunderstanding or at least confusion concerning the terminology and thus meaning of "SIJ" per definition. This often leads to inappropriate comparisons/judgments of methods described in the literature, especially as far as US approaches are concerned.

So for the sake of clarity, what is mainly commented on in the sequel is attributed to the synovial joint or diarthrosis between ilium and sacrum!

Because it is hidden deep in the pelvic framework for most of its extension (see anatomy Figure 5.13), the *SIJ* articular cavity can only be reached under US guidance when entering the joint space in its most *posterior compartment* (Figure 5.41a, b). However, visualisation of the needle within the joint space can not be achieved. As there is potential danger reaching the pelvis and its content through the greater sciatic foramen, correct needle direction and simultaneous demonstration of gluteal surface of ilium is essential! In cases of partial non-fusion of sacral elements near the midline, the *sacral canal* may be reached ultrasonographically quite comparable to US-guided *epidural* approaches elsewhere in the spine (Figure 5.42a, b).

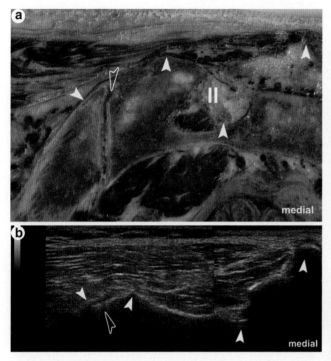

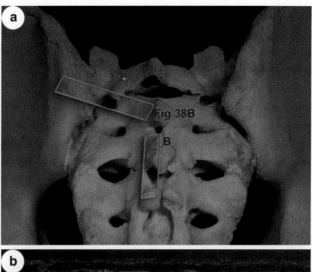

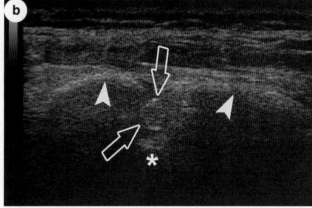

Figure 5.41. (a) Transverse section through the posterior most part of the sacroiliac diarthrosis. The following landmarks (*arrowheads*) seen on this cross section are detectable in US, see corresponding image in (**b**) with same labelling, and their identification is mandatory for safe approaches. From medial to lateral: median sacral crest, second dorsal sacral foramen, lateral sacral crest and gluteal surface of ilium. The entrance into this part of the joint is very small (*open arrowhead*). Note the groove between lateral sacral crest and ilium in the anatomic specimen. If this is the case it may easily be mistaken ultrasonographically as the joint gap! See text for more details.

Figure 5.42. (**a**) Scanning planes of US images in (**b**) and for Figure 5.30b, posterior view of a sacrum with incomplete ossification throughout showing "windows" within the dorsal wall of the sacral canal. (**b**) The bony floor of the sacral canal is clearly seen (above *asterisk*) as well as the terminal part of the dural sac (*open arrows*) reaching far caudally in this individual *White arrowheads* point at equivalent of vertebral laminae.

6

Ultrasound-Guided Third Occipital Nerve and Cervical Medial Branch Nerve Blocks

Andreas Siegenthaler and Urs Eichenberger

Anatomy

Cervical zygapophyseal (facet) joints are diarthrodial joints formed by the superior articular process of one cervical vertebra articulating with the inferior articular process of the vertebrae above at the level of the junction of the lamina and the pedicle. The angulations

U. Eichenberger (✉)
Department of Anesthesiology and Pain Therapy, University Hospital of Bern,
Inselspital, Bern, Switzerland
e-mail: Urs.Eichenberger@insel.ch

S.N. Narouze (ed.), *Atlas of Ultrasound-Guided Procedures in Interventional Pain Management*,
DOI 10.1007/978-1-4419-1681-5_6, © Springer Science+Business Media, LLC 2011

of the facet joints increases caudally, being about 45° to the transverse plane at the upper cervical level to assuming a more vertical position at the upper thoracic level. The superior articular process also faces more posteromedial at the upper cervical level and this changes to more posterolateral at the lower cervical level, with C6 being the most common transition level.[1,2]

Each facet joint has a fibrous capsule and is lined by a synovial membrane. The joint also contains varying amounts of adipose and fibrous tissue forming different types of synovial folds contributing to different pathophysiology for joint dysfunction.[3]

The cervical zygapophysial joints are innervated by articular branches derived from the medial branches of the cervical dorsal rami. The C3–C7 dorsal rami arise from their respective spinal nerves and pass dorsally over the root of their corresponding transverse process. The medial branches of the cervical dorsal rami run transversely across the centroid of the corresponding articular pillars and have a constant relationship with the bone at the dorsolateral aspect of the articular pillar as they are bound to the periosteum by an investing fascia and held in place by the tendon of the semispinalis capitis muscle.[4] Variations in the course of the medial branches are usually distributed across the middle fourth of the height of the articular pillars. The articular branches arise as the nerve approaches the posterior aspect of the articular pillar, one innervating the zygapophysial joint above, and the other innervating the joint below. Consequently, each typical cervical zygapophysial joint below C2-3 has dual innervations, from the medial branch above and below its location.

The medial branches of the C3 dorsal ramus differ in their anatomy. A deep medial branch passes around the waist of the C3 articular pillar similar to other typical medial branches and supplies the C3–C4 zygapophysial joint. The superficial medial branch of C3 is large and known as the third occipital nerve (TON). It curves around the lateral and then the posterior aspect of the C2–C3 zygapophysial joint giving articular branches to the joint. Beyond the C2–C3 zygapophysial joint, the TON becomes cutaneous over the suboccipital region.

Another anatomical exception is the course of the medial branch C7. The C7 medial branch passes more cranial, closer to the foramen of C7, crossing the triangular superior articular process of C7 vertebrae.

Indications for Cervical Medial Branch Block

Cervical facet joints are important in sharing the axial compressive load on the cervical spine along with the intervertebral disk, particularly at higher compressive loads.[5] The facet joint and capsule are also important contributors to the shear strength of the cervical spine and resection, displacement or even facet capsular disruption increases cervical instability.[6,7]

The facet joint and capsule are in close proximity to the semispinalis, multifidus, and rotator neck muscles, and about 23% of the capsule area provides insertion of these muscle fibers contributing to injury with excessive muscle contraction.[8,9] The facet joint and capsule also have been shown to contain nociceptive elements suggesting that they may be an independent pain generator.[10] Facet joint degeneration occurs in elderly almost ubiquitously[11] and the prevalence of facet joint involvement in chronic neck pain has been reported from 35% to 55%,[12,13] making it an important target of interventional pain management.

Cervical facet joint nerve blocks are indicated in axial neck pain not responsive to conservative therapy and with clinical and/or radiological evidence of possible facet joint involvement. Whiplash-associated disorder is a special condition among neck pain patients and a common consequence of different traumatic events, such as car accidents. Excessive facet joint compression and capsular ligament strain have been implicated in neck pain after whiplash injury.[14] Conservative treatment of chronic neck pain following whiplash injury often has poor long-term outcome.[15] Among the possible reasons for this is that an anatomical diagnosis is not made and that treatment does not specifically target the source of pain. Since reliable clinical or radiological signs to identify the responsible joints are lacking, diagnostic blocks of the cervical medial branches are the only validated method to diagnose zygapophysial joint pain.[16,17] Because the false-positive rate of a single block is 38%,[18] a second confirmatory block should be performed on a different day to minimize the chance of obtaining a false-positive response.[19] If diagnostic blocks are used, the source of pain can be traced to one or more of the cervical zygapophysial joints in over 50% of patients.[20] These patients can then be treated by percutaneous radiofrequency neurotomy. Radiofrequency neurotomy, introduced in 1980 by Sluijter and Koetsveld-Baart,[21] has ever since been validated as a very effective therapy for zygapophysial joint pain.[22] Radiofrequency neurotomy is indicated only if a positive response is obtained after both injections. Third occipital neurotomy has been validated as an effective treatment for headache stemming from the C2-3 zygapophysial joint, and mediated by the TON.[23] Furthermore, a recent study showed a positive effect of repetitive therapeutic medial branch blocks with or without steroids.[24]

Why Ultrasound-Guided Facet Nerve Block? The Literature and Our Experience

In a study on volunteers, we demonstrated that it is possible to visualize and block the TON.[25]

Typically, the diagnostic blocks are performed under fluoroscopic (or CT) control. However, the nerves are not visualized by either fluoroscopy or CT. In our study, we tested the hypothesis that the TON, which innervates the C2-3 zygapophysial joint and a small skin area, can be visualized by ultrasound and also blocked by injecting a local anesthetic under ultrasound control. The region of the C2-3 joint was investigated by ultrasound in 14 healthy volunteers, using a 15-MHz transducer. The injection of saline or local anesthetic was performed in a double blind, randomized fashion. The position of the needle was controlled by fluoroscopy. Sensations at the innervated skin area were tested by pinprick and cold. In all 14 volunteers, cervical ultrasound examination was feasible and the TON was successfully visualized in 27 of 28 cases. In most cases, the TON was seen as an oval hypoechoic structure with hyperechoic small spots inside. This is typical for the ultrasound appearance of a peripheral nerve.[26,27]

The median diameter of the TON was 2.0 mm (range, 1.0–3.0) and the nerve was found at a median depth of 20.8 mm (range, 14.0–27.0). Anesthesia of the skin was achieved in all but one case, while no anesthesia was observed after all saline injections. The radiological analysis of the needle positions showed that we localized the C2-3 zygapophysial joint correctly in 27 of 28 cases and revealed that 23 of 28 needle placement were correct (82%).

Although, in the above mentioned study, we reported the feasibility of identifying the TON, there are no other feasibility studies regarding ultrasound-guided lower cervical medial branch block. Nevertheless, the technique has been described.[28,29]

The question regarding the sonographic visibility of all the facet joint supplying nerves is currently being examined in our pain unit, with promising results so far (Siegenthaler et al, unpublished data). In patients suffering from chronic neck pain, the sonographic visibility of the cervical medial branches was described and classified as good in the vast majority of cases. The only exception was the C7 medial branch, which is much more difficult to visualize. The reason for this may be that the C7 medial branch is superimposed by a thicker layer of soft tissue than the medial branches situated more cranially and/or its slightly different anatomical course. The nerves are only about 1–1.5 mm in diameter, the needed high-ultrasound frequency to generate enough resolution to determine such small structures may therefore, in the case of the medial branch C7, not penetrate enough to the target.

Possible Advantages of Ultrasound for Cervical Facet Nerve Blocks

Medial branch blocks are usually performed under fluoroscopic control; however, few pain physicians use computer tomography (CT) as well. The center of the rhomboid-shaped articular pillars (or the superior articular process in the case of C7) serves as bony landmarks and can be easily identified fluoroscopically in a lateral view. There, the medial branches are located in a safe distance from the spinal nerve and the vertebral artery and a needle can be introduced to block the nerves (according to the above mentioned bony landmarks only). Because several blocks are often needed to identify the symptomatic joint, or to rule out zygapophysial joint pain, the procedure may expose patients and personnel to considerable radiation doses.[30] In contrast, ultrasound is not associated with exposure to radiation.

Ultrasound can identify muscles, ligaments, vessels, joints, and bony surfaces. Importantly, thin nerves can be visualized, provided that high-resolution transducers are applied. This characteristic is not shared by either fluoroscopy or CT and is the major reason for the great potential usefulness of ultrasound in interventional pain management. Unlike fluoroscopy and CT, ultrasound does not expose patients and personnel to radiation. Imaging can be performed continuously. The fluid injected is mostly visualized in a real-time fashion. Therefore, if the target nerve is identified, ultrasound provides the unique opportunity to assure spread of the injected solution at the site of block during administration, without radiation exposure and the need of contrast dye injection. Vessels are visualized; most clearly when Doppler sonography is available. Thus, the risk of intravascular injection of local anesthetics or injury of vessels is minimized. Ultrasound is less expensive than CT and, depending on the type of device, may be less expensive than fluoroscopy.

Limitations of Ultrasound

The major limitation of ultrasound is the poor visualization of thin needles. However, the movements of the tissues while advancing the needle provide experienced practitioners with reliable information on the needle tip position. Since bones reflect the ultrasound waves, structures located behind, for examples, osteophytes, are not reliably visualized with ultrasound. The use of high-frequency transducers is mandatory to achieve the appropriate resolution to identify small nerves. However, the higher the used frequency, the lower the ultrasound beam will penetrate into the tissue (possible working depth is limited). This means that it is not possible to visualize thin nerves deeper than a few centimeters from the surface.

Ultrasound-Guided Technique for TON and Cervical Medial Branch Block

Scanning Before Injection

The patient is placed in the left or right lateral position. Usually, we perform an ultrasound examination to identify all important structures prior to the disinfection of the skin and wrapping the ultrasound transducer with a sterile plastic cover.

Identifying the Correct Level: Method 1

Using high-resolution ultrasound imaging (we use a Sequoia 512® Ultrasound System with a 15-MHz high-resolution linear ultrasound transducer, 15L8w, Acuson Corporation, Mountain View, CA) the ultrasound examination is started with the cranial end of the transducer over the mastoid process almost parallel to the underlying spine in a longitudinal plane (Figure 6.1). Moving the transducer slowly anterior and posterior (to the mastoid)

Figure 6.1. To identify the facet joint C2-3, the ultrasound examination is started with the cranial end of the transducer over the mastoid process almost parallel to the underlying spine in a longitudinal plane. The *blue rectangle* shows the transducer position in relation to the underlying spine at this starting point.

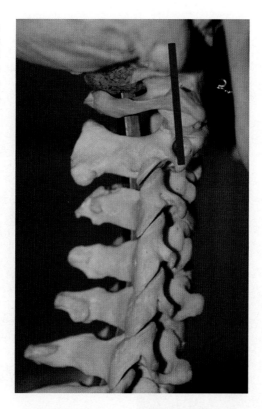

and some millimeter more caudally, the most superficially situated bony landmark of the upper cervical spine, i.e., the transverse process of C1, is visualized. With slight rotations of the transducer the transverse process of C2, about 2 cm more caudally, is searched in the same ultrasound image. All these three bony landmarks are relatively superficial (depending on the habitus of the patient) and produce a bright reflex with the typical dorsal shadowing of bony structures. Between the transverse processes of C1 and C2, 1–2 cm deeper, the pulsation of the vertebral artery can be seen. At this stage, the use of Doppler sonography may facilitate the identification of this important landmark. The vertebral artery crosses the anterior lateral part of articulation of C1-2 at this position.

Moving the transducer about 5–8 mm more posteriorly, the arch of the atlas (C1) and the articular pillar of C2 (cranial part of the facet joint C2-3) in the caudal third of the image are visualized (transducer position as shown in Figure 6.2). Now the transducer, still longitudinal in relation to the neck, can be moved caudally to bring the C2-3 and C3-4 articulations into the center of the ultrasound picture. The approximate position of the ultrasound transducer at this point is illustrated in Figure 6.3 and the obtained ultrasound image is shown in Figure 6.4. Slight rotatory movement of the transducer is needed to identify the TON crossing the articulation of C2-3 at this point. Because it is known that the TON crosses the C2-3 zygapophysial joint in this plane at an average distance of 1 mm from the bone,[31] we search for the typical sonomorphological appearance of a small peripheral nerve at this location. A peripheral nerve crossing the ultrasound plane at an angle of approximately 90°, as in the present case, can be identified better than one running longitudinally along the plane of view. It appears typically as an oval hypoechoic area with hyperechoic spots encircled by a hyperechoic horizon.[26,27,32]

The more caudal cervical medial branches are searched in the same way. Once we have identified the articulation of C2-3, the transducer is slowly moved in a caudal direction. The highest points in the bony reflex of the articular pillars represent the articulations.

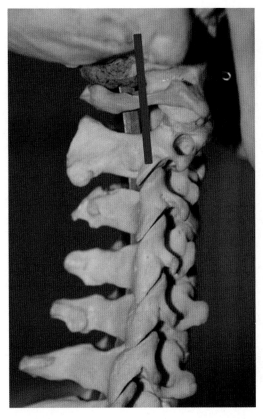

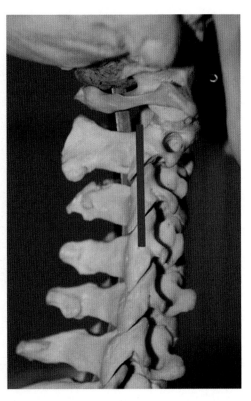

Figure 6.2. From the transducer position shown in Figure 6.1, the transducer is moved about 5–8 mm more posteriorly to the position shown in this image. Know the arch of the atlas (C1) and, in the caudal third of the image, the articular pillar of C2 can be visualized.

Figure 6.3. The final position of the transducer in relation to the underlying cervical spine for the identification of the C2-3 facet joint. The movements of the transducer from the position in Figure 6.1 to the final position in Figure 6.3 are described more extensively in the text.

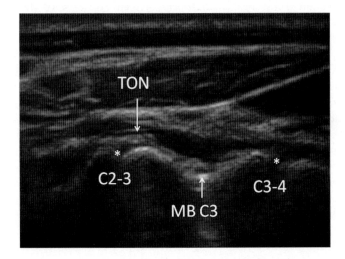

Figure 6.4. Image obtained by a transducer position as shown in Figure 6.3. The third occipital nerve crosses the articulation of C2-3 and the medial branch of C3 crosses at the deepest point between the articulations C2-3 and C3-4. The nerves can be seen with a typical sonomorphological appearance: an *oval* hypoechoic (*black*) structure with hyperechoic (*white*) small spots inside and a hyperechoic horizon around it.

Starting at C2-3 we count the "hills" by moving the transducer – still in longitudinal direction in relation to the neck – caudally until we reach the desired level of the cervical facet joint. With a transducer position as shown in Figures 6.5 and 6.6, you will obtain an image of the level C3-4 and C4-5 as shown in Figure 6.7. Bringing the articulation into the center of the ultrasound picture, we are able to visualize the two medial branches innervating the

Figure 6.5. The transducer position to obtain the image in Figure 6.7 in relation to the underlying cervical spine is shown.

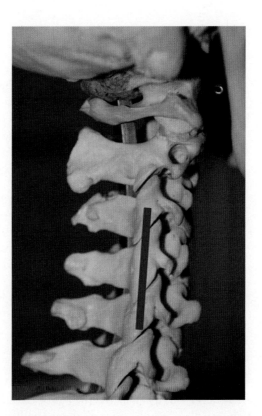

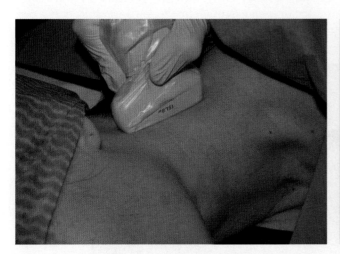

Figure 6.6. The transducer position in relation to the neck to obtain the image in Figure 6.7 is shown.

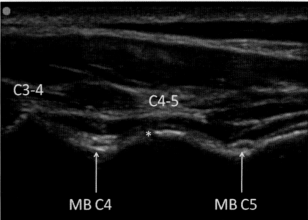

Figure 6.7. Typical white (hyperechoic) reflex of the bony surfaces of the articulations C3-4 and C4-5. The medial branch C4 (MB C4) can be seen at the deepest point between the articulations C3-4 and C4-5, nearly in contact to the bone. The medial branch C5 (MB C5) is seen at the deepest point of the bony surface more caudally of the articulation C4-5.

joint. Only the C2-3 joint is innervated by one single nerve (the TON). All articulations more caudal are innervated by two medial branches, arising out of the two roots, one cranial and one caudal of the articulation. Unlike the TON, the medial branches do not cross over the highest point of the articulation, but at the deepest point of the corresponding articular pillar from anterior to posterior between two articulations and are able to be visualized there (Figure 6.7).

Identifying the correct Level: Method 2

Especially in the lower cervical spine, it is a good alternative to count and identify the roots in the interscalene region and then follow them to the corresponding osseous cervical level. If the visualization of the roots is difficult, first identifying the transverse processes of C5, C6, and C7 may help as anatomic landmarks to find the roots and then follow them more distally. Usually the C6 transverse process is the most prominent one, showing impressive anterior and posterior tubercles (U-shaped) and dorsal shadowing from the bone. Between the two tubercles the anterior part of the nerve root can be seen. Following this root distally one can identify the interscalene region, even if the two interscalene muscles are hardly identified by ultrasound.

At the level of C7, the anterior tubercle is absent and the vertebral artery is usually seen slightly anterior of the root. Figure 6.8 shows the transducer position to obtain an ultrasound image of the root C7 and the vertebral artery (Figure 6.9a). The use of color Doppler is recommended to better identify the vertebral artery (Figure 6.9b). This will help to identify the correct vertebral level and corresponding nerve root, but one must be aware of the possible anatomical variation.

It may be helpful to mark the skin at the level of interest to improve successful identification of the structures after sterile preparation of the work field and the transducer.

Practical Performance of Block

After scanning the neck and identifying the targeted nerves, the skin is disinfected, the transducer is wrapped in a sterile plastic cover, and sterile ultrasound coupling gel is used. The needle is introduced from immediately anterior to the ultrasound probe and slowly advanced perpendicular to the beam ("short axis") as shown in Figure 6.10. We use a short bevel 24-G needle connected over an extension line to a syringe. Injection is performed by a second person holding the syringe. The needle tip is advanced until it is seen

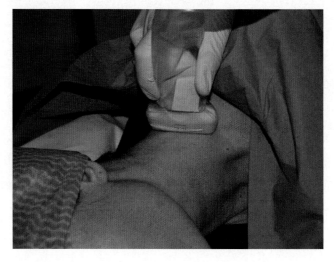

Figure 6.8. Transducer position to scan the root C7 as shown in Figure 6.9a, b for the identification of the vertebral level.

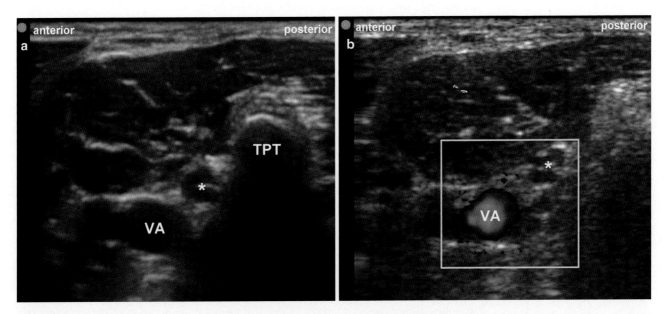

Figure 6.9. (a) Ultrasound image of the root C7 and the vertebral artery some millimeters anteriorly of the root. *Asterisk* root C7, *VA* vertebral artery, *TPT* posterior tubercle of the transverse process of C7. (b) The same ultrasound image as Figure a with the use of Doppler ultrasound.

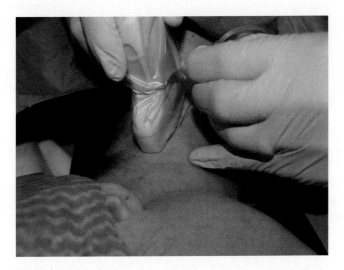

Figure 6.10. Relation needle to transducer to perform an ultrasound-guided cervical medial branch block at the level of C4-5. The transducer is positioned longitudinal to the neck and the needle is introduced immediately anterior to the ultrasound probe and slowly advanced.

to lie just beside the nerve. At this point, increments of 0.1 ml of local anesthetic (LA) are injected, until it reaches the nerve adequately. If necessary, the needle tip is slightly repositioned. The conventional, fluoroscopically guided technique for TON blocks requires needle placements onto three target points, each injected with 0.3 ml (total 0.9 ml) of LA. Our experience showed that using ultrasound guidance 0.5 ml is enough to block the TON. To block the other medial branches usually 0.3 ml of LA is sufficient. The total volume needed is dependent on the spread of LA. We recommend injecting no more than 0.5 ml of LA per nerve, since higher volumes would lower the specificity of the block because of potential anesthesia of other pain relevant structures near the medial branch.

We always introduce the needle from anterior to posterior because all vulnerable structures are situated more anterior to the facet joint line (i.e., vertebral artery and neuroforamen). This lowers the risk of inadvertent puncture of these structures in case the needle tip is not correctly identified. Nevertheless, this procedure is not recommended for people not experienced in ultrasound-guided injections and should be performed only after adequate needle guidance experience and training. As we gain more experience in identifying the course of the nerves by ultrasound, ultrasound-guided radiofrequency ablation (RFA) will become feasible and this may reduce the needed number of lesions. Furthermore, it is possible to bring the RF probes close to the nerve with ultrasound guidance prior to taking an x-ray image, thus reducing the radiation exposure.

Conclusion

This overview illustrates the potentially useful application of ultrasound and describes the technique of TON and cervical medial branch blocks. In contrast to fluoroscopy and CT, ultrasound allows visualization of the cervical medial branches in most patients and thus the local anesthetic can be injected as close as possible to the targeted nerve. However, ultrasound has limitations. Depending on the habitus of patients, it is not possible to visualize the very small nerves in all cases, especially at the C7 level.

Ultrasonography of nerves as small as the cervical medial branches requires excellent anatomical knowledge and experience. The identification of the nerves is frequently difficult. Therefore, adequate training is mandatory before ultrasound is used for this procedure. Lack of training can make the procedure ineffective and unsafe, especially in the neck area which is packed with several vital nearby structures.

Further research in the field should provide evidence that ultrasound is at least equivalent or superior to traditional imaging techniques as fluoroscopy or CT in terms of effectiveness and safety of diagnostic or therapeutic cervical facet nerve interventions.

REFERENCES

1. Pal GP, Routal RV, Saggu SK. The orientation of the articular facets of the zygapophyseal joints at the cervical and upper thoracic region. *J Anat.* 2001;198(pt 4):431–441.
2. Yoganandan N, Knowles SA, Maiman DJ, Pintar FA. Anatomic study of the morphology of human cervical facet joint. *Spine (Phila Pa 1976).* 2003;28(20):2317–2323.
3. Inami S, Kaneoka K, Hayashi K, Ochiai N. Types of synovial fold in the cervical facet joint. *J Orthop Sci.* 2000;5(5):475–480.
4. Bogduk N. The clinical anatomy of the cervical dorsal rami. *Spine.* 1982;7(4):319–330.
5. Teo EC, Ng HW. Evaluation of the role of ligaments, facets and disc nucleus in lower cervical spine under compression and sagittal moments using finite element method. *Med Eng Phys.* 2001;23(3):155–164.
6. Raynor RB, Pugh J, Shapiro I. Cervical facetectomy and its effect on spine strength. *J Neurosurg.* 1985;63(2):278–282.
7. Zdeblick TA, Abitbol JJ, Kunz DN, McCabe RP, Garfin S. Cervical stability after sequential capsule resection. *Spine (Phila Pa 1976).* 1993;18(14):2005–2008.
8. Siegmund GP, Myers BS, Davis MB, Bohnet HF, Winkelstein BA. Mechanical evidence of cervical facet capsule injury during whiplash: a cadaveric study using combined shear, compression, and extension loading. *Spine (Phila Pa 1976).* 2001;26(19):2095–2101.
9. Winkelstein BA, McLendon RE, Barbir A, Myers BS. An anatomical investigation of the human cervical facet capsule, quantifying muscle insertion area. *J Anat.* 2001;198(pt 4):455–461.
10. Kallakuri S, Singh A, Chen C, Cavanaugh JM. Demonstration of substance P, calcitonin gene-related peptide, and protein gene product 9.5 containing nerve fibers in human cervical facet joint capsules. *Spine (Phila Pa 1976).* 2004;29(11):1182–1186.

11. Kettler A, Werner K, Wilke HJ. Morphological changes of cervical facet joints in elderly individuals. *Eur Spine J.* 2007;16(7):987–992.

12. Barnsley L, Lord SM, Wallis BJ, Bogduk N. The prevalence of chronic cervical zygapophysial joint pain after whiplash. *Spine.* 1995;20(1):20–26.

13. Manchikanti L, Boswell MV, Singh V, Pampati V, Damron KS, Beyer CD. Prevalence of facet joint pain in chronic spinal pain of cervical, thoracic, and lumbar regions. *BMC Musculoskelet Disord.* 2004;5:15.

14. Pearson AM, Ivancic PC, Ito S, Panjabi MM. Facet joint kinematics and injury mechanisms during simulated whiplash. *Spine.* 2004;29(4):390–397.

15. Radanov BP, Sturzenegger M, Di Stefano G. Long-term outcome after whiplash injury. A 2-year follow-up considering features of injury mechanism and somatic, radiologic, and psychosocial findings. *Medicine (Baltimore).* 1995;74(5):281–297.

16. Barnsley L, Lord S, Bogduk N. Comparative local anaesthetic blocks in the diagnosis of cervical zygapophysial joint pain. *Pain.* 1993;55(1):99–106.

17. Barnsley L, Bogduk N. Medial branch blocks are specific for the diagnosis of cervical zygapophyseal joint pain. *Reg Anesth.* 1993;18(6):343–350.

18. Barnsley L, Lord S, Wallis B, Bogduk N. False-positive rates of cervical zygapophysial joint blocks. *Clin J Pain.* 1993;9(2):124–130.

19. Bogduk N. International Spinal Injection Society guidelines for the performance of spinal injection procedures. Part 1: zygapophysial joint blocks. *Clin J Pain.* 1997;13(4):285–302.

20. Lord SM, Barnsley L, Wallis BJ, Bogduk N. Chronic cervical zygapophysial joint pain after whiplash. A placebo-controlled prevalence study. *Spine.* 1996;21(15):1737–1745.

21. Sluijter ME, Koetsveld-Baart CC. Interruption of pain pathways in the treatment of the cervical syndrome. *Anaesthesia.* 1980;35(3):302–307.

22. Lord SM, Barnsley L, Wallis BJ, McDonald GJ, Bogduk N. Percutaneous radio-frequency neurotomy for chronic cervical zygapophyseal-joint pain. *N Engl J Med.* 1996;335(23):1721–1726.

23. Govind J, King W, Bailey B, Bogduk N. Radiofrequency neurotomy for the treatment of third occipital headache. *J Neurol Neurosurg Psychiatry.* 2003;74(1):88–93.

24. Manchikanti L, Singh V, Falco FJ, Cash KM, Fellows B. Cervical medial branch blocks for chronic cervical facet joint pain: a randomized, double-blind, controlled trial with one-year follow-up. *Spine.* 2008;33(17):1813–1820.

25. Eichenberger U, Greher M, Kapral S, et al. Sonographic visualization and ultrasound-guided block of the third occipital nerve: prospective for a new method to diagnose C2-C3 zygapophysial joint pain. *Anesthesiology.* 2006,104(2).303–308.

26. Martinoli C, Bianchi S, Dahmane M, Pugliese F, Bianchi-Zamorani P, Valle M. Ultrasound of tendons and nerves. *Eur Radiol.* 2002;12(1):44–55.

27. Silvestri E, Martinoli C, Derchi LE, Bertolotto M, Chiaramondia M, Rosenberg I. Echotexture of peripheral nerves: correlation between US and histologic findings and criteria to differentiate tendons. *Radiology.* 1995;197(1):291–296.

28. Gofeld M. Ultrasonography in pain medicine: a critical review. *Pain Pract.* 2008;8(4):226–240.

29. Siegenthaler A, Narouze S, Eichenberger U. Ultrasound-guided third occipital nerve and cervical medial branch nerve blocks. *Tech Reg Anesth Pain Manag.* 2009;13:128–132.

30. Fishman SM, Smith H, Meleger A, Seibert JA. Radiation safety in pain medicine. *Reg Anesth Pain Med.* 2002;27(3):296–305.

31. Lord SM, McDonald GJ, Bogduk N. Percutaneous radiofrequency neurotomy of the cervical medial branches: a validated treatment for cervical zygapophysial joint pain. *Neurosurg Q.* 1998;8(4):288–308.

32. Fornage BD. Peripheral nerves of the extremities: imaging with US. *Radiology.* 1988;167(1):179–182.

7

Ultrasound-Guided Cervical Zygapophyseal (Facet) Intra-Articular Injection

Samer N. Narouze

Anatomy of the Cervical Facet Joints

Cervical facet joints are diarthrodial joints formed by the superior articular process of one cervical vertebra articulating with the inferior articular process of the vertebrae above at the level of the junction of the lamina and the pedicle. The angulation of the facet joint

S.N. Narouze (✉)
Center for Pain Medicine, Summa Western Reserve Hospital,
1900 23rd Street, Cuyahoga Falls, OH 44223, USA
e-mail: narouzs@hotmail.com

S.N. Narouze (ed.), *Atlas of Ultrasound-Guided Procedures in Interventional Pain Management*,
DOI 10.1007/978-1-4419-1681-5_7, © Springer Science+Business Media, LLC 2011

increases caudally, being about 45° superior to the transverse plane at the upper cervical level to assuming a more vertical position at the upper thoracic level. The superior articular process also faces more posteromedial at the upper cervical level and this changes to more posterolateral at the lower cervical level, with C6 being the most common transition level.[1,2]

Each facet joint has a fibrous capsule and is lined by a synovial membrane. The joint also contains varying amounts of adipose and fibrous tissue forming different types of synovial folds contributing to different pathophysiology for joint dysfunction.[3]

Excessive facet joint compression and capsular ligament strain have been implicated in neck pain after whiplash injury.[4] The facet joint and capsule have been shown to contain nociceptive elements suggesting that it may be an independent pain generator.[5] Facet joint degeneration is more common in the elderly and the prevalence of facet joint involvement in chronic neck pain has been reported to be from 35% to 55%.[6,7]

Indications for Cervical Zygapophyseal Joint Intra-Articular Injection

Facet joint-mediated pain cannot be diagnosed based only on clinical examination or radiological imaging. Cervical facet intra-articular injection has been utilized in the diagnosis and management of facetogenic pain.[8] However, evidence for effective relief of neck pain with cervical zygapophyseal injections is lacking.[9,10] Cervical medial branch block is still considered the gold standard to diagnose pain stemming from the facet joints.[11]

Literature Review of Ultrasound-Guided Cervical Facet Injections

Galiano et al[12] reported the feasibility of ultrasound-guided cervical facet joint intra-articular injections in cadavers using a lateral approach. The facet joints from C2-3 to C6-7 were accurately identified in 36 of 40 cases. CT confirmed needle tip placement inside the joint space. The same group later studied and advocated the use of an ultrasound-guided CT-assisted navigation system as a teaching tool for performing facet injections.[13]

Ultrasound-Guided Technique for Cervical Facet Intra-Articular Injection

Lateral Approach

The patient is placed in the lateral position and the correct cervical level is identified (see Chap. 8). A high-frequency linear transducer is used to obtain a short axis view. The superior articular and the inferior articular processes forming the facet joint appear as hyperechoic signals and the joint space in between as anechoic gap. The needle is inserted at the lateral end of the transducer and advanced from posterior to anterior – in plane – under real-time ultrasonography to the target (joint space).[12]

Posterior Approach

The posterior approach is more practical than the lateral one as the patient is in the prone position and bilateral injections can be performed without the need to change position.

A sagittal scan is obtained first at the midline to identify the correct cervical level. C1 spine has no or rudimentary spinous process and the first identified bifid spinous process belongs to C2 (Figure 7.1). Then after, one can continue counting caudally. A linear or a curved transducer may be used depending on the size of the patient. A longitudinal scan is obtained initially at the midline (spinous process) and then by scanning laterally, one can easily see the lamina and further laterally the facet column will appear in the image as the characteristic "saw sign" (Figure 7.2). If in doubt, one can scan even more laterally till the facet joints are no more in the image and then come back medially toward the facet joints. The inferior articular processes of the level above and the superior articular process of the level below appear as a hyperechoic signals and the joint space appears as anechoic gap in between (Figure 7.3). The needle is then inserted inferior to the caudal end of the

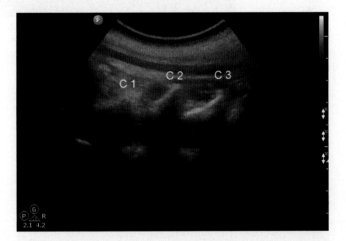

Figure 7.1. A midline longitudinal scan through the cervical spinous processes level. Note that the C1 immediately caudal to the occiput has only a rudimentary spinous process compared to the bifid spinous process of C2.

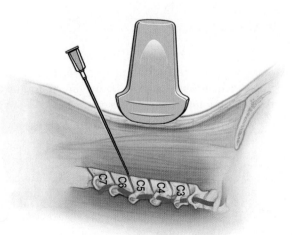

Figure 7.2. The paramedian position of the ultrasound transducer to obtain a sagittal longitudinal scan through the facet column is shown. Needle is advanced in-plane into C5–C6 facet joint. Reprinted with permission, Cleveland Clinic Center for Medical Art & Photography© 2009–2010. All rights reserved.

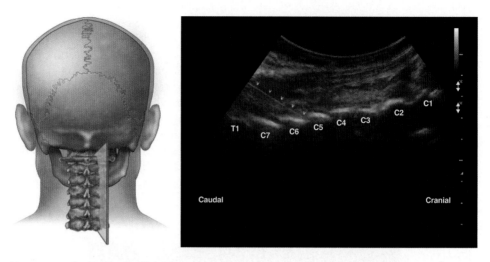

Figure 7.3. Sagittal longitudinal sonogram showing the articular processes of the facet joints as the "saw sign." Reprinted with permission, Cleveland Clinic Center for Medical Art & Photography© 2009–2010. All rights reserved.

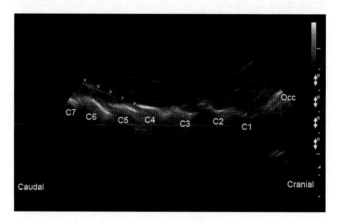

Figure 7.4. Needle is introduced caudal to the transducer and advanced in-plane into the caudal part of the C4–C5 facet joint (*arrow heads*). Occ occiput.

transducer and advanced from caudad to cephalad – in plane – to enter the caudal end of the joint under real-time ultrasonography (Figure 7.4). We believe that this is another advantage of this US approach, as this caudal to cranial direction is matching the caudal angulation of the cervical facet joint, making it easier for the needle to get into the joint space atraumatically.[14]

REFERENCES

1. Pal GP, Routal RV, Saggu SK. The orientation of the articular facets of the zygapophyseal joints at the cervical and upper thoracic region. *J Anat.* 2001;198:431–441.
2. Yoganandan N, Knowles SA, Maiman DJ, Pintar FA. Anatomic study of the morphology of human cervical facet joint. *Spine.* 2003;28:2317–2323.
3. Inami S, Kaneoka K, Hayashi K, Ochiai N. Types of synovial fold in the cervical facet joint. *J Orthop Sci.* 2000;5:475–480.
4. Pearson AM, Ivancic PC, Ito S, Panjabi MM. Facet joint kinematics and injury mechanisms during simulated whiplash. *Spine.* 2004;29:390–397.

5. Kallakuri S, Singh A, Chen C, Cavanaugh JM. Demonstration of substance P, calcitonin gene-related peptide, and protein gene product 9.5 containing nerve fibers in human cervical facet joint capsules. *Spine*. 2004;29:1182–1186.

6. Manchikanti L, Boswell MV, Singh V, Pampati V, Damron KS, Beyer CD. Prevalence of facet joint pain in chronic spinal pain of cervical, thoracic, and lumbar regions. *BMC Musculoskelet Disord*. 2004;5:15.

7. Barnsley L, Lord SM, Wallis BJ, Bogduk N. The prevalence of chronic cervical zygapophysial joint pain after whiplash. *Spine*. 1995;20:20–25.

8. Hove B, Gyldensted C. Cervical analgesic facet joint arthrography. *Neuroradiology*. 1990;32: 456–459.

9. Barnsley L, Lord SM, Wallis BJ, Bogduk N. Lack of effect of intra-articular corticosteroids for chronic pain in the cervical zygapophysial joints. *N Engl J Med*. 1994;330:1047–1050.

10. Carragee EJ, Hurwitz EL, Cheng I, et al. Treatment of neck pain: injections and surgical interventions: results of the Bone and Joint Decade 2000-2010 Task Force on Neck Pain and Its Associated Disorders. *Spine*. 2008;33:S153–S169.

11. Barnsley L, Bogduk N. Medial branch blocks are specific for the diagnosis of cervical zygapophyseal joint pain. *Reg Anesth*. 1993;18:343–50.

12. Galiano K, Obwegeser AA, Bodner G, et al. Ultrasound-guided facet joint injections in the middle to lower cervical spine: a CT-controlled sonoanatomic study. *Clin J Pain*. 2006;22:538–543.

13. Galiano K, Obwegeser AA, Bale R, et al. Ultrasound-guided and CT-navigation-assisted periradicular and facet joint injections in the lumbar and cervical spine: a new teaching tool to recognize the sonoanatomic pattern. *Reg Anesth Pain Med*. 2007;32:254–257.

14. Narouze S, Peng P. Ultrasound-guided interventional procedures in pain medicine: a review of anatomy, sonoanaotmy and procedures. Part II: axial structures. Reg Anesth Pain Med 2010;35(4):386–396.

8

Ultrasound-Guided Cervical Nerve Root Block

Samer N. Narouze

Anatomy of Cervical Nerve Root

The cervical spinal nerve occupies the lower part of the foramen with the epiradicular veins in the upper part. The radicular arteries arising from the vertebral, ascending cervical, and deep cervical arteries lie in close approximation to the spinal nerve.

Huntoon showed, in cadavers, that the ascending and deep cervical arteries may contribute to the anterior spinal artery along with the vertebral artery. Twenty percent of the foramina dissected had the ascending cervical artery or deep cervical artery branches within 2 mm of the needle path for a cervical transforaminal procedure. One third of these vessels entered the foramen posteriorly potentially forming a radicular or a segmental feeder vessel to the spinal cord, making it vulnerable to inadvertent injury or injection even during correct needle placement.[1]

S.N. Narouze (✉)
Center for Pain Medicine, Summa Western Reserve Hospital,
1900 23rd Street, Cuyahoga Falls, OH 44223, USA
e-mail: narouzs@hotmail.com

S.N. Narouze (ed.), *Atlas of Ultrasound-Guided Procedures in Interventional Pain Management*,
DOI 10.1007/978-1-4419-1681-5_8, © Springer Science+Business Media, LLC 2011

Hoeft et al,[2] in a single cadaver study, showed that radicular artery branches from the vertebral artery lie over the most anteromedial aspect of the foramen, while those that arise from the ascending or deep cervical arteries are of greatest clinical significance as they must course medially throughout the entire length of the foramen.

Indications

Cervical nerve root block/transforaminal epidural injections are indicated in cervical radicular pain not responsive to conservative therapy.

Cervical epidural injections can be performed using an interlaminar or a transforaminal approach. As cervical radicular pain is frequently caused by foraminal stenosis, transforaminal approach can maximize the concentration of steroid delivered to the affected nerve roots while reducing the volume of injectate required and was shown to be effective in relieving radicular symptoms.[3,4]

Limitations of the Fluoroscopy-Guided Techniques

Cervical transforaminal injections have been traditionally performed with the use of fluoroscopy or CT. However, there have been few reports of fatal complications in the literature as a result of vertebral artery injury[5,6] and/or infarction of the spinal cord and the brain stem.[7-11] The mechanism of injury was believed to be vasospasm or the particulate nature of the steroid injectate with embolus formation after inadvertent intra-arterial injection.[7,8]

Currently, the guidelines for cervical transforaminal injection technique involve introducing the needle under fluoroscopic guidance into the posterior aspect of the intervertebral foramen just anterior to the superior articular process in the oblique view to minimize the risk of injury to the vertebral artery or the nerve root.[12] Despite strict adherence to these guidelines adverse outcomes have been reported.[7,8] A potential shortcoming of the described fluoroscopic-guided procedure is that the needle may puncture a critical contributing vessel to the anterior spinal artery in the posterior aspect of the intervertebral foramen.[1] Here the ultrasonography may come to play, as it allows for visualization of soft tissues, nerves, and vessels and the spread of the injectate around the nerve, and thus it may be potentially advantageous to fluoroscopy. Ultrasound allows identification of vessels before they are punctured, while fluoroscopy recognizes intravascular injection only after the vessel has been punctured.[13]

Literature Review of Ultrasound-Guided Cervical Nerve Root Block

Galiano et al[14] first described ultrasound-guided cervical periradicular injections in cadavers; however, they were not able to comment on the relevant blood vessels in the vicinity of the vertebral foramen.

Narouze et al[15] reported a pilot study of ten patients who received cervical nerve root injections using ultrasound as the primary imaging tool with fluoroscopy as the control. The radiologic target point was the posterior aspect of the intervertebral foramen just anterior to the SAP in the oblique view, and at the midsagittal plane of the articular pillars in the anteroposterior view (the target point for transforaminal injection).

The needle was exactly at the target point in five patients in the oblique view and in three patients in the AP views. The needle was within 3 mm in all patients in the lateral oblique view and in eight patients in the AP view. In the other two patients, the needle was within 5 mm from the radiologic target as the needle was not introduced into the fora-men intentionally but rather just outside of the foramen as the goal was to perform selec-tive nerve root injection and not a transforaminal injection.

In four patients they were able to identify vessels at the anterior aspect of the foramen, while two patients had critical vessels at the posterior aspect of the foramen and in one patient this artery continued medially into the foramen most likely forming a segmental feeder artery. In these two cases, such vessels could have been injured easily in the pathway of a correctly placed needle under fluoroscopy.

Sonoanatomy of the Cervical Spine and Identification of the Cervical Level

With patients lying in the lateral decubitus position, ultrasound examination is performed using a high-resolution linear array transducer. The transducer is applied transversely to the lateral aspect of the neck to obtain a short axis view of the cervical spine (Figure 8.1). One can easily identify the cervical transverse process with the anterior and posterior tubercles as hyperechoic structures "two-humped camel" sign and the hypoechoic round-to-oval nerve root in between[15] (Figure 8.2). First, the cervical level is determined by identifying the transverse process of the seventh and sixth cervical vertebrae (C7 and C6.) The seventh cervical transverse process (C7) differs from the above levels as it usually has a rudimentary anterior tubercle and one prominent posterior tubercle[16] (Figure 8.3). Then by moving the transducer cranially the transverse process of the sixth cervical spine comes in the image with the characteristic sharp anterior tubercle (Figure 8.4), and then after the consecutive cervical spinal level can be easily identified. At higher levels than C6, the anterior tubercle becomes shorter and equal to the posterior tubercle with a shallow groove in between (Figure 8.2). Another way to determine the cervical spinal level is by following the vertebral artery, which runs anteriorly at the C7 level (Figure 8.3) before it enters the foramen of C6 transverse process in about 90% of cases. However, it enters at C5 or higher in about 10% of cases[17] (Figure 8.5)

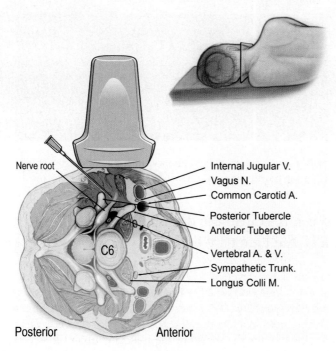

Nerve root

Internal Jugular V.
Vagus N.
Common Carotid A.

Posterior Tubercle
Anterior Tubercle

C6

Vertebral A. & V.
Sympathetic Trunk.
Longus Colli M.

Posterior   Anterior

Figure 8.1. The orientation of the ultrasound transducer to obtain a short axis view at C6 level is shown. Reprinted with permission, Cleveland Clinic Center for Medical Art & Photography© 2008–2010. All rights reserved.

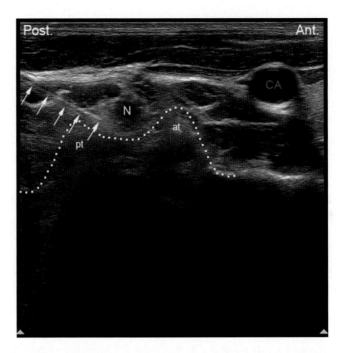

Figure 8.2. Sort-axis transverse ultrasound images showing the anterior tubercle (at) and the posterior tubercle (pt) of the C5 transverse process as the "two-humped camel" sign. *N* nerve root, *CA* carotid artery. *Solid arrows* are pointing to the needle in place at the posterior aspect of the intervertebral foramen. Reprinted with permission, Cleveland Clinic Center for Medical Art & Photography© 2008–2010. All rights reserved.

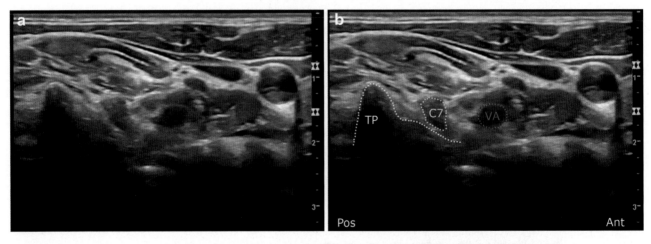

Figure 8.3. (**a, b**) Short-axis transverse ultrasound image showing the pt of the C7 transverse process. Note the vertebral artery (VA) is anterior to the C7 nerve root. No anterior tubercle. (Reprinted with permission from Ohio Pain and Headache Institute).

Ultrasound-Guided Technique for Cervical Selective Nerve Root Block

Once the appropriate spinal level is identified, a 22-gauge blunt-tip needle can be introduced under real-time ultrasound guidance from posterior to anterior with an in-plane technique to target the corresponding cervical nerve root (from C3–C8) at the external foraminal opening between the anterior and posterior tubercles of the transverse process (Figure 8.2). One can successfully monitor the spread of the injectate around the cervical nerve with real-time ultrasonography and the absence of such spread around the nerve root may suggest unsuspected or inadvertent intravascular injection. However, it is difficult to monitor the

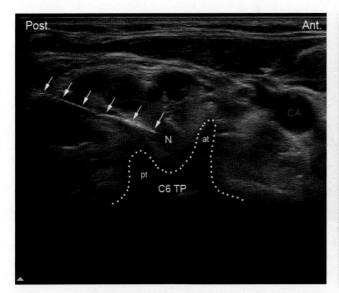

Figure 8.4. Short-axis transverse ultrasound image showing the sharp anterior tubercle (at) of the C6 transverse process (C6tp). *N* nerve root, *CA* carotid artery, *pt* posterior tubercle. *Solid arrows* are pointing to the needle in place at the posterior aspect of the intervertebral foramen. Reprinted with permission, Cleveland Clinic Center for Medical Art & Photography© 2008–2010. All rights reserved.

Figure 8.5. Short-axis transverse ultrasound image showing the sharp anterior tubercle (at) of the C6 transverse process and the vertebral artery (VA) is anterior. *N* nerve root, *CA* carotid artery, *pt* posterior tubercle. Reprinted with permission, Cleveland Clinic Center for Medical Art & Photography© 2008–2010. All rights reserved.

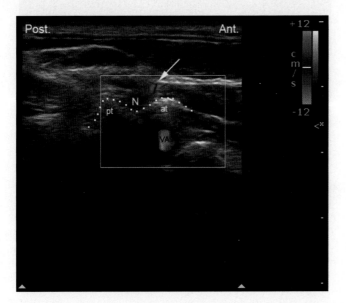

Figure 8.6. Short-axis transverse ultrasound image with color Doppler showing a small artery at the anterior aspect of the intravertebral foramen. *at* anterior tubercle, *pt* posterior tubercle, *VA* vertebral artery. (Reprinted with permission from Ohio Pain and Headache Institute).

spread of the injectate through the foramen into the epidural space because of the bony drop out artifact of the transverse process. We therefore refer to this approach as a "cervical selective nerve root block" rather than cervical transforaminal epidural injection.

The author believes that visualization of such small vessels (radicular arteries) may be very challenging especially in obese patients and requires special training and expertise. Real-time fluoroscopy with contrast injection and digital subtraction – when available – should still be used with ultrasound as an adjunct to help identifying blood vessels in the vicinity of the foramen (Figures. 8.6–8.8).

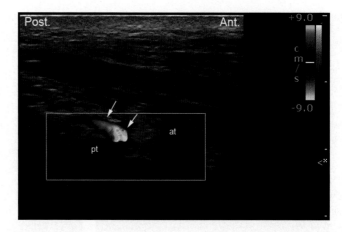

Figure 8.7. Short-axis transverse ultrasound image with color Doppler showing a small vessel at the posterior aspect of the intravertebral foramen. *at* anterior tubercle, *pt* posterior tubercle. (Reprinted with permission from Ohio Pain and Headache Institute).

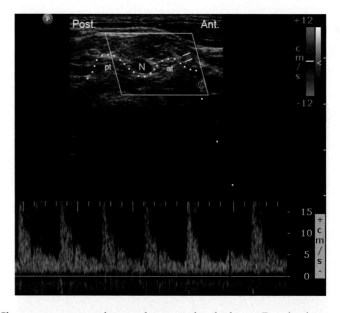

Figure 8.8. Short-axis transverse ultrasound image with pulsed-wave Doppler showing arterial perfusion in a small vessel at the anterior aspect of the intervertebral foramen. *N* nerve root, *VA* vertebral artery, *at* anterior tubercle, *pt* posterior tubercle. Reprinted with permission, Cleveland Clinic Center for Medical Art & Photography© 2008–2010. All rights reserved.

REFERENCES

1. Huntoon MA. Anatomy of the cervical intervertebral foramina: vulnerable arteries and ischemic neurologic injuries after transforaminal epidural injections. *Pain.* 2005;117:104–111.
2. Hoeft MA, Rathmell JP, Monsey RD, Fonda BJ. Cervical transforaminal injection and the radicular artery: variation in anatomical location within the cervical intervertebral foramina. *Reg Anesth Pain Med.* 2006;31:270–274.
3. Kolstad F, Leivseth L, Nygaard OP. Transforaminal steroid injections in the treatment of cervical radiculopathy: a prospective outcome study. *Acta Neurochir.* 2005;147:1065–1070.
4. Slipman CW, Lipetz JS, Jackson HB, Rogers DP, Vresilovic EJ. Therapeutic selective nerve root block in the nonsurgical treatment of atraumatic cervical spondylotic radicular pain: a retrospective analysis with independent clinical review. *Arch Phys Med Rehabil.* 2000;81:741–746.

5. Wallace MA, Fukui MB, Williams RL, Ku A, Baghai P. Complications of cervical selective nerve root blocks performed with fluoroscopic guidance. *AJR Am J Roentgenol.* 2007;188:1218–1221.

6. Rozin L, Rozin R, Koehler SA, et al. Death during transforaminal epidural steroid nerve root block (C7) due to perforation of the left vertebral artery. *Am J Forensic Med Pathol.* 2003; 24:351–355.

7. Tiso RL, Cutler T, Catania JA, Whalen K. Adverse central nervous system sequelae after selective transforaminal block: the role of corticosteroids. *Spine J.* 2004;4:468–474.

8. Baker R, Dreyfuss P, Mercer S, Bogduk N. Cervical transforaminal injections of corticosteroids into a radicular artery: a possible mechanism for spinal cord injury. *Pain.* 2003;103:211–215.

9. Muro K, O'Shaughnessy B, Ganju A. Infarction of the cervical spinal cord following multilevel transforaminal epidural steroid injection: case report and review of the literature. *J Spinal Cord Med.* 2007;30(4):385–388.

10. Brouwers PJ, Kottink EJ, Simon MA, Prevo RL. A cervical anterior spinal artery syndrome after diagnostic blockade of the right C6-nerve root. *Pain.* 2001;91:397–399.

11. Beckman WA, Mendez RJ, Paine GF, Mazzilli MA. Cerebellar herniation after cervical transforaminal epidural injection. *Reg Anesth Pain Med.* 2006;31:282–285.

12. Rathmell JP, Aprill C, Bogduk N. Cervical transforaminal injection of steroids. *Anesthesiology.* 2004;100:1595–1600.

13. Narouze S, Peng PWH. Ultrasound-guided interventional procedures in pain medicine: a review of anatomy, sonoanaotmy and procedures. Part II: axial structures. *Reg Anesth Pain Med.* 2010;35(4):386–396.

14. Galiano K, Obwegeser AA, Bodner G, et al. Ultrasound-guided periradicular injections in the middle to lower cervical spine: an imaging study of a new approach. *Reg Anesth Pain Med.* 2005;30:391–396.

15. Narouze S, Vydyanathan A, Kapural L, Sessler D, Mekhail N. Ultrasound-guided cervical selective nerve root block: a fluoroscopy-controlled feasibility study. *Reg Anesth Pain Med.* 2009;34:343–348.

16. Martinoli C, Bianchi S, Santacroce E, Pugliese F, Graif M, Derchi LE. Brachial plexus sonography: a technique for assessing the root level. *AJR Am J Roentgenol.* 2002;179:699–702.

17. Matula C, Trattnig S, Tschabitscher M, Day JD, Koos WT. The course of the prevertebral segment of the vertebral artery: anatomy and clinical significance. *Surg Neurol.* 1997;48:125–131.

9

Ultrasound-Guided Thoracic Paravertebral Block

Manoj Kumar Karmakar

M.K. Karmakar (✉)
Department of Anaesthesia and Intensive Care, The Chinese University of Hong Kong, Prince of Wales
Hospital, 32 Ngan Shing Street, Shatin, New Territories, Hong Kong
e-mail: karmakar@cuhk.edu.hk

S.N. Narouze (ed.), *Atlas of Ultrasound-Guided Procedures in Interventional Pain Management*,
DOI 10.1007/978-1-4419-1681-5_9, © Springer Science+Business Media, LLC 2011

Introduction

Thoracic paravertebral block (TPVB) is the technique of injecting local anesthetic alongside the thoracic vertebral body close to where the spinal nerves emerge from the intervertebral foramen. This produces unilateral (ipsilateral), segmental, somatic, and sympathetic nerve blockade in multiple contiguous thoracic dermatomes,[1,2] which is effective for managing acute and chronic pain of unilateral origin from the thorax and abdomen.[3] Recently, TPVB has also been used for surgical anesthesia in patients undergoing inguinal herniorrhaphy[4] and breast surgery[5,6] with improved postoperative outcomes.[3]

Anatomy

The thoracic paravertebral space (TPVS) is a wedge-shaped space located on either side of the vertebral column (Figure 9.1).[3] Anterolaterally it is bound by the parietal pleura (PP) while the superior costotransverse ligament (SCL), which extends from the lower border of the transverse process above to the upper border of the transverse process below, forms the posterior border (Figures 9.1 and 9.2).[3] The base of the wedge is formed by the posterolateral surface of the vertebral body, intervertebral disk, and the intervertebral foramen with its contents.[3] Interposed between the PP and the SCL is fibroelastic structure the "endothoracic fascia"[3,7,8] which is the deep fascia of the thorax (Figures 9.1–9.3)[3,7,8] and lines the inside of the chest wall. A layer of loose areolar tissue the "subserous fascia" is present between the PP and the endothoracic fascia (Figures 9.1 and 9.2).[3,7] The endothoracic fascia thus divides the TPVS into two potential fascial compartments, the anterior "extrapleural paravertebral compartment" and the posterior "subendothoracic paravertebral compartment" (Figure 9.1). The TPVS contains fatty tissue within which lie the intercostal nerve, the dorsal rami, the intercostal vessels, and the sympathetic chain. The TPVS communicates with the contiguous space above and below, the epidural space medially, the intercostal space laterally, the contralateral paravertebral space via the prevertebral and epidural route, and inferiorly (the lower TPVS's) with the retroperitoneal space posterior to the fas-

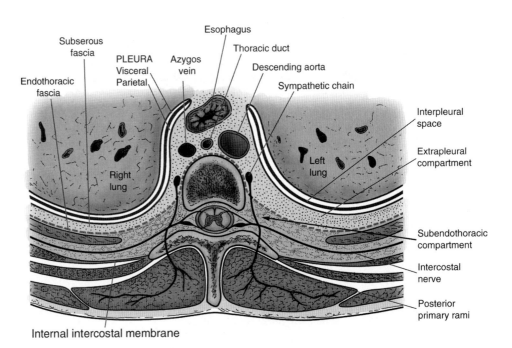

Figure 9.1. Anatomy of the thoracic paravertebral space (TPVS).

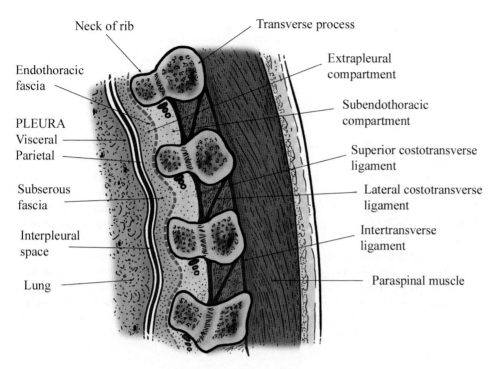

Figure 9.2. Sagittal section through the TPVS.

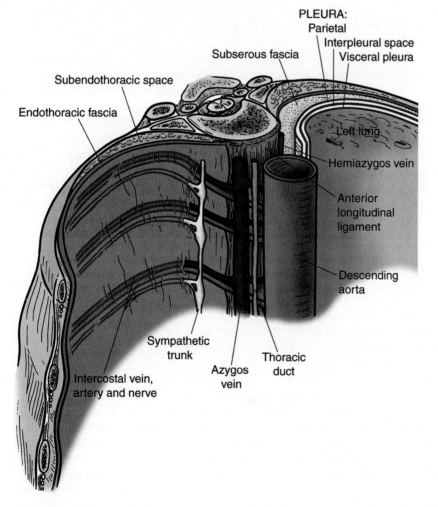

Figure 9.3. The endothoracic fascia and its relations to the TPVS.

cia transversalis via the medial and lateral arcuate ligaments.[3,8,9] The cranial extension of the TPVS is still not defined but we have observed spread of radiocontrast medium to the cervical paravertebral region on chest radiograph after thoracic paravertebral injection.

Mechanism of Blockade

The exact mechanism by which a thoracic paravertebral injection produces ipsilateral, segmental, thoracic anesthesia, and analgesia is still not clear. A thoracic paravertebral injection may remain localized to the space injected[10] or it may spread to contiguous spaces above and below,[8,11,12] the intercostal space laterally,[3,11–13] the epidural space medially,[11,13] or a combination of the above.[3] This is how the ipsilateral somatic and sympathetic nerves, including the posterior primary ramus, at multiple contiguous thoracic levels are affected.[3] The role of epidural spread in the extension of sensory blockade after thoracic paravertebral injection is still not clear. Varying degrees of epidural spread have been shown to occur in majority (70%) of patients.[13] However, the volume of injectate that enters the epidural space is only a small fraction of the total injectate[12] and confined to the side of the injection.[13] Sensory blockade is also unilateral and greater after epidural spread than after paravertebral spread only.[13] Current evidence therefore suggests that epidural spread after thoracic paravertebral injection contributes to the extension of a TPVB.[3]

Techniques of TPVB

There are several different techniques of performing TPVB and can be performed with the patient in the sitting, lateral decubitus (with the side to be blocked uppermost), or prone position.[3] The technique that is most frequently used involves eliciting "loss of resistance."[14] At the appropriate dermatome under aseptic precautions, a 22-G Tuohy needle (for a single-shot injection) or a 18- or 16-G Tuohy needle, if a catheter is to be inserted, is introduced 2.5 cm lateral to the highest point of the spinous process and advanced perpendicular to the skin in all planes until the transverse process is contacted. For safety, it is imperative to locate the transverse process before the needle is advanced any further to avoid deep needle insertion and possible inadvertent pleural puncture. Once the transverse process is located, the needle is withdrawn to the subcutaneous tissue and readvanced in a cephalad direction to pass through the space between the two transverse processes until loss of resistance is elicited as the needle traverses the SCL, usually within 1.5–2 cm from the transverse process. Occasionally a subtle pop may also be felt. Unlike epidural space location, the loss of resistance felt as the needle enters the TPVS is subjective and indefinite.[14–16] More often it is usually a change of resistance rather than a definite give. It is the author's experience that the loss of resistance is best appreciated if one uses a glass syringe filled with air. Luyet et al[17] have recently demonstrated the presence of a gap between the medial and lateral portions of the SCL in cadavers, which they propose is a possible reason for not being able to elicit a loss of resistance in all cases.[17]

Alternatively for TPVB the block needle may also be advanced by a fixed predetermined distance (1–2 cm) once the needle is walked of the transverse process without eliciting loss of resistance.[18] This variation has been used very effectively with minimal complications including pneumothorax.[18] Other techniques that have been used to perform TPVB include "the medial approach," "pressure measurement technique," "paravertebral–peridural block," "fluoroscopy guidance," and "paravertebral catheter placement under direct vision at thoracotomy."[3] It is not known whether advancing the needle superior to or inferior to the transverse process affects the overall extent and quality of TPVB.[3]

Ultrasound-Guided TPVB

TPVB is traditionally performed using surface anatomical landmarks and although it is a blind technique, it is technically simple,[3] has a high success rate,[3,5,19,20] and the overall complication rate is relatively low.[3,5,19–21] Recently, there has been an increase in interest in the use of ultrasound for peripheral[22–24] and central neuraxial blocks.[25–27] However, data on the use of ultrasound for TPVB are limited with only a few publications on the subject to date.[17,28–32]

Pusch et al[32] used ultrasound to measure the distance from the skin to the transverse process and pleura in women who were scheduled to receive a single-shot TPVB at T4 for breast surgery and found a good correlation between needle insertion depth from the skin to the transverse process and that measured using ultrasound.[32] They also found a good correlation between ultrasound measured distance from the skin to the PP and the eventual distance from the skin to the paravertebral space that was measured after needle placement.[32] Hara et al were the first group to describe ultrasound-guided (USG) TPVB (single shot), which they successfully performed in 25 women undergoing breast surgery.[31] They performed a sagittal scan over the paravertebral area at the T4 level and were able to delineate the transverse processes, the ligaments (intertransverse and costotransverse ligaments), and the pleura and were also able to measure the distance from the skin to these structures before block placement.[31] The block needle was inserted, under ultrasound guidance, in the short axis of the ultrasound beam (out-of-plane technique) until it contacted the transverse process.[31] Loss of resistance to saline was then elicited by advancing the needle above the transverse process, without ultrasound guidance, and the spread of the local anesthetic injection was visualized in real time using ultrasound.[31] Hara et al report turbulence at the level of the injection in all (100%) cases and forward displacement of the parietal pleura in four (16%) cases.[31] Since all the injections resulted in a successful block these sonographic changes may be considered as objective evidence of a correct paravertebral injection during USG TPVB. Another interesting observation that Hara et al made in their cohort of patients is that while they were able to delineate the parietal pleura at the T4 level in all their patients it was not possible to do so at the T1 level in any patient.[31] The exact reason for this difference is not clear but may be related to the greater depth to the paravertebral space in the upper thoracic region compared to the midthoracic region[33] and the use of high-frequency ultrasound which lacks penetration and thus lacks the ability to visualize structures at a depth such as the pleura. Future research should investigate whether low-frequency ultrasound, which penetrates deeper into tissues, can circumvent this problem in the upper thoracic region.

Luyet et al recently described a cadaver study in which they investigated the feasibility of performing USG TPVB and catheter placement.[17] The authors performed a sagittal scan of the paravertebral region at the midthoracic level (T4–T8) using low-frequency ultrasound (2–5 MHz).[17] They were able to delineate the underlying paravertebral anatomy (transverse process, costotransverse ligament, and pleura) and observed that the best views of the paravertebral anatomy were obtained with the transducer tilted slightly obliquely, i.e., with the upper part of the transducer directed slightly medially in the sagittal axis.[17] An 18-G Tuohy needle was then inserted in the plane of the ultrasound beam (in-plane technique) and advanced under ultrasound guidance to the TPVS.[17] Correct position of the needle in the paravertebral space was confirmed by injecting saline and observing distension of the paravertebral space,[17] similar to that reported by Hara et al[31] A catheter was then inserted through the Tuohy needle and 10 ml of a dilute contrast medium was injected via the catheter after which axial CT scans of the thoracic spine was performed. The catheter itself could not be visualized and various types of contrast spread were noted on the CT scans: paravertebral, epidural (only), intercostal, prevertebral, and pleural.[17] The incidence of pleural puncture (5%) with the US technique described[17] appears to be higher than that reported after landmark-based techniques (pleural puncture 1.1%).[21] However, before we make any conclusion we must bear in mind that this was a cadaver study and the results may not translate into clinical practice. Further clinical research evaluating the technique of USG paravertebral catheter placement as described by Luyet et al[17] is warranted.

Shibata and Nishiwaki[30] and Ben-Ari et al[28] describe an intercostal approach to the paravertebral space. While there are minor differences in the two approaches described above,[28,30] it basically involves performing a transverse scan of the paravertebral region with a high-frequency linear transducer at the desired level and advancing the block needle from a lateral to medial direction in the plane of the ultrasound beam[28,30] until the tip of the block needle is confirmed to be in the apex of the TPVS.[28,30] On a transverse sonogram the apex of TPVS is identified as a wedge-shaped hypoechoic space between the hyperechoic parietal pleura anteriorly and the internal intercostal membrane posteriorly and is continuous laterally with the posterior intercostal space.[30] Therefore, local anesthetic injected into the posterior intercostal space can spread medially to the TPVS. A correct injection is confirmed by observing anterior displacement of the parietal pleura[28,30] and widening of the apex of the TPVS. Shibata and Nishiwaki[30] suggest that since the block needle is inserted tangential to the pleura this technique should reduce the risk of pleural puncture.[30] However, it is our experience that this approach causes significant pain and discomfort to the patients during needle insertion, particularly when one performs the multiple injection TPVB for breast surgery despite using a fine bore block needle (22 G). This may be due to the greater distance that the block needle has to traverse before it enters the TPVS when compared to a traditional landmark-based injection. Therefore, one should consider sedation and analgesia for patient comfort when using this approach for block or catheter placement. Moreover, since the block needle is advanced in the direction of the intervertebral foramen there is need for larger trials to determine the incidence of complications with this intercostal approach because central neuraxial complications after TPVB are more common with a medially directed needle.[3]

More recently O'Riain et al[29] in a cadaver and clinical study described an in-plane technique of performing USG TPVB. A high-frequency linear transducer (10–5 MHz) was positioned at a point 2.5 cm later to the tip of the spinous process in the longitudinal axis producing a paramedian sagittal scan of the TPVS.[29] The authors describe the contiguous transverse processes as two dark lines.[29] The PP was deep to the transverse process and also seen as a hyperechoic structure that moved with respiration.[29] The SCL was less well defined but was seen as a collection of linear echogenic bands interspersed with hypoechoic areas between two contiguous transverse processes.[29] The TPVS was seen as a hypoechoic space between the SCL and PP.[29] For the block, the midpoint of the transducer was positioned midway between two contiguous transverse processes and a Tuohy needle (18 G) was inserted in-plane and in a cephalad orientation until it traversed the SCL.[29] Saline was injected to confirm the needle position by demonstrating anterior displacement of the PP and to facilitate catheter placement.[29] The authors comment that it was difficult to track the tip of the advancing needle, which they attribute to the acute angle of needle insertion.[29] Nevertheless, they were able to successfully place a paravertebral catheter in eight of the ten attempts in the cadavers and all patients in the clinical study ($n = 9$) had evidence of thoracic wall anesthesia and provided postoperative analgesia.[29]

Other than the data described above, the author is not aware of any other published data describing the sonoanatomy relevant for TPVB or the technique of performing real-time USG TPVB in the clinical setting. The following section is a summary of the author's work on USG TPVB.

Sonoanatomy Relevant for TPVB

Basic Considerations

An ultrasound scan for TPVB can be performed in the transverse (axial scan) or longitudinal (sagittal scan) axis with the patient in the sitting (author's preference), lateral decubitus, or prone position. The prone position is useful in patients presenting for a chronic pain procedure when fluoroscopy may also be used in conjunction with ultrasound imaging. Currently, there are no data demonstrating an optimal axis for the scan or the intervention. It is often a matter of individual preference and experience. The transducer used for the ultrasound scan depends on the body habitus of the patient. High-frequency ultrasound provides better resolution than low-frequency ultrasound but its penetration is poor. Moreover, if one has to scan at a depth using high-frequency ultrasound then the field of vision is also significantly narrow. Under such circumstances it may be preferable to use a low-frequency ultrasound transducer (2–5 MHz) with a divergent beam and a wide field of vision. The author prefers to use a high-frequency linear transducer (13–6 MHz) for scanning the thoracic paravertebral region because the transverse process, costotransverse ligament, and the pleura in the midthoracic region are located at a relatively shallow depth in patients that he cares for in his clinical practice. It is also the author's practice to perform a scout (preview) scan before the ultrasound-guided intervention. The objectives of the scout scan is to preview the anatomy, identify any underlying asymptomatic abnormality or variation, optimize the image, measure relevant distances to the transverse process and pleura, and identify the best possible location and trajectory for needle insertion. A liberal amount of ultrasound gel is applied to the skin over the thoracic paravertebral region at the level of injection for acoustic coupling prior to the scan and sterile ultrasound gel must be used during the USG intervention. The ultrasound image is optimized by making the following adjustments on the ultrasound unit: (a) selecting an appropriate preset (small parts or musculoskeletal preset), (b) setting an appropriate scanning depth (4–6 cm), (c) selecting the "General" optimization (midfrequency range) option of the broadband transducer, (d) adjusting the "focus" to the right depth corresponding to the area of interest, and finally (e) manually adjusting the "gain," "dynamic range" map, and "compression" settings to obtain the best possible image. Compound imaging and tissue harmonic imaging when available are useful in improving the quality of the images.

Transverse Scan of the Thoracic Paravertebral Region

For a transverse scan of the thoracic paravertebral region, the ultrasound transducer is positioned lateral to the spinous process with the orientation marker directed to the right side of the patient (Figure 9.4). On a transverse sonogram the paraspinal muscles are clearly delineated and lie superficial to the transverse process (Figures 9.5 and 9.6). The transverse process is seen as a hyperechoic structure, anterior to which there is a dark

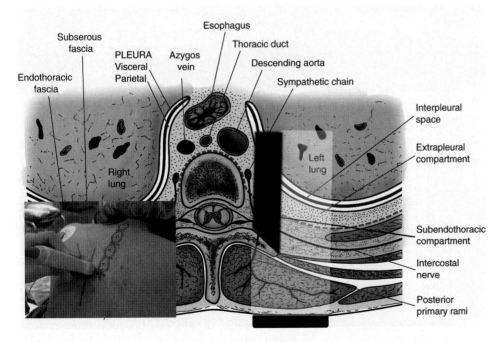

Figure 9.4. The orientation of the ultrasound transducer and how the ultrasound beam is insonated during a transverse scan of the thoracic paravertebral region is shown. The transverse process (TP) usually casts an acoustic shadow (represented in *black*), which obscures the ultrasound visibility of the TPVS. Picture in the inset shows the position of the ultrasound transducer relative to the spine.

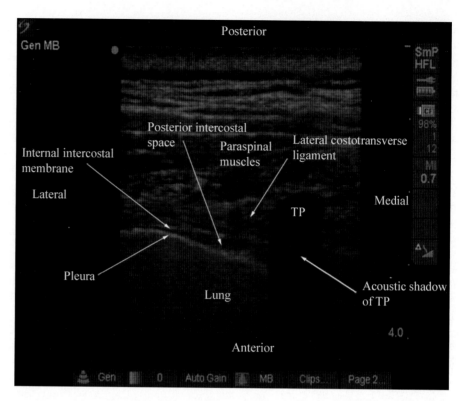

Figure 9.5. Transverse sonogram of the thoracic paravertebral region with the ultrasound beam being insonated over the transverse process. Note how the acoustic shadow of the TP obscures the TPVS. The hypoechoic space between the parietal pleura and the lateral costotransverse ligament and internal intercostals membrane laterally represents the apex of the TPVS or the medial limit of the posterior intercostal space.

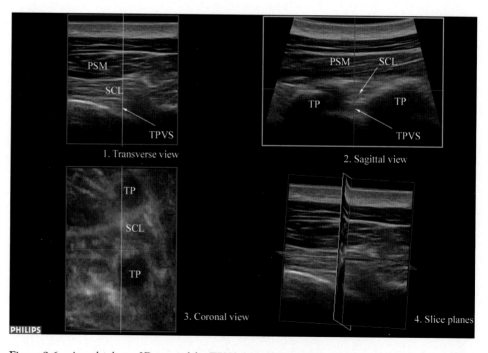

Figure 9.6. A multiplanar 3D view of the TPVS. Note how the three slice planes (*red* – transverse, *green* – sagittal, and *blue* – coronal) are obtained. *PSM* paraspinal muscles, *SCL* superior costotransverse ligament, *TPVS* thoracic paravertebral space, *TP* transverse process.

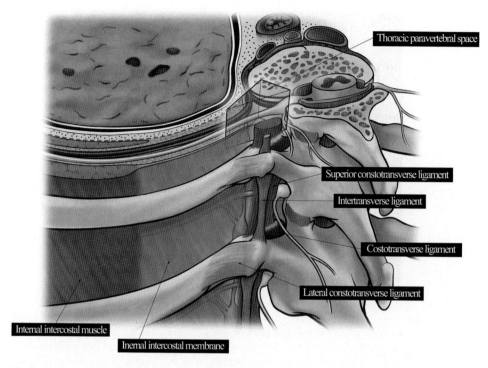

Figure 9.7. Anatomy of the thoracic paravertebral region showing the various paravertebral ligaments and their anatomical relations to the TPVS.

acoustic shadow which completely obscures the TPVS (Figure 9.5). Lateral to the transverse process the hyperechoic pleura that moves with respiration and exhibits the typical "lung sliding sign,"[34] which is the sonographic appearance of the pleural surfaces moving relative to each other within the thorax, is seen. Comet tail artifacts, which are reverberation artifacts, may also be seen deep to the pleura and within the lung tissue, and are often synchronous with respiration.[34] A hypoechoic space is also seen between the parietal pleura and the internal intercostal membrane (Figures 9.5 and 9.6), which is the medial extension of the internal intercostal muscle and is continuous medially with the SCL (Figure 9.7). This hypoechoic space represents the medial limit of the posterior intercostal space or the apex of the TPVS and the two communicate with each other (Figures 9.5–9.7). Therefore, local anesthetic injected medially into the TPVS can often be seen to spread laterally to distend this space or vice versa; local anesthetic injected laterally into this space can spread medially to the paravertebral space and is the basis of the intercostal approach for USG TPVB[28,30] where the needle is inserted in the plane of the US beam from a lateral to medial direction (see below, *Technique 3*). From the scan position described above (i.e., over the transverse process), if one slides the transducer slightly cranially or caudally, it is possible to perform a transverse scan of the paravertebral region with the ultrasound beam being insonated between the two transverse processes. The ultrasound signal is now not impeded by the transverse process or the costotransverse junction and parts of the parietal pleura and the "true" TPVS can now be faintly visualized (Figures 9.6 and 9.8). The SCL which forms the posterior border of the TPVS is also visible and it blends laterally with the internal intercostal membrane, which forms the posterior border of the posterior intercostal space (Figure 9.8). The communication between the TPVS and the posterior intercostal space is also clearly seen (Figure 9.8).

Sagittal Scan of the Thoracic Paravertebral Region

During a sagittal scan of the thoracic paravertebral region the ultrasound transducer is positioned 2–3 cm lateral to the midline with its orientation marker directed cranially

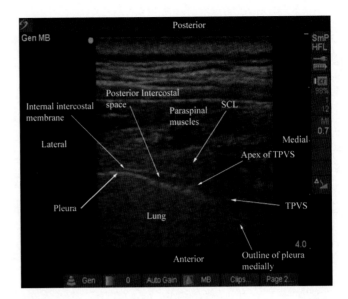

Figure 9.8. Transverse sonogram of the thoracic paravertebral region with the ultrasound beam being insonated between two adjacent transverse processes. Note that the acoustic shadow of the transverse process is now less obvious and parts of the TPVS and the anteromedial reflection of the pleura are now visible. The superior costotransverse ligament (SCL) which forms the posterior border of the TPVS is also visible and it blends laterally with the internal intercostal membrane, which forms the posterior border of the posterior intercostal space. The communication between the TPVS and the posterior intercostal space is also clearly seen.

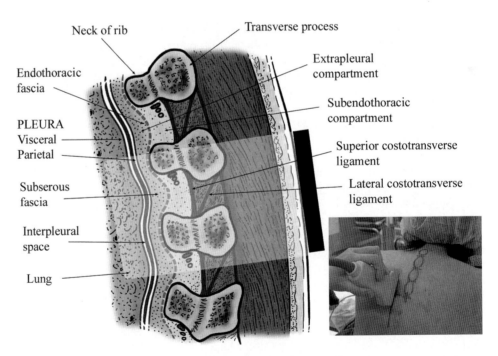

Figure 9.9. The orientation of the ultrasound transducer and how the ultrasound beam is insonated during a paramedian sagittal scan of the thoracic paravertebral region is shown. The picture in the inset shows the position of the ultrasound transducer relative to the spine during the scan.

(Figure 9.9). On a sagittal sonogram the transverse processes are seen as hyperechoic and rounded structures deep to the paraspinal muscles and they cast an acoustic shadow anteriorly (Figures 9.10 and 9.11). In between the acoustic shadows of two adjacent transverse processes there is an acoustic window produced by reflections from the SCTL

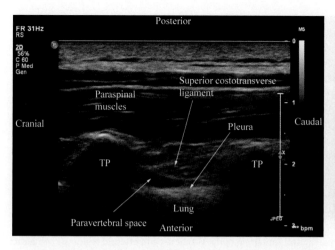

Figure 9.10. Paramedian sagittal sonogram of the thoracic paravertebral region. Note that although the pleura and the TPVS are visible they are not clearly delineated. *TP* transverse process.

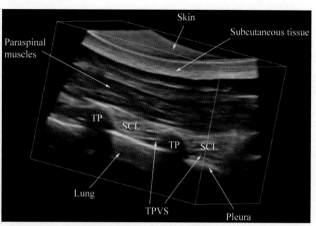

Figure 9.11. A rendered 3D view of the TPVS. The acquired 3D volume has been rendered such that the sagittal anatomy of the TPVS is being visualized from the lateral (intercostal space) side. Note the apical part of the TPVS is clearly delineated between the SCL and the parietal pleura.

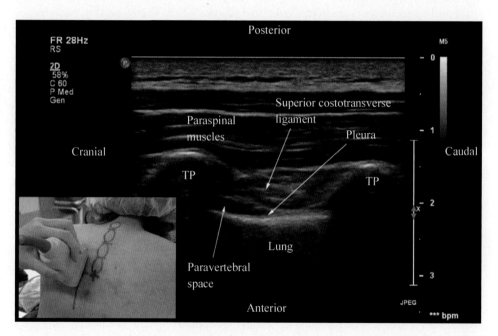

Figure 9.12. Paramedian oblique sagittal sonogram of the thoracic paravertebral region. The picture in the inset shows how the transducer is tilted slightly laterally (outward) during the scan. Note the pleura, SCL, and the TPVS are now clearly delineated (same patient as in Fig. 9.10). *TP* transverse process, *IIM* internal intercostal membrane.

and intertransverse ligaments, the paravertebral space and its contents, the PP and lung tissue (in a posterior to anterior direction) (Figures 9.10 and 9.11). It is the author's observation that the pleura and the paravertebral space are not clearly delineated in a true sagittal scan (Figure 9.9), which may be due to the loss of spatial resolution at the depth or due to "anisotropy," because the ultrasound beam is not being insonated at right angles to the pleura due to its anteromedial reflection close to the vertebral bodies. In a recent investigation, our group has demonstrated objectively that the ultrasound visibility of the SCL, the paravertebral space, and the pleura is better when the ultrasound beam is insonated in a slightly oblique axis, i.e., with the ultrasound transducer tilted slightly laterally or outward (data to be published) (Figure 9.12). The author believes by

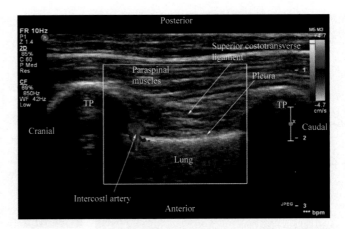

Figure 9.13. Paramedian oblique sagittal sonogram of the thoracic paravertebral region showing the color Doppler signal from the intercostal artery in the paravertebral space. *TP* transverse process.

doing so the ultrasound beam encounters less bony obstruction from the transverse processes and the beam is also more at right angles to the pleura explaining why the paravertebral space and parietal pleura are better visualized (Figure 9.12). Therefore, the "paramedian oblique sagittal axis" is in the author's opinion the optimal axis for ultrasound imaging of the TPVS. However, this only allows one to visualize the apical part of the paravertebral space. Moreover, with current ultrasound technology the author has not been able to visualize the intercostal nerve in the paravertebral space but the intercostal vessels are more readily visible using Doppler ultrasound (Figure 9.13).

Techniques of USG TPVB

Today there are no data or consensus on the best or safest approach for USG TPVB. Real-time USG TPVB can be performed using any one of the three different approaches described below.

Transverse Scan with Short-Axis Needle Insertion (Technique 1)

In this technique, a transverse scan of the thoracic paravertebral region at the desired level is performed as described above and the block needle is inserted in the short axis of the ultrasound beam (Figure 9.14). During the scout scan the depth to the transverse process and pleura is determined. The direction of needle insertion with this approach is similar to that when one performs a TPVB using surface anatomical landmarks. Since the needle is inserted in the short axis, it is visualized only as a bright spot and the aim of this approach is to guide the needle to the TP. Once the TP is contacted the needle is slightly withdrawn and readvanced by a predetermined distance of 1.5 cm so as to pass under the transverse process into the TPVS. After negative aspiration for blood or CSF, the calculated dose of local anesthetic is injected in aliquots. Following the injection it is common to see widening of the apex of the TPVS and anterior displacement of the pleura by the local anesthetic (Figure 9.14). The local anesthetic may also spread to the posterior intercostal space laterally. Widening of the contiguous paravertebral spaces by the injected local anesthetic can also be visualized on a sagittal scan.

Paramedian Oblique Sagittal Scan with In-Plane Needle Insertion (Technique 2)

In this approach, a paramedian oblique sagittal scan is performed as described above (Figure 9.12) and the block needle is inserted in the plane of the ultrasound beam

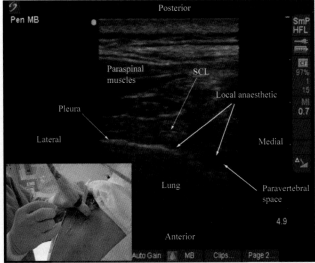

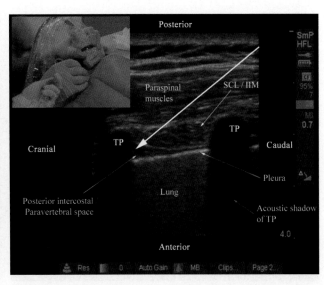

Figure 9.14. Ultrasound-guided TPVB using a transverse scan in which the block needle is inserted in the short axis of the ultrasound plane (Technique 1). Note the widening of the paravertebral space and anterior displacement of the pleura by the local anesthetic on the transverse sonogram. The local anesthetic is also seen to spread to the posterior intercostal space laterally. The picture in the inset shows how the transducer is oriented and the direction in which the needle is inserted. *SCL* superior costotransverse ligament.

Figure 9.15. Ultrasound-guided TPVB using a paramedian oblique sagittal scan (Technique 2). The *long white arrow* represents the direction in which the needle is inserted and the picture in the inset shows how the block needle is inserted in the long axis of the ultrasound plane. Visualizing the block needle with this approach can be very challenging. *TP* transverse process, *SCL* superior costotransverse ligament, *IIL* internal intercostal membrane.

(Figure 9.15). It is the author's experience that, although the block needle is inserted in the plane of the ultrasound beam, it is often quite challenging to visualize the needle with this approach. This is in agreement with that reported by O'Riain et al.[29] This may be because the block needle is often inserted at quite an acute angle and the ultrasound beam is also insonated with a slight oblique (outward) tilt for optimal visibility of the TPVS. Therefore, it is the author's practice to advance the block needle under ultrasound guidance to contact the lower border of the TP after which the needle is slightly withdrawn and readvanced so as to pass under the lower border of the TP. A test bolus of normal saline (2–3 ml) is then injected and sonographic evidence (described above) is sought to ensure that the tip of the needle is in the TPVS. A calculated dose of local anesthetic is then injected in aliquots. Following the injection it is common to see anterior displacement of the pleura, widening of the paravertebral space, and an increased echogenicity of the pleura (Figure 9.16) that are objective signs of a correct injection into the TPVS. The author has also observed, in real time, the spread of the injected local anesthetic to the contiguous paravertebral spaces (Figure 9.16) confirming previous reports that the contiguous TPVSs communicate with each other.[3]

Transverse Scan with In-Plane Needle Insertion or the Intercostal Approach to the TPVS (Technique 3)

In this approach, a transverse scan is performed as described above (Figure 9.5) and the block needle is inserted in the plane of the ultrasound beam from a lateral to medial direction (Figure 9.17) until the tip of the block needle is seen to lie in the posterior intercostal space or the apex of the TPVS. A test bolus of normal saline (2–3 ml) is then injected and sonographic evidence (described above) is sought to ensure that the tip of the needle is in the apical part of the TPVS. A calculated dose of local anesthetic is then slowly injected in aliquots. It is common to see widening of the paravertebral space and anterior displace-

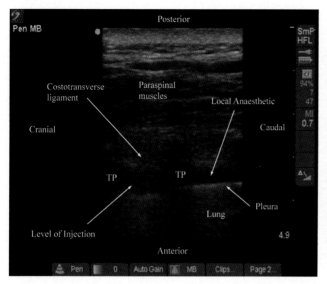

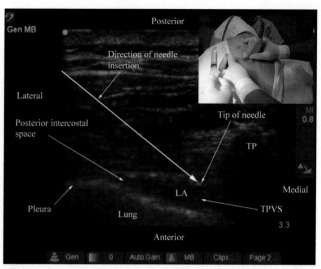

Figure 9.16. Paramedian oblique sagittal sonogram of the TPVS after local anesthetic injection (Technique 2). Note the widening of the paravertebral space and displacement of the pleura. The local anesthetic is also seen to have spread to the contiguous paravertebral space from the level of injection. *TP* transverse process.

Figure 9.17. Transverse sonogram of the TPVS after local anesthetic injection (Technique 3). Note the widening of the paravertebral space, anterior displacement of the pleura, and spread of local anesthetic (LA) to the posterior intercostal space laterally. The *long white arrow* represents the direction in which the block needle is inserted. The picture in the inset shows how the block needle is inserted in the plane of the ultrasound beam from a lateral to medial direction. *TP* transverse process, *TPVS* thoracic paravertebral space.

ment of the parietal pleura during the injection (Figure 9.17). Compared with the other techniques described above the block needle is best visualized with this approach since it is inserted in the plane of the ultrasound beam. However, since the needle is inserted from a lateral to medial direction, i.e., toward the intervertebral foramen it may predispose to a higher incidence of epidural spread or inadvertent intrathecal injection.[3] Further research is required to confirm the safety and efficacy of this technique in clinical practice. Furthermore, since the block needle traverses the greatest amount of soft tissue this approach also appears to cause the greatest amount of discomfort and pain to the patient during block placement and necessitates large doses of intravenous sedation and analgesia during multilevel paravertebral injections.

Conclusion

Recent improvements in ultrasound technology and image processing capabilities of ultrasound machines have made it possible to image parts of the TPVS. Being able to delineate the relevant anatomy of the TPVS before and during a TPVB in real time may offer several advantages. Ultrasound is noninvasive, safe, simple to use, involves no radiation, and appears to be a promising alternative to traditional landmark-based techniques for TPVB. Using ultrasound one is able to preview the paravertebral anatomy prior to block placement and determine the depth to the transverse process and pleura. The latter defines the maximum safe depth for needle insertion and may help reduce the incidence of pleural puncture. Ultrasound guidance during TPVB also allows the block needle to be advanced accurately to the TPVS and visualize the distribution of the local anesthetic during the injection in real time. This may translate into improved technical outcomes, higher success rates, and reduced needle-related complications. However, there is a need to establish an optimal axis for ultrasound imaging and needle insertion because visualization of the block needle during USG TPVB can be quite challenging. Ultrasound is also an excellent teaching tool for demonstrating the anatomy relevant for TPVB and has the potential to improve the learning curve of this technique. Currently, there are limited data on the use of ultrasound for TPVB and further research is warranted to establish its role in clinical practice.

Acknowledgment

All figures in this article have been reproduced with permission from http://www.aic.cuhk.edu.hk/usgraweb.

REFERENCES

1. Cheema SP, Ilsley D, Richardson J, Sabanathan S. A thermographic study of paravertebral analgesia. *Anaesthesia*. 1995;50:118–121.
2. Karmakar MK, Critchley LA, Ho AM, Gin T, Lee TW, Yim AP. Continuous thoracic paravertebral infusion of bupivacaine for pain management in patients with multiple fractured ribs. *Chest*. 2003;123:424–431.
3. Karmakar MK. Thoracic paravertebral block. *Anesthesiology*. 2001;95:771–780.
4. Wassef MR, Randazzo T, Ward W. The paravertebral nerve root block for inguinal herniorrhaphy – a comparison with the field block approach. *Reg Anesth Pain Med*. 1998;23:451–456.
5. Coveney E, Weltz CR, Greengrass R, et al. Use of paravertebral block anesthesia in the surgical management of breast cancer: experience in 156 cases. *Ann Surg*. 1998;227:496–501.
6. Klein SM, Bergh A, Steele SM, Georgiade GS, Greengrass RA. Thoracic paravertebral block for breast surgery. *Anesth Analg*. 2000;90:1402–1405.
7. Karmakar MK, Chung DC. Variability of a thoracic paravertebral block. Are we ignoring the endothoracic fascia? *Reg Anesth Pain Med*. 2000;25(3):325–327.
8. Karmakar MK, Kwok WH, Kew J. Thoracic paravertebral block: radiological evidence of contralateral spread anterior to the vertebral bodies. *Br J Anaesth*. 2000;84(2):263–265.
9. Karmakar MK, Gin T, Ho AM. Ipsilateral thoraco-lumbar anaesthesia and paravertebral spread after low thoracic paravertebral injection. *Br J Anaesth*. 2001;87:312–316.
10. MacIntosh RR, Mushin WW. Observations on the epidural space. *Anaesthesia*. 1947;2:100–104.
11. Conacher ID, Kokri M. Postoperative paravertebral blocks for thoracic surgery. A radiological appraisal. *Br J Anaesth*. 1987;59:155–161.
12. Conacher ID. Resin injection of thoracic paravertebral spaces. *Br J Anaesth*. 1988;61:657–661.
13. Purcell-Jones G, Pither CE, Justins DM. Paravertebral somatic nerve block: a clinical, radiographic, and computed tomographic study in chronic pain patients. *Anesth Analg*. 1989;68:32–39.
14. Eason MJ, Wyatt R. Paravertebral thoracic block-a reappraisal. *Anaesthesia*. 1979;34:638–642.
15. Richardson J, Cheema SP, Hawkins J, Sabanathan S. Thoracic paravertebral space location. A new method using pressure measurement. *Anaesthesia*. 1996;51:137–139.
16. Richardson J, Lonnqvist PA. Thoracic paravertebral block. *Br J Anaesth*. 1998;81:230–238.
17. Luyet C, Eichenberger U, Greif R, Vogt A, Szucs FZ, Moriggl B. Ultrasound-guided paravertebral puncture and placement of catheters in human cadavers: an imaging study. *Br J Anaesth*. 2009;102:534–539.
18. Greengrass R, O'Brien F, Lyerly K, et al. Paravertebral block for breast cancer surgery. *Can J Anaesth*. 1996;43:858–861.
19. Kirvela O, Antila H. Thoracic paravertebral block in chronic postoperative pain. *Reg Anesth*. 1992;17:348–350.
20. Tenicela R, Pollan SB. Paravertebral-peridural block technique: a unilateral thoracic block. *Clin J Pain*. 1990;6:227–234.
21. Lonnqvist PA, MacKenzie J, Soni AK, Conacher ID. Paravertebral blockade. Failure rate and complications. *Anaesthesia*. 1995;50:813–815.
22. Abrahams MS, Aziz MF, Fu RF, Horn JL. Ultrasound guidance compared with electrical neurostimulation for peripheral nerve block: a systematic review and meta-analysis of randomized controlled trials. *Br J Anaesth*. 2009;102:408–417.
23. Chin KJ, Chan V. Ultrasound-guided peripheral nerve blockade. *Curr Opin Anaesthesiol*. 2008;21:624–631.

24. Marhofer P, Greher M, Kapral S. Ultrasound guidance in regional anaesthesia. *Br J Anaesth.* 2005;94:7–17.
25. Grau T, Leipold RW, Conradi R, Martin E, Motsch J. Ultrasound imaging facilitates localization of the epidural space during combined spinal and epidural anesthesia. *Reg Anesth Pain Med.* 2001;26:64–67.
26. Grau T, Leipold RW, Fatehi S, Martin E, Motsch J. Real-time ultrasonic observation of combined spinal-epidural anaesthesia. *Eur J Anaesthesiol.* 2004;21:25–31.
27. Karmakar MK, Li X, Ho AM, Kwok WH, Chui PT. Real-time ultrasound-guided paramedian epidural access: evaluation of a novel in-plane technique. *Br J Anaesth.* 2009;102:845–854.
28. Ben-Ari A, Moreno M, Chelly JE, Bigeleisen PE. Ultrasound-guided paravertebral block using an intercostal approach. *Anesth Analg.* 2009;109:1691–1694.
29. O'Riain SC, Donnell BO, Cuffe T, Harmon DC, Fraher JP, Shorten G. Thoracic paravertebral block using real-time ultrasound guidance. *Anesth Analg.* 2010;110:248–251.
30. Shibata Y, Nishiwaki K. Ultrasound-guided intercostal approach to thoracic paravertebral block. *Anesth Analg.* 2009;109:996–997.
31. Hara K, Sakura S, Nomura T, Saito Y. Ultrasound guided thoracic paravertebral block in breast surgery. *Anaesthesia.* 2009;64:223–225.
32. Pusch F, Wildling E, Klimscha W, Weinstabl C. Sonographic measurement of needle insertion depth in paravertebral blocks in women. *Br J Anaesth.* 2000;85(6):841–843.
33. Naja MZ, Gustafsson AC, Ziade MF, et al. Distance between the skin and the thoracic paravertebral space. *Anaesthesia.* 2005;60:680–684.
34. Lichtenstein DA, Menu Y. A bedside ultrasound sign ruling out pneumothorax in the critically ill. Lung sliding. *Chest.* 1995;108:1345–1348.

10

Ultrasound-Guided Lumbar Zygapophysial (Facet) Nerve Block

David M. Irwin and Michael Gofeld

Introduction

The concept of blocking spinal nerves is validated by relieving the pain transmitted by that nerve. Similarly, blocking a painful structure (e.g., inflamed joint) should provide at least temporal alleviation of pain. Diagnostic and therapeutic lumbar zygapophysial (facet) nerve and joint interventions are among the most commonly performed injections in pain management. Traditionally, fluoroscopic guidance is required to ensure precise needle position-

M. Gofeld (✉)
Department of Anesthesia and Pain Medicine, University of Washington School of Medicine,
4225 Roosevelt Way NE, Seattle, WA 98105, USA
e-mail: gofeld@u.washington.edu

S.N. Narouze (ed.), Atlas of Ultrasound-Guided Procedures in Interventional Pain Management,
DOI 10.1007/978-1-4419-1681-5_10, © Springer Science+Business Media, LLC 2011

ing and to exclude intravascular injection. Since the procedure is considered to be a low-risk intervention, utilization of ultrasound guidance is thought to be an attractive alternative to fluoroscopy mainly because it renders no ionizing radiation to the patient and medical personnel and helps identify soft tissue targets. In addition, ultrasound-guided procedures are essentially "office-based" and do not require a radiology suite or operating room.

Anatomy

The lumbar vertebrae, L3–L5, are most frequently involved in spinal pathology because these vertebrae carry the majority of body weight and are subject to the largest stress forces along the spine. Each vertebra is connected to the adjacent level by the intervertebral disk anteriorly and the zygapophysial or facet joints in the posterior. The vertebral body is a thin rim of dense cortical bone encompassing the trabecular inner milieu. The pedicles are two short rounded processes that extend posteriorly from lateral margin of the dorsal vertebral body. The laminae are two flattened plates of bone extending medially from the pedicles to form the posterior wall of the vertebral foramen. The ligamentum flavum anchors the posterior wall of each vertebra. As the nerve root exits the foramen, it divides into ventral and dorsal rami. Dorsal ramus gives off three branches, the medial, intermediate, and lateral branches. Each facet joint is innervated by the medial branch at the corresponding level and from the level above. Medial branches travel in the groove formatted by the corresponding superior articular process (SAP) and the transverse process or may lie slightly cephalad at the base of the SAP. The L5 medial branch is an articular nerve network with variable pathway, and, therefore the L5 dorsal ramus is targeted. This nerve is constantly located at the root of the S1 SAP and the sacral ala. Anatomic variations of the lumbar spine can pose a challenge during image-guided zygapophysial nerve and joint injection. Variations, including scoliosis, the sixth lumbar vertebrae, sacralization of the fifth lumbar vertebra, and pseudoarthrosis, can lead to erroneous and incorrect level of needle placement. Thus, it is imperative to review prior imaging studies when planning an interventional procedure.

Literature Review

Over the past decade, ultrasonography has been introduced in regional anesthesia to visualize paraspinal and neuroaxial structures. Grau and Arzola demonstrated that the distance to the epidural space can be measured by ultrasound (US) in obstetric anesthesia.[1,2] In 2008, Lee concluded that preprocedure spinal sonography may prevent inadvertent dural puncture by revealing aberrant anatomy of the lumbar spine and ligamentum flavum.[3] In 2009, Luyet published his techniques for ultrasound-assisted paravertebral punctures and catheter placement on human cadavers.[4] First publication related to ultrasound-guided pain management procedures described a periarticular injection of lumbar zygapophysial joints.[5] The method was recently validated in 2007, when Galiano et al concluded that the US approach to the lumbar facet joints is feasible with minimal risks in a large majority of patients and results in a significant reduction of procedure duration vs. CT-controlled interventions.[6]

Lumbar zygapophysial joint pain is routinely diagnosed by the analgesic blockade of the sensory nerves.[7] US guidance of such injections has been studied on healthy volunteers[8] and validated against CT.[6,9] In the recently published clinical study with fluoroscopic control,[10] all 101 needles were placed at the correct lumbar segment, and 96 (95%) of the needles were in the correct position. Two injections were associated with an intravascular spread of the contrast dye. Mean pain score on the visual analog scale was reduced from 52 before to 16 after blockade.[10] The study had several limitations, in particular, a relatively low body mass index (BMI) of the study patients, which might have allowed good visualization of the spine and ultimately resulted in high technical success. In addition, patients with the pain related to the lumbosacral zygapophysial joint were excluded from the study,[10] and, therefore, L5 dorsal ramus block has not been evaluated. However, in the earlier study by Greher et al,[9] US imaging was of an adequate quality in a patient with BMI 36 kg/m², thus obesity was deemed as a nonabsolute contraindication. Recently, Rauch et al concluded that medial branch blocks cannot be performed by US guidance in obese patients.[11] US applications in chronic spinal pain imaging and guidance continue to remain in an emerging stage. Their place in diagnostic and therapeutic injections has yet to be established as standard of care.

Scanning Technique

With the patient in the prone position, a pillow is placed under the abdomen to diminish lumbar lordosis. A 3–8 MHz curvilinear US probe is utilized to perform the examination. US scanning of the spine requires following a particular sequence in image acquisition to obtain optimal views of the soft tissues (paraspinous muscles, ligaments, dura) and vertebrae. Liberal amount of ultrasound gel is applied on the skin. Starting at the sacrum, longitudinal scanning begins with the transducer positioned at the midline. In patients with scoliosis, medial or lateral tilting may be required to obtain an optimal view (Figure 10.1). Skin marking can be done with a pen alongside the transducer to help localize spinal levels and provide "reference points" of anatomic structures. Once the longitudinal midline images are obtained, the transducer is gently shifted laterally until a "saw-tooth" hyperechoic line is seen (Figure 10.2). This bony structure represents the superior and inferior articular processes; however, the joint space cannot be seen on that view. Shifting the probe further laterally reveals a hyperechoic dotted line. These are the transverse processes with the hypoechoic soft tissue between them (Figure 10.3). The most caudal wide bone shadow in this view typically represents the sacrum.

After completion of the longitudinal scanning, for a second time starting at the sacrum, axial (short axis) sonography is performed. The first distinct midline bony protuberance is the S1 median crest of the sacrum (Figure 10.4). The transducer is then moved cephalad until a deep hyperechoic structure is seen. This normally corresponds to the L5/S1 intrathecal space (Figure 10.5). Typically, a hyperechoic enhancement of the signal is seen when US is passed through the cerebrospinal fluid and reflects off the ventral dura and the posterior longitudinal ligament. Sometimes, particularly in young patients, two hyperechoic lines can be seen, these represent the posterior dura and the ventral dura.

Next midline hyperechoic signal, cephalad to the intrathecal space, is the L5 spinous process. At any lumbar level two axial views can be obtained: the "interlaminar window" (Figure 10.5) and the "spinous process/lamina window" (Figure 10.6). (Note: At the

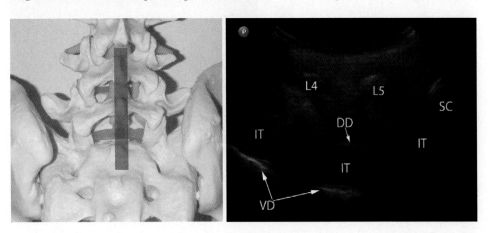

Figure 10.1. *Left*: Midline position of the transducer (*semitransparent red rectangle*). *Right*: Sonographic long-axis view of the lumbar spine showing the L4 (L4) and L5 (L5) spinous processes, median S1 crest (SC), the hyperechoic lines of dorsal (DD) and ventral (VD) dura and the hypoechoic intrathecal space (IT).

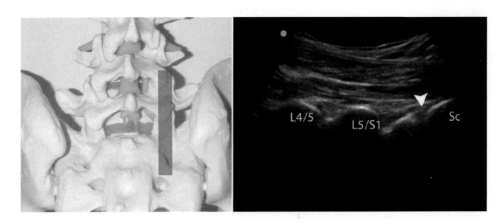

Figure 10.2. *Left:* Paramedian position of the transducer (*semitransparent red rectangle*). *Right:* Sonographic long-axis view of the lumbar spine with the L4/5 (L4/5) and L5/S1 (L5/S1) zygapophysial joint contours and the S1 (*arrowhead*) dorsal foramen. The joint gap is not visible in this view.

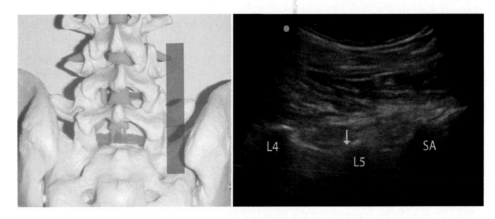

Figure 10.3. *Left:* Lateral position of the transducer (*semitransparent red rectangle*). *Right:* Sonographic long-axis view showing the L4 (L4) and L5 (L5) transverse processes and the sacral ala (SA). Upper edge of the transverse process, or the sacral ala, immediately lateral to the superior articular process (*arrow*) is the correct anatomical target.

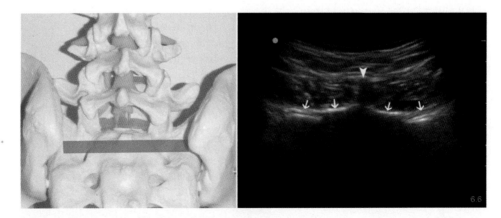

Figure 10.4. *Left:* Axial position of the transducer (*semitransparent red rectangle*). *Right:* Sonographic short-axis view of the sacrum showing the S1 median crest (*arrowhead*) and the hyperechoic surface (*arrows*) of the sacrum.

"spinous process/lamina" position the facet joint cannot be seen. Instead the exiting ventral ramus is occasionally visible.) It is advisable to continue cephalad scanning and identify all lumbar spinous processes and correlate those with the previously performed skin marking. This correlation will prevent injections at an erroneous level. When the transducer is

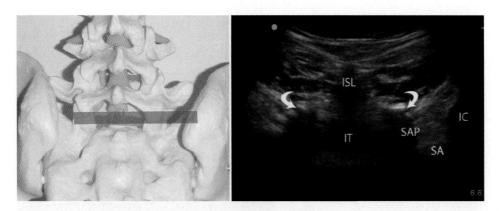

Figure 10.5. *Left*: Axial position of the transducer (*semitransparent red rectangle*). *Right*: Sonographic short-axis view of the lumbosacral segment showing the hypoechoic L5/S1 interspinous ligament (ISL), L5/S1 zygapophysial joints (*curved arrows*), the intrathecal space (IT), the S1 superior articular process (SAP), the sacral ala (SA), and the iliac crest (IC).

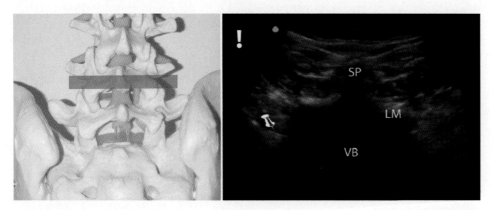

Figure 10.6. *Left*: Axial position of the transducer (*semitransparent red rectangle*). *Right*: Sonographic short-axis view of the L4 vertebra (bone window): L4 (SP) spinous process and L4 lamina (LM) are completely shadowing the L4 vertebral body (VB). Intrathecal space and the transverse process are not visible at this view. Exiting L4 nerve root is seen on the left (*pin arrow*).

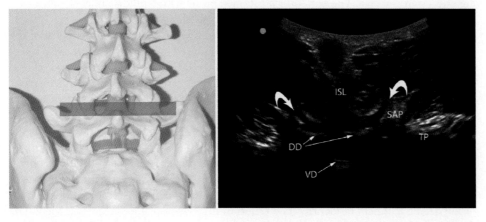

Figure 10.7. *Left*: Axial position of the transducer (*semitransparent red rectangle*). *Right*: Sonographic short-axis view of the L4/5 segment showing the hypoechoic L4/5 interspinous ligament (ISL), L4/5 zygapophysial joints (*curved arrows*), the dorsal (DD) and ventral (VD) dura, the L5 SAP, and the L4 transverse process (TP).

firmly positioned at the desired level, a three-step shadow of the lumbar vertebra will become evident: the most superficial hyperechoic structure is the interspinous ligament or the spinous process, with the zygapophysial joint positioned just inferiorly and lateral to it and the transverse process located further inferiorly and laterally (Figure 10.7). Fine tuning

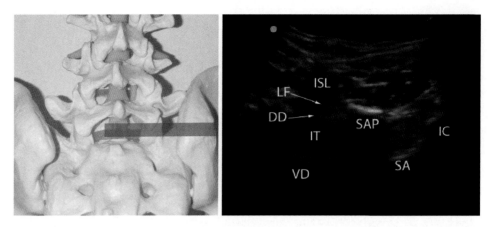

Figure 10.8. *Left*: Axial position of the transducer (*semitransparent red rectangle*). *Right*: Sonographic short-axis right-sided view of the lumbosacral segment showing the hypoechoic L5/S1 interspinous ligament (ISL), the ligamentum flavum (LF), the dorsal (DD) and ventral (VD) dura, the intrathecal space (IT), the right S1 superior articular process (SAP), the sacral ala (SA), and the iliac crest (IC).

of the probe will help to "open the joint" and to visualize the angle between the superior articular and transverse processes. The later is the anatomical target for the medial branch block (L1–L4). At the L5/S1 level, junction of the S1 SAP with the sacral ala should be targeted. Iliac crest is typically seen laterally to the sacral ala (Figure 10.8).

Injection Technique

Lumbar (L1–L4) Zygapophysial Medial Branch and L5 Dorsal Ramus Nerve Block

An antiseptic is utilized to prepare the skin at the block area. The US transducer is covered by a sterile sleeve. The patient is positioned prone with a pillow under the abdomen to diminish the lumbar lordosis. Sterile ultrasound gel should be used.

The procedure begins with longitudinal scanning of the midline, starting from the sacrum as described above. The transducer is then rotated to obtain the short axis view of the desired level. The previously described three-step shadow of the lumbar vertebra is obtained. Depth is measured and the insertion angle is estimated (Figure 10.9). A block needle is inserted immediately next to the lateral edge of the transducer and advanced in-plane until it contacts the bony surface at the root of the corresponding SAP (Figure 10.10). The L5 dorsal ramus block can be technically challenging due to high iliac crest. If the iliac crest is obscuring the view, the injection may be done using an out-of-plane approach (see below). Once the bone contact is made, the transducer is rotated sagittally to obtain the longitudinal view, and positioned paravertebrally at the "transverse processes" plane. The shadows of the transverse processes and/or the sacral ala should be localized. Agitation of the needle will help to identify its position in this out-of-plane sonographic view. The needle tip must be seen at the upper part of the transverse process or the sacral ala (Figure 10.11). If the needle did not contact the bone at the predetermined depth, the longitudinal view should clarify the needle tip position relative to the transverse process. In this case, the needle tip will be seen somewhat below or above the bone shadow. Failure to recognize the tip position may result in transforaminal advancement of the needle and injury of the exiting nerve root.

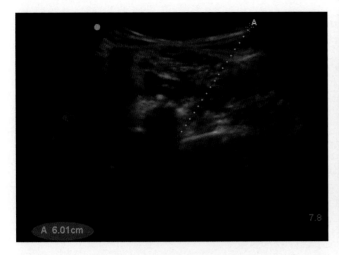

Figure 10.9. Short-axis view of a lumbar vertebra: lateral to the midline transducer positioning improves visualization of the target and decreases injection angle. The skin to target distance (*dotted line*) is 6 cm.

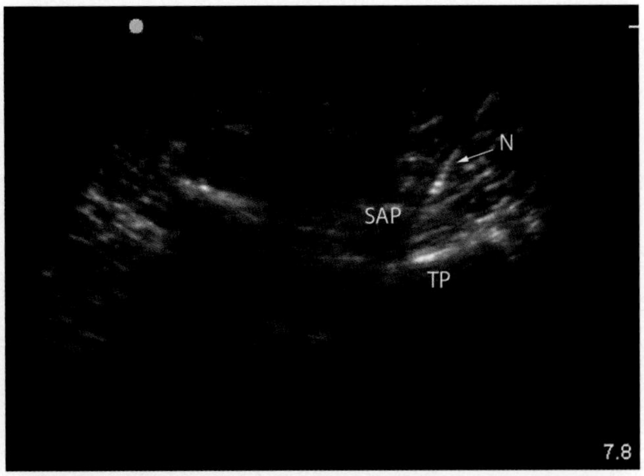

Figure 10.10. The needle (N) is positioned using the short-axis in-plane approach to the angle between transverse (TP) and superior articular (SAP) processes.

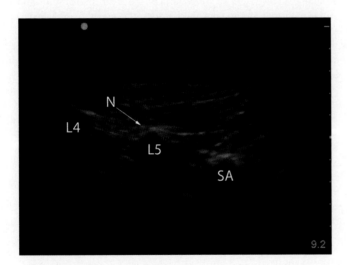

Figure 10.11. Final checkup of the needle tip (N) positioning at the upper part of the L5 transverse process (L5) is done utilizing long-axis out-of-plane view.

After verification of the needle position, 0.5 ml of local anesthetic is injected. It is utmost important to visualize the tip during injection. High-resolution US allows observation of a hypoechoic expansion produced by the injectate. Failure to identify this phenomenon indicates an improper needle placement or intravascular injection.

When the L5 dorsal ramus block is performed in an out-of-plane approach, the transducer is positioned at the level L5/S1 at the short axis. The root of the S1 SAP (the angle between S1 SAP and the sacral ala) is kept in the middle of image. The block needle is inserted immediately caudad to the midpoint of the transducer and advanced in the caudocephalad direction until the tip contacts the target, S1/sacral ala junction (Figure 10.8). The longitudinal view should be applied to verify that the tip is not positioned beyond the sacral ala into the L5/S1 intervertebral foramen.

Limitations of Ultrasound-Guided Zygapophysial Nerve and Joint Injection

US guidance provides a feasible alternative to radiologic image-guided lumbar zygapophysial (facet) nerve and joint interventions. However, US guidance may not provide clear image acquisition in patients whose anatomic features pose particular challenges (e.g., obesity, severe degenerative changes, malformations). In addition, US cannot clearly detect an intravascular injection or inadvertent foraminal spread. Lastly, one of the largest limiting factors is the level of expertise and training of the sonographer.

REFERENCES

1. Grau T, Leipold RW, Horter J, et al. The lumbar epidural space in pregnancy: visualization by ultrasonography. *Br J Anaesth.* 2001;86:798–804.
2. Arzola C, Davies S, Rofaeel A, et al. Ultrasound using the transverse approach to the lumbar spine provides reliable landmarks for labor epidurals. *Anesth Analg.* 2007;104:1188–1192.
3. Lee Y, Tanaka M, Carvalho JC. Sonoanatomy of the lumbar spine in patients with previous unintentional dural punctures during labor epidurals. *Reg Anesth Pain Med.* 2008;33:266–270.
4. Luyet C, Eichenberger U, Greif R, et al. Ultrasound-guided paravertebral puncture and placement of catheters in human cadavers: an imaging study. *Br J Anaesth.* 2009;102:534–539.
5. Küllmer K, Rompe JD, Löwe A, et al. Ultrasound image of the lumbar spine and the lumbosacral transition. Ultrasound anatomy and possibilities for ultrasonically-controlled facet joint infiltration. *Z Orthop Ihre Grenzgeb.* 1997;135:310–314.
6. Galiano K, Obwegeser AA, Walch C, et al. Ultrasound-guided versus computed tomography-controlled facet joint injections in the lumbar spine: a prospective randomized clinical trial. *Reg Anesth Pain Med.* 2007;32:317–322.
7. Boswell MV, Shah RV, Everett CR, et al. Interventional techniques in the management of chronic spinal pain: evidence-based practice guidelines. *Pain Physician.* 2005;8:1–47.
8. Greher M, Scharbert G, Kamolz LP, et al. Ultrasound-guided lumbar facet nerve block: a sonoanatomic study of a new methodologic approach. *Anesthesiology.* 2004;100:1242–1248.
9. Greher M, Kirchmair L, Enna B, et al. Ultrasound-guided lumbar facet nerve block: accuracy of a new technique confirmed by computed tomography. *Anesthesiology.* 2004;101:1195–1200.
10. Shim JK, Moon JC, Yoon KB, et al. Ultrasound-guided lumbar medial-branch block: a clinical study with fluoroscopy control. *Reg Anesth Pain Med.* 2006;31:451–454.
11. Rauch S, Kasuya Y, Turan A, et al. Ultrasound-guided lumbar medial-branch block in obese patients: a fluoroscopically confirmed clinical feasibility study. *Reg Anesth Pain Med.* 2009; 34:340–342.

11

Ultrasound-Guided Lumbar Nerve Root (Periradicular) Injections

Klaus Galiano and Hannes Gruber

Introduction

Lumbar periradicular infiltrations (nerve root blocks) are well established in the diagnosis and management of lumbar radiculopathy.[1] Lumbar periradicular injections are preferentially performed as fluoroscopically or computed tomography (CT) controlled interventions.[2,3] However, both guidance modalities have significant radiation exposure, at least in part, expensive equipment. As an alternative guidance method, ultrasound (US) imaging is also applicable for spinal infiltrations[4-8] and for lumbar periradicular injections.[9]

K. Galiano (✉)
Department of Neurosurgery, Innsbruck Medical University, TILAK,
Anichstrasse 35, Innsbruck 6020, Austria
e-mail: klaus.galiano@i-med.ac.at

S.N. Narouze (ed.), *Atlas of Ultrasound-Guided Procedures in Interventional Pain Management*,
DOI 10.1007/978-1-4419-1681-5_11, © Springer Science+Business Media, LLC 2011

Ultrasound-Guided Technique

A standard US device with a broadband curved array transducer working at 2–5 MHz is usually used. The patients are positioned prone. To reduce lumbar lordosis, a cushion should be placed under the abdomen. The image gain should be set to maximum penetration as only the bony surfaces are of interest for the depictions. A posterior paravertebral parasagittal sonogram is first obtained to identify the different spinal levels (Figure 11.1). Then a transverse sonogram is obtained at the desired level (see previous chapter). The spinous process and adjacent structures (lamina of vertebral arch, zygapophyseal articulations, inferior and superior facet, transverse process, and vertebral isthmus) have to be clearly delineated with Figure 11.2.

Once the correct level is identified in the sagittal plane, the transducer is rotated and the corresponding spinous process is traced until the lamina can be delineated. The lamina should be demonstrated in their entire length to assess their lower margin. The next slit laterally is the facet joint space. Starting from this imaging, the intervertebral foramen and the corresponding spinal nerve can be traced[9] (Figure 11.2).

The nerve root leaves the neuroforamen under the ligament between the transverse processes. The needle should be advanced very slowly when approaching the neuroforamen and going under the transverse processes, because radicular pain can be provoked. Sometimes the nerve root in the neuroforamen cannot be clearly depicted. In this case, we try to demonstrate both adjacent transverse processes before advancing the needle tip very slowly toward the neuroforamen. On approaching the nerve root, the patients will feel slight paresthesia along the corresponding nerve root territory (clinical control), at which point the needle is slightly withdrawn and the medication delivered.

We recommend the "in-plane-technique" in which the whole needle path is under control at any time and no mismatch between needle, needle tip, and target is actually possible (Figure 11.3).

Limitations of the Ultrasound-Guided Technique

For a successful infiltration, two conditions are required: a clear depiction of the target and a clear delineation of the needle (tip) directed to the target. Therefore, the first step is to

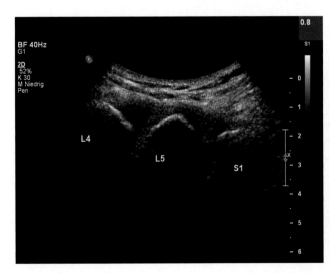

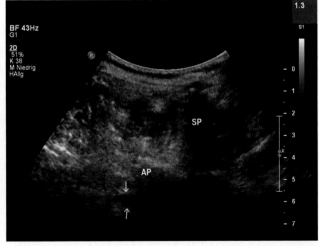

Figure 11.1. Sagittal sonogram of the lumbar spine. *S1* superficial part of spinous process S1, *L5* superficial part of spinous process L5, *L4* superficial part of spinous process L4.

Figure 11.2. Axial transverse sonogram of the intervertebral foramen at L4–L5 level. *Arrows* point at the exiting nerve root. *SP* spinal process, *AP* articular process.

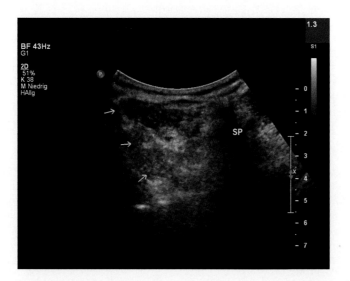

Figure 11.3. Axial transverse sonogram of the intervertebral foramen at L4–L5 level showing the needle in plan targeting the neuroforamen.

adjust the US modalities for the lumbar approach. To visualize the bony surfaces, a hard image (maximum penetration gain) has to be captured by using an appropriate setting with modified gain and persistence. Otherwise, the patient's tissue shows up differently, compromising the sonoanatomy and the possibility to achieve clear sonographic images. In our experience, the depiction of the target can be particularly demanding in patients with an altered fatty muscle consistency. Such tissue is like foam plastic and cannot be penetrated by the US signal, which results in a low picture quality. Obviously, in obese patients or subjects with prior lumbar surgery (distinct scar formation, instrumentation, laminectomy), to date, the US approach cannot be recommended. Keeping the needle tip in the viewing field as the needle is advanced toward the target requires some practice. Failing to do so was the most common mistake observed in residents being trained on US-guided peripheral nerve blocks. Persistent failure to visualize the needle tip was documented even after performing more than 100 US-guided peripheral nerve blocks, suggesting that experienced practitioners can also face substantial difficulties. Needle advancements and/or drug injections without adequate needle tip visualization may result in unintentional vascular or neural injuries. Using surrogate markers of tip location, such as tissue movement (jiggling the needle in small, controlled, in-out movements) and hydrolocation (rapid injection of small amount of fluid, 0.5–1 ml), are sometimes very helpful.[10] A promising feature to visualize the needle tip might be the development of needles with a sensor in the needle tip. This sensor would be recognized by the US technology and reported in real time in the sonographic picture. Nevertheless, this technique and its practical impact still have to be evaluated.

In our experience, lumbar spinal periradicular infiltrations are feasible in most patients. However, intravascular injections cannot be reliably recognized in all patients as the ultrasound will lack enough resolution at such depth.

REFERENCES

1. Ng L, Chaudhary N, Sell P. The efficacy of corticosteroids in periradicular infiltration for chronic radicular pain: a randomized, double blind, controlled trial. *Spine*. 2005;30:857–862.
2. Gangi A, Dietemann JL, Mortazavi R, et al. CT-guided interventional procedures for pain management in the lumbosacral spine. *Radiographics*. 1998;18:621–633.
3. Derby R, Kine G, Saal JA, et al. Response to steroid and duration of radicular pain as predictors of surgical outcome. *Spine*. 1992;17:S176–S183.

4. Galiano K, Obwegeser AA, Bodner G, et al. Ultrasound guidance for facet joint injections in the lumbar spine: a computed tomography-controlled feasibility study. *Anesth Analg.* 2005; 101:579–583.

5. Galiano K, Obwegeser AA, Bodner G, et al. Ultrasound-guided periradicular injections in the middle to lower cervical spine: an imaging study of a new approach. *Reg Anesth Pain Med.* 2005;30:391–396.

6. Galiano K, Obwegeser AA, Bodner G, et al. Ultrasound-guided facet joint injections in the middle to lower cervical spine: a CT-controlled sonoanatomic study. *Clin J Pain.* 2006;22: 538–543.

7. Galiano K, Obwegeser AA, Bale R, et al. Ultrasound-guided and CT-navigation assisted periradicular and facet joint injections in the lumbar and cervical spine: a new teaching tool to recognize the sonoanatomic pattern. *Reg Anesth Pain Med.* 2007;32:254–257.

8. Galiano K, Obwegeser AA, Walch C, et al. Ultrasound-guided versus computed tomography-controlled facet joint injections in the lumbar spine: a prospective randomized clinical trial. *Reg Anesth Pain Med.* 2007;32:317–322.

9. Galiano K, Obwegeser AA, Bodner G, et al. Real-time sonographic imaging for periradicular injections in the lumbar spine: a sonographic anatomic study of a new technique. *J Ultrasound Med.* 2005;24:33–38.

10. Chin KJ, Perlas A, Chan VW, et al. Needle visualization in ultrasound guided regional anesthesia: challenges and solutions. *Reg Anesth Pain Med.* 2008;33:532–544.

12

Ultrasound-Guided Central Neuraxial Blocks

Manoj Kumar Karmakar

M.K. Karmakar (✉)
Department of Anaesthesia and Intensive Care, The Chinese University of Hong Kong, Prince of Wales
Hospital, 32 Ngan Shing Street, Shatin, New Territories, Hong Kong
e-mail: karmakar@cuhk.edu.hk

S.N. Narouze (ed.), *Atlas of Ultrasound-Guided Procedures in Interventional Pain Management*,
DOI 10.1007/978-1-4419-1681-5_12, © Springer Science+Business Media, LLC 2011

Introduction

Central neuraxial blocks (CNBs; spinal and epidural) are techniques that are frequently used for anesthesia or analgesia in the perioperative period and for managing chronic pain. Success of these techniques depends on one's ability to accurately locate the epidural or the intrathecal space. Traditionally, CNBs are performed using surface anatomical landmarks, fascial clicks, visualizing the free flow of cerebrospinal fluid (CSF) and "loss of resistance." Although anatomical landmarks are useful they are often difficult to locate or palpate in patients with obesity,[1] edema in their backs, and underlying spinal deformity or after spinal surgery. Even in the absence of the above, a given intervertebral space is accurately identified in only 30%[2,3] of cases and anesthesiologists very frequently incorrectly identify a space higher than intended,[2,4,5] which has been attributed as a cause for injury of the conus medullaris[4] or spinal cord[6] after spinal anesthesia. This error is exaggerated by obesity[2] and as one tries to locate an intervertebral space in the upper spinal levels.[2,4,5] Therefore, the Tuffier's line, a surface anatomical landmark, that is ubiquitously used during CNB is not a reliable landmark.[5] Moreover, because of the blind nature of the landmark-based techniques, it is not possible for the operator to predict the ease or difficulty of needle placement prior to skin puncture. Data from the UK indicate that 15% of spinal anesthetics are technically difficult,[7] 10% require more than five attempts[7], and a failed CNB can occur in 5% of patients below the age of 50.[8] Multiple attempts at needle placement can lead to pain and discomfort to the patient, injury to soft tissue structures that lie in the path of the advancing needle, and may rarely result in complications, such as dural puncture, postdural puncture headache, or epidural hematoma. Therefore, any method that can reduce technical difficulties or assist the operator during CNB is desirable.

Various imaging modalities (CT scan, MRI, and fluoroscopy) have been used to improve precision and accuracy during peripheral nerve blockade,[9] chronic pain interventions,[10] and lumbar puncture.[11] However, this is not practical in the operating room environment because it involves transfer of the patient to the radiology suite, availability of a trained radiologist to interpret the images, and exposure to radiation and/or contrast medium with their attendant risks. Recent years have seen an increase in interest in the use of ultrasound (US) for interventions in regional anesthesia[12] and pain medicine. There is evidence that peripheral nerve blocks that are performed with US, when compared with peripheral nerve stimulation, take less time to perform, require fewer needle passes, require less local anesthetic dosage, has a faster onset, produce superior quality of sensory blockade, last longer in duration, is less likely to fail, and also reduces inadvertent vascular puncture.[12,13] When used for chronic pain interventions US may eliminate or reduce exposure to radiation, something that may be welcomed by pain physicians. The US machine is gradually becoming an integral part of the armamentarium of an anesthesiologist and an increasing number of peripheral nerve blocks are being performed with US assistance or real-time guidance. The same may also be true in pain medicine as pain physicians are embracing the US machine and performing pain interventions under ultrasound guidance[14,15] or in conjunction with fluoroscopy.[16] US may also offer other advantages when used for CNB. It is noninvasive, safe, simple to use, can be quickly performed, does not involve exposure to radiation, provides real-time images, is free from adverse effects, and may also be beneficial in patients with abnormal or variant spinal anatomy. In this chapter, the author reviews our current understanding of spinal sonography and its applications for CNB.

History

Published literature suggests that Bogin and Stulin were the first to report the use of US for central neuraxial interventions.[17] They used ultrasound to perform lumbar puncture and described their experience, in the Russian literature, in 1971.[17] Porter et al in 1978 used US to image the lumbar spine and measure the diameter of the spinal canal in diagnostic radiology.[18] Cork et al were the first group of anesthesiologists to use US to locate the landmarks relevant for epidural anesthesia.[19] Despite the poor quality of the US images in 1980,

Cork et al's report was able to define, although for the skeptic not very convincingly, the lamina, ligamentum flavum, transverse process, spinal canal, and the vertebral body.[19] Thereafter, US was used mostly to preview the spinal anatomy and measure the distances from the skin to the lamina and epidural space before epidural puncture.[20,21] Grau et al from Heidelberg in Germany conducted a series of investigations, between 2001 and 2004, to evaluate the utility of US for epidural access,[22–28] which significantly improved our understanding of spinal sonography. Grau et al also describe a two-operator technique of real-time US visualization, through a paramedian sagittal axis, of an advancing epidural needle that was inserted through the midline during a combined spinal epidural procedure.[29] It appears that the quality of US imaging that was available at the time hindered widespread acceptance and further research in this area. Recent improvements in US technology allow us to image the spine and neuraxial structures with improved clarity and the authors group from the Chinese University of Hong Kong has recently published their experience on real-time ultrasound-guided (USG) epidural access performed by a single operator.[30]

Ultrasound Imaging of the Spine

Basic Considerations

The neuraxial structures are located at a depth that necessitates the use of low-frequency US (2–5 MHz) and curved array transducers for US imaging of the spine. Low-frequency US provides good penetration but lacks spatial resolution at the depths (5–7 cm) at which the neuraxial structures are located. Nevertheless, high-frequency US has also been used to image the spine.[31,32] Although high-frequency US provides better resolution than low-frequency US, it lacks penetration, which seriously limits its usage other than for imaging superficial structures of the spine.[31,32] Moreover, the field of vision with a high-frequency linear transducers is also very limited compared to that of a low-frequency curved array transducer which produces a divergent beam with a wide field of vision. The latter is particularly useful during USG interventions of the spine (see below). Besides, the bony framework of the spine also does not lend to optimal conditions for US imaging of the neuraxial structures because it reflects majority of the incident US energy before it even reaches the spinal canal. Moreover, the acoustic shadow of the bony structures of the spine produces a narrow acoustic window for imaging. This often results in US images of variable quality. However, recent improvements in US technology, image processing capabilities of US machines, the availability of compound imaging, and the development of new scan protocols (see below) have significantly improved our ability to image the spine. Today it is possible to accurately identify the neuraxial anatomy relevant for CNB.[30,33] Also of note is that technology that was once only available in the high-end cart-based US systems are now available in portable US devices making them adequate for spinal sonography and USG CNB.

Axis of Scan

An US scan of the spine can be performed in the transverse (axial scan)[33,34] or longitudinal (sagittal)[30] axis with the patient in the sitting,[24,25,29,33] lateral decubitus,[30] or prone[16] position. The sagittal scan is performed either through the midline (midline sagittal or median scan) or through a paramedian [paramedian sagittal scan (PMSS)] location. The prone position is useful in patients presenting for a chronic pain procedure when fluoroscopy may also be used in conjunction with US imaging.[16] Since the bony framework of the spine wraps around the neuraxial structures, they can only be optimally visualized, within the spinal canal, if the US beam is insonated through the widest acoustic window available. Grau et al have demonstrated that the PMSS plane is better than the median transverse or median sagittal plane for visualizing the neuraxial structures.[22] There are also proponents of the transverse axis for US imaging the spine.[34] In fact the two axis of scan complement each other during an US examination of the spine.[34] In a recent investigation the authors group objectively compared the visibility of neuraxial structures when the spine was imaged in the paramedian sagittal and paramedian oblique sagittal axis, i.e., with the transducer tilted slightly medially during the scan (Figure 12.1). The medial tilt is done to ensure that the incident US beam enters the spinal canal through the widest part of the interlaminar space and not the lateral sulcus. Neuraxial structures were significantly better visualized in the PMOS scans (data to be published) and therefore the PMOS axis is the author's preferred axis for imaging during USG CNB in the lumbar region (see below).

Liberal amounts of US gel are applied to the skin over the area of interest prior to the scout (preview) scan for acoustic coupling. The objective of the scout scan is to preview the anatomy, optimize the image, identify any underlying asymptomatic abnormality or variation, measure relevant distances to the lamina, ligamentum flavum, or dura, and identify the best possible location and trajectory for needle insertion. The US image is optimized by making the following adjustments on the US unit: (a) selecting an appropriate preset (can be customized), (b) setting an appropriate scanning depth (6–10 cm) depending on the body habitus of the patient, (c) selecting the "General" optimization (midfrequency range) option of the broadband transducer, (d) adjusting the "focus" to a depth corresponding to the area of interest, and finally (e) manually adjusting the "gain," "dynamic range," and "compression" settings to obtain the best possible image. Compound imaging and selecting an appropriate "map" when available are also useful in improving the quality of the images. Once an optimal image is obtained, the position of the transducer is marked on the patients' back using a skin marking pen to ensure that the transducer is returned to the same position after sterile preparations are made before the intervention. This also circumvents the need to repeat the scout scan routine to identify a given intervertebral space.

Spinal Sonoanatomy

Currently, there are limited data on spinal sonography or on how to interpret US images of the spine. Even recent textbooks of regional anesthesia have very limited or no information

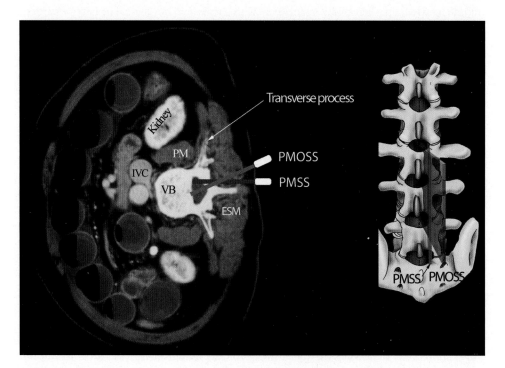

Figure 12.1. Paramedian sagittal scan of the lumbar spine. The paramedian sagittal axis of scan (PMSS) is represented by the red color and the paramedian oblique sagittal axis of scan (PMOS) is represented by the blue color. Note how the PMOSS is tilted slightly medially. This is done to ensure that majority of the ultrasound energy enters the spinal canal through the widest part of the interlaminar space. (Reproduced with permission from www.aic.cuhk.edu.hk/usgraweb).

on this subject. Moreover, while the landscape of regional anesthesia is changing and US guidance for peripheral nerve blocks is becoming an integral part of regional anesthetic practice, it may be fair to say that, there are few anesthesiologists or pain physicians who currently use US for CNB.[35] This is quite interesting when there is evidence to suggest that US improves technical and clinical outcomes during CNB,[26,29] and emergency physicians are able to interpret US images of the spine[1,31] and are performing lumbar puncture in the accident and emergency department using US.[1,31,32] Even after the National Institute of Clinical Excellence (NICE) in the United Kingdom (UK) recommended that ultrasound be used for epidural insertions,[36] 97% of respondents to a survey in the UK had never used US to image the epidural space.[35] The reason for this paucity of data or a lack of interest in the use of US for imaging the spine and performing central neuraxial interventions is not clear, but the author believes that it may be due to a lack of understanding of spinal sonoanatomy. Today there are models to learn musculoskeletal US imaging techniques (human volunteers), the sonoanatomy relevant for peripheral nerve blocks (human volunteers or cadavers), and the required interventional skills (tissue mimicking phantoms, fresh cadavers); however, when it comes to learning spinal sonoanatomy or the interventional skills required for USG CNBs, there are very few models or tools available today for this purpose.

The Water-Based Spine Phantom

Let us consider that the spine is made up of bone and soft tissue. If one is able to accurately identify the osseous elements of the spine then one should be able to identify the gaps in the bony framework, i.e., the interlaminar space or the interspinous space, through which the US beam can be insonated to visualize the neuraxial structures within the spinal canal and/or insert a needle during US-assisted or -guided CNB. The author and his group have recently described using a "water-based spine phantom" to study the osseous anatomy of the spine (Figure 12.2a).[37] This is based on a model previously described by Greher et al to study the osseous anatomy relevant for USG lumbar facet nerve block.[15] The "water-based spine phantom" is prepared by immersing a commercially available lumbosacral spine model (Sawbones, Pacific Research Laboratories, Inc., Vashon, WA) in water (Figure 12.2a) and scanning it in the transverse and sagittal axis through the water. We have found that each osseous element of the spine has a "signature" appearance (Figures 12.2–12.4) and they are comparable to that seen in vivo (Figures 12.3 and 12.4). Being able to recognize these patterns is in the author's opinion the first step toward learning how to interpret US images of the spine. Representative US images of the spinous process (Figure 12.2b, c), L5/S1 interlaminar space or gap (Fig. 12.3a, b), lamina (Fig. 12.3c, d) articular process of the facet joint (Figures 12.2d and 12.3a), and the transverse process (Figure 12.4c) from the "water-based spine phantom" are presented in Figures 12.2–12.4. Another important feature of the phantom described above is that one is able to see through the water, so it is possible to validate the sonographic appearance of a target osseous structure by performing the scan with a marker (e.g., a needle) in contact with it.

Ultrasound Imaging of the Sacrum

US imaging of the sacrum is usually performed to identify the sonoanatomy relevant for a caudal epidural injection.[16] Since the sacrum is a superficial structure a high-frequency linear array transducer is used for the scan.[16] The patient is positioned in the lateral or prone position with a pillow under the abdomen to flex the lumbosacral spine. On a transverse sonogram of the sacrum at the level of the sacral hiatus, the sacral cornua are seen as two hyperechoic reversed U-shaped structures,[16] one on either side of the midline (Figure 12.5). Connecting the two sacral cornua and deep to the skin and subcutaneous tissue is a hyperechoic band, the sacrococcygeal ligament (Figure 12.5). Anterior to the sacrococcygeal ligament is another hyperechoic linear structure, which represents the posterior surface of the sacrum (Figure 12.5). The hypoechoic space between the sacrococcygeal ligament and the bony posterior surface of the sacrum is the sacral hiatus (Figure 12.5).[16]

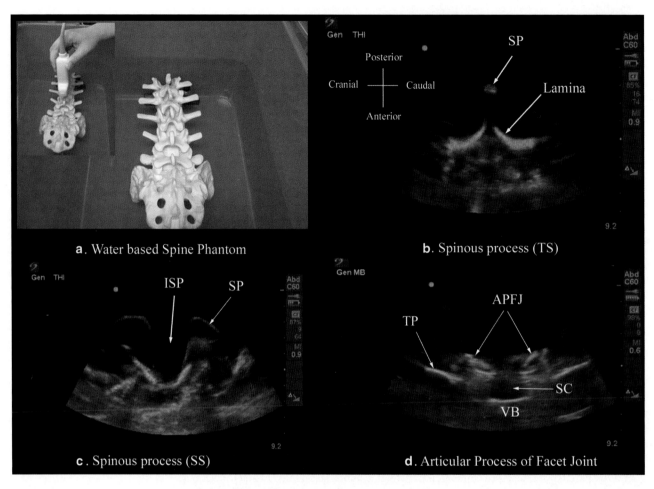

Figure 12.2. The water-based spine phantom (**a**) and sonograms of the spinous process in the transverse (**b**) and sagittal (**c**) axes, and a scan through the interspinous space (**d**). *SP* spinous process, *ISP* interspinous space, *TP* transverse process, *APFJ* articular process of the facet joints, *SC* spinal canal, *VB* vertebral body, *TS* transverse scan, *SS* sagittal scan. (Reproduced with permission from www.aic.cuhk.edu.hk/usgraweb).

The two sacral cornua and the posterior surface of the sacrum produce a pattern on the sonogram that we refer to as the "frog eye sign" because of its resemblance to the eyes of a frog. On a sagittal sonogram of the sacrum at the level of the sacral cornua, the sacrococcygeal ligament, the base of sacrum, and the sacral hiatus are also clearly visualized (Figure 12.6).

Above the sacral hiatus on a sagittal sonogram the sacrum is identified as a flat hyperechoic structure with a large anterior acoustic shadow (Figure 12.6).[3] If one slides the transducer cephalad, maintaining the same orientation, a dip or gap is seen between the sacrum and the L5 lamina (PMSS), which is the L5/S1 intervertebral space[3,30] and is also referred to as the L5/S1gap (Figures 12.3a, b and 12.7).[30] This is the sonographic landmark that is often used to identify a specific lumbar intervertebral space (L4/L5, L3/L4, etc.) by counting upward.[3,30] US is more accurate than palpation in identifying a given lumbar intervertebral space.[3] However, since US localization of the lumbar intervertebral spaces relies on one's ability to locate the L5/S1 gap on the sonogram, there are limitations of this method in the presence of a sacralized L5 vertebra or a lumbarized S1 vertebra when the L4/L5 interspace may be misinterpreted as the L5/S1 gap. Since it is not possible to predict the presence of the above without alternative imaging (x-ray, CT, or MRI), the L5/S1 gap is still a useful sonographic landmark when used for USG CNB although one must bear in mind that occasionally the identified intervertebral level may be off by one or two intervertebral levels.

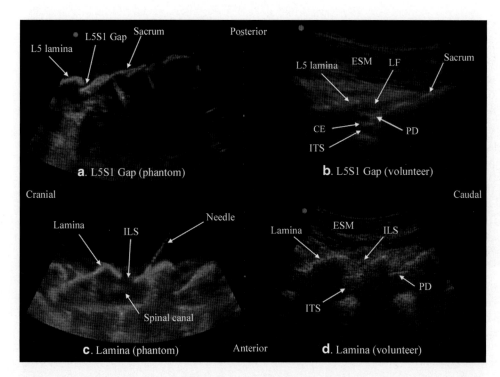

Figure 12.3. Paramedian sagittal sonogram of the L5/S1 interlaminar space or gap (**a**) and the lamina of the lumbar vertebra (**c**) from the water-based spine phantom and corresponding images from volunteers (**b, d**). Note the similarities in the sonographic appearances of the osseous elements in the phantom and volunteers. *ESM* erector spinae muscle, *LF* ligamentum flavum, *PD* posterior dura, *CE* cauda equina, *ITS* intrathecal space, *ILS* interlaminar space. (Reproduced with permission from www.aic.cuhk.edu.hk/usgraweb).

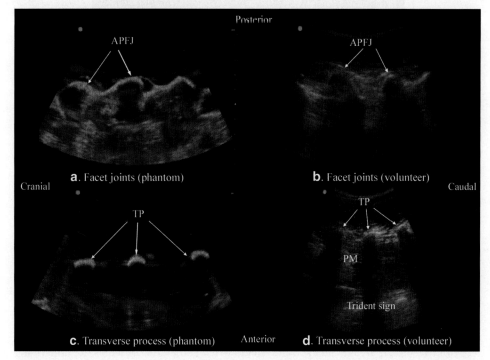

Figure 12.4. Paramedian sagittal sonogram of the articular process of the facet joints (**a**) and transverse process (**c**) from the water-based spine phantom and corresponding images from volunteers (**b, d**). Once again note the similarities in the sonographic appearances of the osseous elements in the phantom and volunteers. *APFJ* articular process of the facet joints, *TP* transverse process, *PM* psoas major muscle. (Reproduced with permission from www.aic.cuhk.edu.hk/usgraweb).

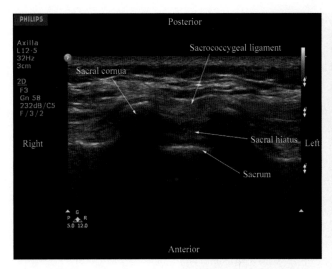

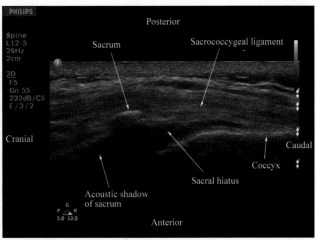

Figure 12.5. Transverse sonogram of the sacrum at the level of the sacral hiatus. Note the two sacral cornua and the hyperechoic sacrococcygeal ligament that extends between the two sacral cornua. The hypoechoic space between the sacrococcygeal ligament and the posterior surface of the sacrum is the sacral hiatus. (Reproduced with permission from www.aic.cuhk.edu.hk/usgraweb).

Figure 12.6. Sagittal sonogram of the sacrum at the level of the sacral hiatus. Note the hyperechoic sacrococcygeal ligament which extends from the sacrum to the coccyx and the acoustic shadow of the sacrum which completely obscures the sacral canal. (Reproduced with permission from www.aic.cuhk.edu.hk/usgraweb).

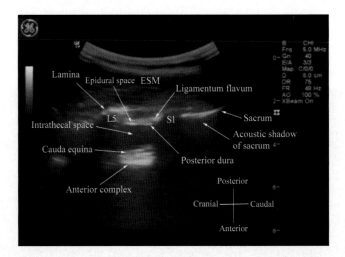

Figure 12.7. Paramedian sagittal sonogram of the lumbosacral junction. The posterior surface of the sacrum is identified as a flat hyperechoic surface with a large acoustic shadow anterior to it. The dip or gap between the sacrum and the lamina of L5 is the L5/S1 intervertebral space. *ESM* erector spinae muscle. (Reproduced with permission from www.aic.cuhk.edu.hk/usgraweb).

Ultrasound Imaging of the Lumbar Spine

For a transverse scan of the lumbar spine the US transducer is positioned over the spinous process with the patient in the sitting or lateral position. On a transverse sonogram the spinous process is seen as a hyperechoic reflection under the skin and subcutaneous tissue, anterior to which there is a dark acoustic shadow that completely obscures the underlying spinal canal and thus the neuraxial structures (Figure 12.8). Therefore, this view is not ideal for imaging the neuraxial structures but is useful for identifying the midline when the spinous processes cannot be palpated (obesity and in those with edema in their backs).[34] If one now slides the transducer slightly cranially or caudally it is possible to perform a transverse scan of the lumbar spine with the US beam being insonated through the interspinous space (interspinous view) (Figure 12.9). Since the US signal is now not impeded by the spinous process, the ligamentum flavum, posterior dura, thecal sac, and the anterior complex (discussed below) are visualized in the midline (from a posterior to anterior direction) within the spinal canal and laterally the articular process of the facet joints (APFJ) and the transverse processes are visible (Figure 12.9). The resultant sonogram produces a pattern which Carvalho likens to a "flying bat."[34] The interspinous view can also be used to determine whether there is any rotation in the vertebra such as in scoliosis. Normally the APFJs on either side of the spine are symmetrically located (Figure 12.9). However, if they are asymmetrically located or either one of the articular processes is not visible then one should suspect rotation of the spine (provided the transducer is correctly positioned and aligned) as in scoliosis and anticipate a potentially difficult spinal or epidural.

For a sagittal scan of the lumbar spine, the author prefers to position the patient in the left lateral position with the knees and hip slightly flexed (Figure 12.10). The transducer is positioned 1–2 cm lateral to the spinous process (midline) at the lower back on the nondependent side with its orientation marker directed cranially. The transducer is also tilted slightly medially during the scan[30] so that the US beam is insonated in a PMOS plane (Figure 12.10, inset). During the scout scan the L3/4 and L4/5 interlaminar space is located as described above. On a PMOS sonogram of the lumbar spine the erector spinae muscles are clearly delineated and lie superficial to the lamina. The lamina appears hyperechoic and is the first osseous structure visualized (Figure 12.10). Since bone impedes the passage of US there is an acoustic shadow anterior to each lamina. The sonographic appearance of the lamina produces a pattern that resembles the head and neck of a horse which we refer to as the "horse head sign" (Figures 12.3c, d and 12.10). The interlaminar space is the gap between the adjoining lamina. In contrast, the articular processes of the facet joints appear as one continuous hyperechoic wavy line with no intervening gaps as seen at the level of the lamina (Figure 12.4a, b), and are the usual clues to differentiate the lamina from the articular processes. The APFJ in a sagittal sonogram produces a pattern that resembles multiple camel humps which we refer to as the "camel hump sign"

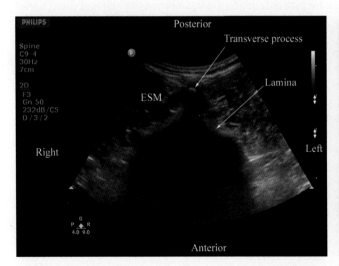

Figure 12.8. Transverse sonogram of the lumbar spine with the transducer positioned directly over the spinous process. Note the acoustic shadow of the spinous process which completely obscures the spinal canal and the neuraxial structures. *ESM* erector spinae muscle. (Reproduced with permission from www.aic.cuhk.edu.hk/usgraweb).

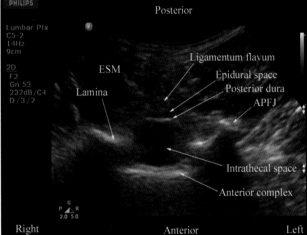

Figure 12.9. Transverse sonogram of the lumbar spine with the transducer positioned such that the ultrasound beam is insonated through the interspinous space. The ligamentum flavum, epidural space, posterior dura, intrathecal space, and anterior complex are now visible within the spinal canal in the midline and the APFJ and the TP are visible laterally. Note how the articular processes of the facet joints (APFJ) on either side are symmetrically located. *ESM* erector spinae muscle. (Reproduced with permission from www.aic.cuhk.edu.hk/usgraweb).

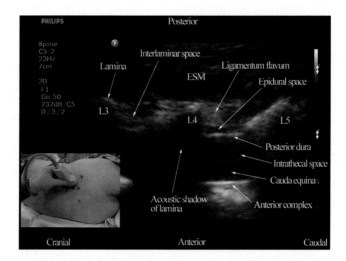

Figure 12.10. Paramedian oblique sagittal sonogram of the lumbar spine at the L3/4 and L4/5 level. Note the hypoechoic epidural space (few millimeters wide) between the hyperechoic ligamentum flavum and the posterior dura. The intrathecal space is the anechoic space between the posterior dura and the anterior complex in the sonogram. The cauda equina nerve fibers are also seen as hyperechoic, longitudinal structures within the thecal sac. Picture in the inset shows how the transducer is positioned on the nondependent side of the back and how it is tilted slightly medially during the scan. *ESM* erector spinae muscle, *L3* lamina of L3 vertebra, *L4* lamina of L4 vertebra, *L5* lamina of L5 vertebra. (Reproduced with permission from www.aic.cuhk.edu.hk/usgraweb).

(Figure 12.4a, b). In between the dark acoustic shadows of adjacent lamina there is a rectangular area in the sonogram where the neuraxial structures are visualized (Figure 12.10).[30] This is the "acoustic window" and results from reflections of the US signal from the neuraxial structures within the spinal canal. The ligamentum flavum is also hyperechoic and is often seen as a thick band across two adjacent lamina (Figure 12.10). The posterior dura is the next hyperechoic structure anterior to the ligamentum flavum and the epidural space is the hypoechoic area (few millimeters wide) between the ligamentum flavum and the posterior dura (Figure 12.10).[30] The thecal sac with the CSF is the anechoeic space anterior to the posterior dura. The cauda equina, which is located within the thecal sac, is often seen as multiple horizontal hyperechoic shadows within the anechoeic thecal sac (Figure 12.10)[30] and their location can vary with posture. Pulsations of the cauda equina are also identified in some patients. The anterior dura is also hyperechoic, but it is often difficult to differentiate it from the posterior longitudinal ligament and the vertebral body or the intervertebral disc as they are of the same echogenicity (isoechoeic) and very closely apposed to each. This often results in a single, composite, hyperechoic reflection anteriorly that is also referred to as the "anterior complex" (Figure 12.10).

Ultrasound Imaging of the Thoracic Spine

US imaging of the thoracic spine is more demanding because of the acute angulation of the spinous processes and the narrow interspinous spaces. This results in a narrow acoustic window for US imaging with limited visibility of the neuraxial structures (Figure 12.11).[25] US imaging of the thoracic spine can be performed via the transverse (median transverse scan)[25] or paramedian[25] axis with the patient in the sitting or lateral decubitus position. Grau et al performed US imaging of the thoracic spine at the T5/6 level in young volunteers and compared these images with MRI images of the spine at the same level.[25] They observed that the US scans in the transverse axis produced the best images of the neuraxial structures[25] and the epidural space was best visualized in the paramedian scans.[25] However, compared to the MRI images, which were easier to interpret, US had limited ability to delineate the epidural space or the spinal cord but was better than MRI in

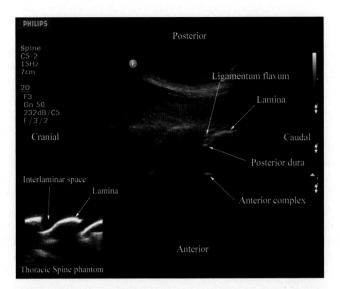

Figure 12.11. Paramedian oblique sagittal sonogram of the midthoracic spine. Note the narrow acoustic window through which the posterior dura and anterior complex are visible. Picture in the inset shows a sagittal sonogram of the thoracic spine from the water-based spine phantom. *ILS* interlaminar space. (Reproduced with permission from www.aic.cuhk.edu.hk/usgraweb).

demonstrating the dura.[25] As in the lumbar region the lamina in the thoracic region is also hyperechoic but the acoustic window for visualizing the neuraxial structures is very narrow (Figure 12.11). Despite this the posterior dura, which is also hyperechoic, is consistently visualized through the narrow interlaminar spaces but the epidural space is more difficult to delineate (Figure 12.11).

Ultrasound-Guided CNB

US is commonly used to preview the spinal anatomy prior to performing a traditional epidural access using "loss-of-resistance."[19,24,26,29,33] Real-time USG epidural access, as a two-operator[29] or as a single operator[30] technique, has also been described in the literature. The patient can be positioned in the sitting, lateral, or prone position during a USG CNB. The author believes that for maximum manual dexterity the patient should be positioned such that the operator can use the dominant hand to perform the intervention and use the nondominant hand to hold the US transducer and perform the scan. Although liberal amounts of US gel is used for acoustic coupling during the scout scan it is the author's practice not to apply US gel directly on to the patients' skin over the area scanned during USG CNB.[30] Normal saline solution, which is applied using sterile swabs, is used as an alternative coupling agent[30] with the aim to keep the area under the footprint of the transducer moist. This is done because there are no data demonstrating the safety of US gel on the meninges or central neuraxial structures. Therefore, while preparing the US transducer a thin layer of sterile US gel from a disposable sachet is applied directly on to the footprint of the transducer, which is then covered with a sterile-transparent dressing, making sure that no air is trapped between the footprint and the dressing. The transducer and cable are then covered with a sterile plastic sleeve. Since no US gel is applied on the skin, as expected, there is a slight deterioration in the quality of the US image compared to that obtained during the scout scan, but this can be easily compensated by manually adjusting the overall gain and compression settings.[30] All these additional steps bring about changes in our routine practice, which may increase the potential for infection via contamination during the preparation of the equipment. Therefore, strict asepsis must be maintained during any USG CNB.

Caudal Epidural Injection

Caudal epidural injections (steroids or local anesthetics) are frequently performed for pain management. For a USG caudal epidural injection, a transverse or sagittal scan is performed at the level of the sacral hiatus. Since the sacral hiatus is a superficial structure, high-frequency (6–13 MHz) linear array transducer is commonly used for the scan as described above (Figures 12.5 and 12.6). The block needle can be inserted in the short (out of plane) or long axis (in-plane) of the US plane. For a long-axis needle insertion (author's preference) a sagittal scan is performed (Figure 12.6) and the passage of the block needle through the sacrococcygeal ligament into the sacral canal is visualized in real time (Figure 12.12). However, since the sacrum impedes the passage of the US beam there is a large acoustic shadow anteriorly (Figures 12.6 and 12.12), which makes it impossible to visualize the tip of the needle or the spread of the injectate within the sacral canal. Moreover an inadvertent intravascular injection, which is reported in 5–9% of such procedures, cannot be detected using US. So in clinical practice one still has to rely on clinical signs such as the "pop" or "give" as the needle traverses the sacrococcygeal ligament, ease of injection, absence of subcutaneous swelling, "whoosh test," nerve stimulation, or the assessment of the clinical effects of the injected drug to confirm correct needle placement. Chen et al describe using fluoroscopy after contrast injection to confirm the position of a caudal needle that was placed under US guidance and report a 100% success rate.[16] This is encouraging considering that even in experienced hands there is a failure to successfully place a needle in the caudal epidural space is as high as 25%.[16,38] More recently, Chen et al[39] have described US imaging as a screening tool for caudal epidural injections.[39] In their cohort of patients the mean diameter of the sacral canal at the sacral hiatus was 5.3 ± 2 mm and the distance between the sacral cornua (bilateral) was 9.7 ± 1.9 mm.[39] Chen et al also identified that sonographic features such as a closed sacral hiatus and a sacral diameter of around 1.5 mm have a greater probability for a failed caudal epidural injection.[39] Based on the published data one can conclude that US, despite its limitation, may be useful as an adjunct tool for caudal epidural needle placement and has the potential to improve technical outcomes, minimize failure rates and exposure to radiation in the chronic pain setting, and therefore deserves further investigation in the future.

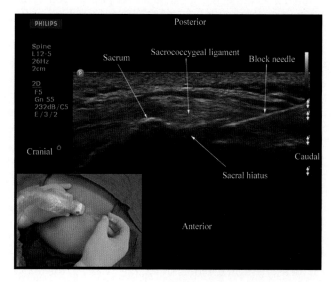

Figure 12.12. Sagittal sonogram of the sacrum at the level of the sacral hiatus during a real-time ultrasound guided caudal epidural injection. Note the hyperechoic sacrococcygeal ligament and the block needle that has been inserted in the plane (in-plane) of the ultrasound beam. Picture in the inset shows the position and orientation of the transducer and the direction in which the block needle is inserted. (Reproduced with permission from www.aic.cuhk.edu.hk/usgraweb).

Lumbar Epidural Injection

During lumbar epidural access US imaging can be used to preview the underlying spinal anatomy[24,26,29] or to guide the needle in real time.[30] As described above real-time US guidance for epidural access is performed either as a two-operator[29] or as a single operator[30] technique. In the former technique that was described by Grau et al for combined spinal epidural anesthesia the first operator performs the US scan via the paramedian axis while the second operator performs the epidural access via the midline using the traditional "loss-of-resistance" technique.[29] Grau et al were able to visualize the advancing needle in all their cases despite the axis of the US scan and the needle insertion being different.[29] Moreover, they were also able to visualize the dural puncture in all their patients and dural tenting in a few cases during the needle-through-needle spinal puncture.[29] Recently, we have described the successful use of real-time US guidance in conjunction with loss of resistance to saline for paramedian epidural access, performed by a single operator, with the epidural needle inserted in the plane of the US beam.[30] As a result it is possible to visualize the advancing needle in real time until it is seen to engage in the ligamentum flavum (Figure 12.13). We were able to circumvent the need for a second operator (additional hands), to perform the LOR, by using the Episure™ AutoDetect™ syringe (Indigo Orb, Inc., Irvine, CA), which is a new LOR syringe with an internal compression spring that applies constant pressure on the plunger (Figure 12.14, inset).[40] We were also able to demonstrate objective changes within the spinal canal, at the level of needle insertion, immediately after the loss of resistance to saline in majority (>50%) of our patients.[30] Anterior displacement of the posterior dura and widening of the posterior epidural space were the most frequently visualized changes within the spinal canal, but compression of the thecal sac was also seen in a few patients (Figure 12.14).[30] These are objective signs of a correct epidural injection and have previously been described in children.[41] The neuraxial changes that occur within the spinal canal following the "loss-of-resistance" to saline may have

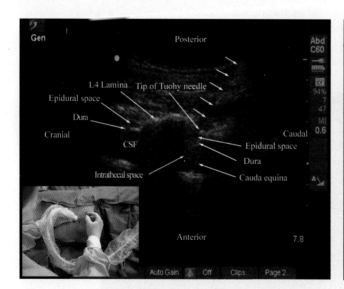

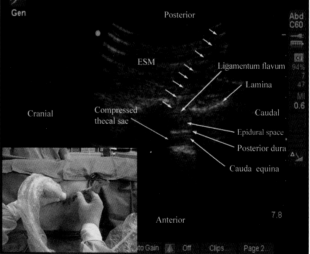

Figure 12.13. Paramedian oblique sagittal sonogram of the lumbar spine during real-time ultrasound-guided paramedian epidural access. The tip of the Tuohy needle (*short white arrows*) is seen embedded in the ligamentum flavum. Picture in the inset shows the position and orientation of the transducer and the direction in which the Tuohy needle is inserted (in-plane) during the epidural access. *CSF* cerebrospinal fluid. (Reproduced with permission from www.aic.cuhk.edu.hk/usgraweb).

Figure 12.14. Paramedian oblique sagittal sonogram of the lumbar spine showing the sonographic changes within the spinal canal after the "loss-of-resistance" to saline. Note the anterior displacement of the posterior dura, widening of the posterior epidural space, and compression of the thecal sac. The cauda equina nerve roots are also now better visualized within the compressed thecal sac in this patient. Picture in the inset shows how the Episure™ AutoDetect™ syringe was used to circumvent the need for a third hand for the "loss-of resistance." (Reproduced with permission from www.aic.cuhk.edu.hk/usgraweb).

clinical significance and are discussed in detail in our report.[30] Despite our success with real-time USG epidural access, we have not been able to visualize an indwelling epidural catheter to date in adults. However, we have occasionally observed changes within the spinal canal, e.g., anterior displacement of the posterior dura and widening of the posterior epidural space, after an epidural bolus injection via the catheter. These are surrogate markers of the location of the catheter tip and of limited value in clinical practice. Our observations are in agreement with the experience of Grau[27] and may be related to the small diameter and poor echogenicity of conventional epidural catheters that are in use today. There is a need to develop new epidural catheter designs with improved echogenicity.

Thoracic Epidural Injection

There are no published data on USG thoracic epidural blocks. This may be due to the poor US visibility of the neuraxial structures in the thoracic region (refer above) and the associated technical difficulties. However, despite the narrow acoustic window; the lamina, the interlaminar space, and the posterior dura are consistently visualized using the paramedian axis (Figure 12.11). The epidural space is more difficult to delineate but is also best visualized in a paramedian scan (Figure 12.11).[25] As a result the author has been using an US-assisted technique to perform thoracic epidural catheterization via the paramedian window. In this approach, the patient is positioned in the sitting position and a paramedian oblique sagittal scan (PMOS) is performed at the desired thoracic level with the orientation marker of the transducer directed cranially (Figure 12.15). Under strict aseptic precautions (described above) the Tuohy needle is inserted via the paramedian axis in real time and in the plane of the ultrasound beam (Figure 12.15). The needle is steadily advanced until it is seen to contact the lamina or enter the interlaminar space. Since the lamina is relatively superficial in the thoracic region, it is possible to visualize the advancing Tuohy needle in real time (Figure 12.15). Once the tip of the Tuohy needle is in contact with the lamina or in the interlaminar space, the author puts the US transducer down and uses the traditional loss-of-resistance to saline technique to access the epidural space. Preliminary experience with this approach indicates that US may improve the likelihood of thoracic epidural access on the first attempt. Research comparing the US-assisted technique described above with the traditional approach is planned at the author's institution.

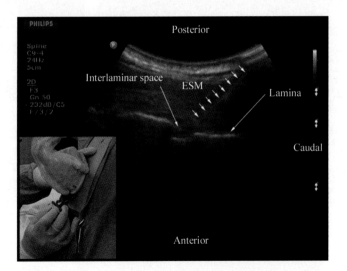

Figure 12.15. Paramedian oblique sagittal sonogram of the thoracic spine during an ultrasound-assisted paramedian epidural access. The Tuohy needle (*short white arrows*) has been inserted in the plane of the ultrasound beam and its tip is seen in the interlaminar space. Picture in the inset shows the patient in the sitting position and how the transducer is positioned and oriented. Also note the direction in which the Tuohy needle is inserted (in-plane) during the paramedian epidural access. *ESM* erector spinae muscle. (Reproduced with permission from www.aic.cuhk.edu.hk/usgraweb).

Spinal Injection

There are very limited data in the anesthesia or pain medicine literature on the use of US for spinal (intrathecal) injections[42,43] although it has been shown to be useful for lumbar punctures by radiologists[44] and emergency physicians.[32] Majority of the data are in the form of case reports.[42,43,45,46] Yeo and French, in 1999, were the first to describe the successful use of US to assist spinal injection in a patient with abnormal spinal anatomy.[46] They used US to locate the vertebral midline in a parturient with severe scoliosis with Harrington rods in situ.[46] Yamauchi et al describe using US to preview the neuraxial anatomy and measure the distance from the skin to the dura in a postlaminectomy patient before the intrathecal injection was performed under x-ray guidance.[45] Costello and Balki used US to facilitate spinal injection by locating the position of the L5/S1 space in a parturient with poliomyelitis and previous Harrington rod instrumentation of the spine.[42] Prasad et al report using US to assist spinal injection in a patient with obesity, scoliosis, and multiple previous back surgery with instrumentation.[43] More recently, Chin et al[47] have described real-time ultrasound-guided spinal anesthesia in two patients with abnormal spinal anatomy (one had lumbar scoliosis and the other had undergone spinal fusion surgery at the L23 level).

The Evidence

Currently, there are limited outcome data on the use of ultrasound for CNB. Majority of data are from its use in the lumbar region with limited data from the thoracic region. Most studies to date have evaluated the utility of performing a prepuncture US scan or scout scan. A scout scan allows one to identify the midline[34] and accurately determine the interspace for needle insertion,[3,30] which are useful in patients in whom anatomical landmarks are difficult to palpate, such as in those with obesity,[1,23] edema in the back, or abnormal anatomy (scoliosis,[23,48] postlaminectomy surgery,[45] or spinal instrumentation).[42,43,46] It also allows the operator to preview the neuraxial anatomy,[24,26,29,30,33] identify asymptomatic spinal abnormalities such as in spina bifida,[49] accurately predict the depth to the epidural space[19,20,24,26] including in the obese,[50] identify ligamentum defects,[51] and determine the optimal site and trajectory for needle insertion.[26,27]

Cumulative evidence suggests that when an US examination is performed before the epidural puncture it improves the success rate of epidural access on the first attempt,[24] reduces the number of puncture attempts[23,24,26,29] or the need to puncture multiple levels,[24,26,29] and also improves patient comfort during the procedure.[26] Preliminary data suggest that this may also be true in patients with presumed difficult epidural access such as in those with a history of difficult epidural access, obesity, and kyphosis or scoliosis of the lumbar spine.[23] When used for obstetric epidural anesthesia, it also improves the quality of analgesia, reduces side effects, and improves patient satisfaction.[23,28] There are also data demonstrating that a scout scan improves the learning curve of epidural blocks in parturients.[28] Currently, there are very limited data evaluating real-time US guidance for epidural access,[29,30] but preliminary results indicate that it also improves technical outcomes.[29] Research in this area is ongoing at the author's institution.

Education and Training

Learning USG CNB techniques takes time and patience. In the author's experience, irrespective of the technique used, USG CNB and in particular real-time USG CNB are advanced techniques and by far the most difficult USG interventions. It also demands a high degree of manual dexterity, hand–eye coordination, and an ability to conceptualize

2D information into a 3D image. Therefore, before attempting to perform a USG CNB the operator should have a sound knowledge of the basics of US, be familiar with spinal sonography and sonoanatomy, and have the necessary interventional skills. It is advisable to start by attending a course or workshop that is tailor-made for this purpose where one can learn the basic scanning techniques, spinal sonoanatomy, and the required interventional skills. Further experience of spinal sonography can also be acquired in volunteers. It appears that anesthesiologists with no prior experience in using US for CNB require more than the following: reading published educational material, attending a lecture and demonstration workshop, and performing 20 supervised scans, to become competent in US assessment of the lumbar spine.[52] Today there are very few models (phantoms) for practicing USG central neuraxial interventions. The authors group has been using anesthetized pigs and more recently a pig carcass model to acquire the skills necessary for USG central neuraxial interventions. Once the basic skills are attained it is best to start by performing USG spinal injections, under supervision, before progressing on to performing epidurals. Real-time USG epidurals can be technically demanding even for an experienced operator. If there is no experience in USG CNB locally then it is advisable to visit a center where such interventions are practiced. Today it is also not known how many such interventions need to be performed before one becomes proficient in performing real-time USG CNB. Further research in this area is warranted.

Conclusion

USG CNB is a promising alternative to traditional landmark-based techniques. It is non-invasive, safe, simple to use, and can be quickly performed. It also does not involve exposure to radiation, provides real-time images, and is free from adverse effects. With recent improvements in ultrasound technology and image processing capabilities of US machines, today it is possible to visualize neuraxial structures using US and this has significantly improved our understanding of spinal sonoanatomy. US imaging has been used to assist or guide CNB in the sacral, lumbar, and thoracic regions. Majority of the outcome data are from its application in the lumbar region and there are limited data on its use in the thoracic region. A prepuncture (scout) scan allows the operator to preview the spinal anatomy, identify the midline, accurately predict the depth to the epidural space, identify any rotational deformity in the spine, and determine the optimal site and trajectory for needle insertion. US imaging when used during CNB also improves the success rate of epidural access on the first attempt, reduces the number of puncture attempts or the need to puncture multiple levels, and also improves patient comfort during the procedure. The same may also apply in patients with presumed difficult epidural access and difficult spines. It is an excellent teaching tool for demonstrating the anatomy of the spine, and improves the learning curve of epidural blocks in parturients. US also assists in performing CNB in patients who in the past may have been considered unsuitable for such procedures, e.g., in those with abnormal spinal anatomy. However, US guidance for CNB is still in its infancy and evidence to support its use is sparse. There is also a paucity of data on the use of ultrasound for CNB in pain medicine. The author envisions that as ultrasound technology continues to improve and as more anesthesiologists and pain physicians embrace this technology and acquire the necessary skills to perform USG interventions, USG CNB will no doubt become more widespread and may become the standard of care in the future.

Acknowledgment

All the figures have been reproduced with permission from www.aic.cuhk.edu.hk/usgraweb.

REFERENCES

1. Stiffler KA, Jwayyed S, Wilber ST, Robinson A. The use of ultrasound to identify pertinent landmarks for lumbar puncture. *Am J Emerg Med.* 2007;25:331–334.

2. Broadbent CR, Maxwell WB, Ferrie R, Wilson DJ, Gawne-Cain M, Russell R. Ability of anaesthetists to identify a marked lumbar interspace. *Anaesthesia.* 2000;55:1122–1126.

3. Furness G, Reilly MP, Kuchi S. An evaluation of ultrasound imaging for identification of lumbar intervertebral level. *Anaesthesia.* 2002;57:277–280.

4. Holmaas G, Frederiksen D, Ulvik A, Vingsnes SO, Ostgaard G, Nordli H. Identification of thoracic intervertebral spaces by means of surface anatomy: a magnetic resonance imaging study. *Acta Anaesthesiol Scand.* 2006;50:368–373.

5. Reynolds F. Damage to the conus medullaris following spinal anaesthesia. *Anaesthesia.* 2001;56:238–247.

6. Hamandi K, Mottershead J, Lewis T, Ormerod IC, Ferguson IT. Irreversible damage to the spinal cord following spinal anesthesia. *Neurology.* 2002;59:624–626.

7. Tarkkila P, Huhtala J, Salminen U. Difficulties in spinal needle use. Insertion characteristics and failure rates associated with 25-, 27- and 29-gauge Quincke-type spinal needles. *Anaesthesia.* 1994;49:723–725.

8. Seeberger MD, Lang ML, Drewe J, Schneider M, Hauser E, Hruby J. Comparison of spinal and epidural anesthesia for patients younger than 50 years of age. *Anesth Analg.* 1994;78:667–673.

9. Klaastad O, Lilleas FG, Rotnes JS, Breivik H, Fosse E. Magnetic resonance imaging demonstrates lack of precision in needle placement by the infraclavicular brachial plexus block described by Raj et al. *Anesth Analg.* 1999;88:593–598.

10. Perello A, Ashford NS, Dolin SJ. Coeliac plexus block using computed tomography guidance. *Palliat Med.* 1999;13:419–425.

11. Eskey CJ, Ogilvy CS. Fluoroscopy-guided lumbar puncture: decreased frequency of traumatic tap and implications for the assessment of CT-negative acute subarachnoid hemorrhage. *AJNR Am J Neuroradiol.* 2001;22:571–576.

12. Marhofer P, Greher M, Kapral S. Ultrasound guidance in regional anaesthesia. *Br J Anaesth.* 2005;94:7–17.

13. Abrahams MS, Aziz MF, Fu RF, Horn JL. Ultrasound guidance compared with electrical neurostimulation for peripheral nerve block: a systematic review and meta-analysis of randomized controlled trials. *Br J Anaesth.* 2009;102:408–417.

14. Gofeld M, Christakis M. Sonographically guided ilioinguinal nerve block. *J Ultrasound Med.* 2006;25:1571–1575.

15. Greher M, Scharbert G, Kamolz LP, et al. Ultrasound-guided lumbar facet nerve block: a sonoanatomic study of a new methodologic approach. *Anesthesiology.* 2004;100:1242–1248.

16. Chen CP, Tang SF, Hsu TC, et al. Ultrasound guidance in caudal epidural needle placement. *Anesthesiology.* 2004;101:181–184.

17. Bogin IN, Stulin ID. Application of the method of 2-dimensional echospondylography for determining landmarks in lumbar punctures. *Zh Nevropatol Psikhiatr Im S S Korsakova.* 1971;71:1810–1811.

18. Porter RW, Wicks M, Ottewell D. Measurement of the spinal canal by diagnostic ultrasound. *J Bone Joint Surg Br.* 1978;60-B:481–484.

19. Cork RC, Kryc JJ, Vaughan RW. Ultrasonic localization of the lumbar epidural space. *Anesthesiology.* 1980;52:513–516.

20. Currie JM. Measurement of the depth to the extradural space using ultrasound. *Br J Anaesth.* 1984;56:345–347.

21. Wallace DH, Currie JM, Gilstrap LC, Santos R. Indirect sonographic guidance for epidural anesthesia in obese pregnant patients. *Reg Anesth.* 1992;17:233–236.

22. Grau T, Leipold RW, Horter J, Conradi R, Martin EO, Motsch J. Paramedian access to the epidural space: the optimum window for ultrasound imaging. *J Clin Anesth.* 2001;13:213–217.

23. Grau T, Leipold RW, Conradi R, Martin E. Ultrasound control for presumed difficult epidural puncture. *Acta Anaesthesiol Scand.* 2001;45:766–771.

24. Grau T, Leipold RW, Conradi R, Martin E, Motsch J. Ultrasound imaging facilitates localization of the epidural space during combined spinal and epidural anesthesia. *Reg Anesth Pain Med.* 2001;26:64–67.

25. Grau T, Leipold RW, Delorme S, Martin E, Motsch J. Ultrasound imaging of the thoracic epidural space. *Reg Anesth Pain Med.* 2002;27:200–206.

26. Grau T, Leipold RW, Conradi R, Martin E, Motsch J. Efficacy of ultrasound imaging in obstetric epidural anesthesia. *J Clin Anesth*. 2002;14:169–175.

27. Grau T. The evaluation of ultrasound imaging for neuraxial anesthesia. *Can J Anaesth*. 2003;50: R1–R8.

28. Grau T, Bartusseck E, Conradi R, Martin E, Motsch J. Ultrasound imaging improves learning curves in obstetric epidural anesthesia: a preliminary study. *Can J Anaesth*. 2003;50:1047–1050.

29. Grau T, Leipold RW, Fatehi S, Martin E, Motsch J. Real-time ultrasonic observation of combined spinal-epidural anaesthesia. *Eur J Anaesthesiol*. 2004;21:25–31.

30. Karmakar MK, Li X, Ho AM, Kwok WH, Chui PT. Real-time ultrasound-guided paramedian epidural access: evaluation of a novel in-plane technique. *Br J Anaesth*. 2009;102:845–854.

31. Ferre RM, Sweeney TW. Emergency physicians can easily obtain ultrasound images of anatomical landmarks relevant to lumbar puncture. *Am J Emerg Med*. 2007;25:291–296.

32. Peterson MA, Abele J. Bedside ultrasound for difficult lumbar puncture. *J Emerg Med*. 2005;28: 197–200.

33. Arzola C, Davies S, Rofaeel A, Carvalho JC. Ultrasound using the transverse approach to the lumbar spine provides reliable landmarks for labor epidurals. *Anesth Analg*. 2007;104:1188–1192.

34. Carvalho JC. Ultrasound-facilitated epidurals and spinals in obstetrics. *Anesthesiol Clin*. 2008;26:145–158.

35. Mathieu S, Dalgleish DJ. A survey of local opinion of NICE guidance on the use of ultrasound in the insertion of epidural catheters. *Anaesthesia*. 2008;63:1146-1147.

36. National Institute for Clinical Excellence. Guidance on ultrasound guided catheterisation of the epidural space. Interventional Procedure Guidance No 249, January 2008. http://www.nice. org.uk.

37. Karmakar MK, Li X, Kwok WH, Ho AM, Ngan Kee WD. The "water-based-spine-phantom" – a small step towards learning the basics of spinal sonography. *Brit J Anaesth*. 2009;E-letters. http:// bja.oxfordjournals.org/cgi/qa-display/short/brjana_el;4114.

38. Tsui BC, Tarkkila P, Gupta S, Kearney R. Confirmation of caudal needle placement using nerve stimulation. *Anesthesiology*. 1999;91:374–378.

39. Chen CP, Wong AM, Hsu CC, et al. Ultrasound as a screening tool for proceeding with caudal epidural injections. *Arch Phys Med Rehabil*. 2010;91:358–363.

40. Habib AS, George RB, Allen TK, Olufolabi AJ. A pilot study to compare the Episure Autodetect syringe with the glass syringe for identification of the epidural space in parturients. *Anesth Analg*. 2008;106:541–543.

41. Rapp HJ, Folger A, Grau T. Ultrasound-guided epidural catheter insertion in children. *Anesth Analg*. 2005;101:333–339.

42. Costello JF, Balki M. Cesarean delivery under ultrasound-guided spinal anesthesia [corrected] in a parturient with poliomyelitis and Harrington instrumentation. *Can J Anaesth*. 2008;55:606–611.

43. Prasad GA, Tumber PS, Lupu CM. Ultrasound guided spinal anesthesia. *Can J Anaesth*. 2008;55:716–717.

44. Coley BD, Shiels WE, Hogan MJ. Diagnostic and interventional ultrasonography in neonatal and infant lumbar puncture. *Pediatr Radiol*. 2001;31:399-402.

45. Yamauchi M, Honma E, Mimura M, Yamamoto H, Takahashi E, Namiki A. Identification of the lumbar intervertebral level using ultrasound imaging in a post-laminectomy patient. *J Anesth*. 2006;20:231–233.

46. Yeo ST, French R. Combined spinal-epidural in the obstetric patient with Harrington rods assisted by ultrasonography. *Br J Anaesth*. 1999;83:670–672.

47. Chin KJ, Chan VW, Ramlogan R, Perlas A. Real-time ultrasound-guided spinal anesthesia in patients with a challenging spinal anatomy: two case reports. *Acta Anaesthesiol Scand*. 2010;54: 252–255.

48. McLeod A, Roche A, Fennelly M. Case series: ultrasonography may assist epidural insertion in scoliosis patients. *Can J Anaesth*. 2005;52:717–720.

49. Asakura Y, Kandatsu N, Hashimoto A, Kamiya M, Akashi M, Komatsu T. Ultrasound-guided neuroaxial anesthesia: accurate diagnosis of spina bifida occulta by ultrasonography. *J Anesth*. 2009;23:312–313.

50. Balki M, Lee Y, Halpern S, Carvalho JC. Ultrasound imaging of the lumbar spine in the transverse plane: the correlation between estimated and actual depth to the epidural space in obese parturients. *Anesth Analg*. 2009;108:1876–1881.

51. Lee Y, Tanaka M, Carvalho JC. Sonoanatomy of the lumbar spine in patients with previous unintentional dural punctures during labor epidurals. *Reg Anesth Pain Med*. 2008;33:266–270.

52. Margarido CB, Arzola C, Balki M, Carvalho JC. Anesthesiologists' learning curves for ultrasound assessment of the lumbar spine. *Can J Anaesth*. 2010;57:120-126.

13

Ultrasound-Guided Caudal, Ganglion Impar, and Sacroiliac Joint Injections

Amaresh Vydyanathan and Samer N. Narouze

S.N. Narouze (✉)
Center for Pain Medicine, Summa Western Reserve Hospital, 1900 23rd St,
Cuyahoga Falls, OH 44223, USA
e-mail: narouzs@hotmail.com

S.N. Narouze (ed.), *Atlas of Ultrasound-Guided Procedures in Interventional Pain Management*,
DOI 10.1007/978-1-4419-1681-5_13, © Springer Science+Business Media, LLC 2011

Ultrasound-Guided Caudal Epidural Injections

Anatomy

The sacrum and coccyx are formed by the fusion of eight vertebrae (five sacral and three coccygeal vertebrae). There is a natural defect resulting from incomplete fusion of the lower portion of S4 and entire S5 in the posterior midline. This defect is termed the sacral hiatus and is covered by the sacrococcygeal ligament. The hiatus is bounded laterally by the sacral cornua, and the floor is comprised of the posterior aspect of the sacrum.[1,2] The epidural space extends from the base of the skull to the level of the sacral hiatus. It is the space confined between the dura mater and the ligamentum flavum and surrounds the dural sac. It is divided into anterior and posterior compartments and bounded anteriorly by the posterior longitudinal ligaments, laterally by the pedicles and neural foramina, and posteriorly by the ligamentum flavum. The epidural space contains the spinal nerve roots and the spinal artery that pass through the neural foramina and the epidural venous plexus. Below the level of S2, where the dura terminates, the epidural space continues as the caudal epidural space that can be accessed via the sacral hiatus which is covered by the sacrococcygeal membrane. The sacral epidural canal contains the sacral and coccygeal roots, spinal vessels, and the filum terminale. The epidural venous plexus is concentrated in the anterior space in the caudal epidural canal.[1,3,4]

Indications for Caudal Epidural Injection

Caudal injections are usually performed as a diagnostic or therapeutic intervention in various lumbosacral pain syndromes especially in cases of spinal stenosis and postlaminectomy syndrome where lumbar epidural access is more difficult or not desirable.

Limitations of the Landmark "Blind" Technique

Anatomical variations of the sacrum and the contents within the sacral canal pose a challenge during caudal epidural steroid injections. Variations in sacral anatomy have been reported to be as high as 10%[5] and resulted in misplaced needles in 25.9% of caudal epidural injections performed by experienced physicians without fluoroscopic guidance.[6]

Inadvertent intravascular injection has been reported to range from 2.5% to 9%[5–7] and negative needle aspiration for blood has been shown to be neither sensitive nor specific.[7,8] Intravascular injection is also more likely in elderly patients as the epidural venous plexus may continue inferior to the S4 segment in these patients.[9] This provides the rational for the need of performing caudal epidural injections with real-time imaging guidance, in order to maximize the outcome and minimize the complications.[10]

Literature Review of Ultrasound-Guided Caudal Epidural Injections

Klocke et al[11] first described the use of ultrasound imaging in performing caudal epidural steroid injections and they found it particularly useful in moderately obese patients or patients who are unable to position prone. Lower frequency transducers (2–5 MHz) in obese patients were required to achieve adequate penetration. Chen et al[12] evaluated ultrasound guidance in performing caudal epidural steroid injections in 70 patients with lumbosacral neuritis. They used a high-frequency transducer (5–12 MHz) to identify the sacral hiatus. The needle position was then confirmed by contrast fluoroscopy. They had a 100% success rate in needle placement but observed that the needle tip was no longer visualized after needle advancing into the sacral epidural space secondary to the bony artifacts. This eliminated the possibility of identifying a dural tear or intravascular placement other than needle aspiration. This led Yoon et al[10] to evaluate the use of color Doppler ultrasonography for caudal injections to identify intravascular placement. They injected 5 ml of the injectate while observing the flow spectrum in color Doppler mode. They defined the injection as successful if unidirectional flow (observed as one dominant color) of the solution was observed with color Doppler through the epidural space, with no flows being observed in other directions (observed as multiple colors). The correct placement of the needle was then verified by contrast fluoroscopy. In three patients, including two with positive Doppler spectrum, the contrast dye was outside of the epidural space.

Ultrasound-Guided Caudal Injection Is Better than the "Blind" Technique

A retrospective study of caudal injections in 83 pediatric patients comparing the accuracy of caudal needle placement with the "swoosh" test, 2D transverse ultrasonographic evidence of turbulence within the caudal space, and color flow Doppler concluded that ultrasonography is superior to the "swoosh" test as an objective confirmatory technique during caudal block placement in children.[13] They found the presence of turbulence during injection within the caudal space to be the best single indicator of block success.

Ultrasound-Guided Technique for Caudal Epidural Injection

With the patient in the prone position, the sacral hiatus is palpated and a linear high-frequency transducer (or curved low frequency transducer in obese patients) is placed transversely in the midline to obtain a transverse view of the sacral hiatus.[12] The bony prominences of the two sacral cornua appear as two hyperechoic reversed U-shaped structures. Between the two cornua, two hyperechoic band-like structures, the sacrococcygeal ligament superiorly and the dorsal bony surface of the sacrum inferiorly can be identified and the sacral hiatus is the hypoechoic area in between (Figure 13.1). A 22-gauge needle is then inserted between the two cornua into the sacral hiatus. A "pop" or "give" is usually felt when the sacrococcygeal ligament is penetrated. The transducer is then rotated 90° to obtain a longitudinal view of the sacrum and sacral hiatus and the needle is advanced into the sacral canal under real-time sonographic guidance (Figures 13.2 and 13.3).

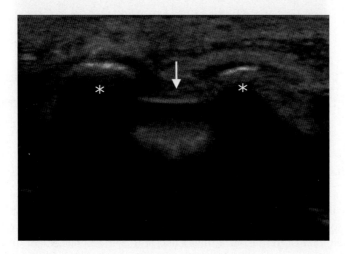

Figure 13.1. Short-axis sonogram showing the two sacral cornua (*asterisk*) as two hyperechoic reversed U-shaped structures. *Arrows* point at the sacrococcygeal ligament covering the sacral hiatus. Reprinted with permission from Ohio Pain and Headache Institute.

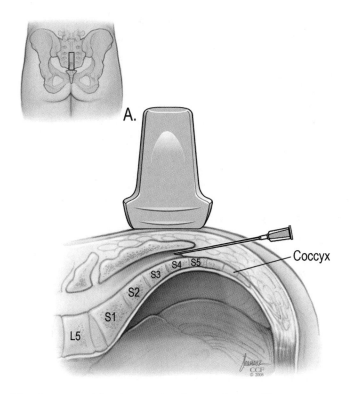

Figure 13.2. The placement of the ultrasound probe over the sacral hiatus to obtain a longitudinal scan is shown. Reprinted with permission, Cleveland Clinic Center for Medical Art & Photography© 2008–2010. All rights reserved.

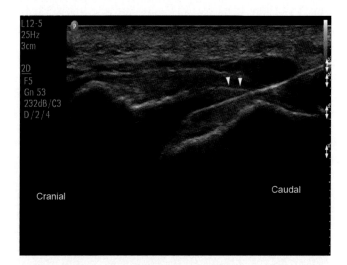

Figure 13.3. Long axis sonogram showing the needle (in plane) inside the caudal epidural space. *Arrow heads* pointing at the sacrococcygeal ligament. Reprinted with permission, Cleveland Clinic Center for Medical Art & Photography© 2008–2010. All rights reserved.

Limitations of the Ultrasound-Guided Technique

In adults, it is usually difficult to follow the needle inside the sacral canal secondary to the bony artifacts from the sacrum and accordingly a dural puncture or intravascular placement cannot be readily identified. As negative aspiration is not reliable, we recommend test dose injection first to rule out intravascular or intrathecal placement. Injection is carried out under real-time sonographic guidance with monitoring of the turbulence in the sacral canal and the spread of the injectate cephalad. Color Doppler mode may be used to

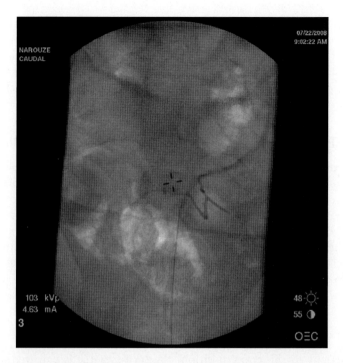

Figure 13.4. AP x-ray showing intravascular spread of the contrast agent during caudal epidural injection. Reprinted with permission from Ohio Pain and Headache Institute.

facilitate this as discussed above,[10] but it is very unreliable as turbulence from the injectate can be interpreted as flow in many directions and can be misinterpreted as intravascular injection. Contrast fluoroscopy remains the best tool to evaluate inadvertent intravascular needle placement in this area (Figure 13.4). Ultrasound can be used if fluoroscopy is unavailable or contraindicated or as an adjunct to guide needle placement into the sacral canal in difficult patients.

Ultrasound-Guided Ganglion Impar Block

Anatomy

The ganglion impar is a solitary neural structure located anterior to the sacrococcygeal joint (SCJ). It represents the fusion of the caudal end of the bilateral sympathetic chains. The ganglion impar innervates the perineum, distal rectum, anal canal, distal urethra, scrotum, distal third of the vagina, and the vulva.[14,15]

Indications

Ganglion impar (ganglion of Walther or sacrococcygeal ganglion) block is used in the diagnosis and management of visceral or sympathetic-maintained pain in the perineal and coccygeal areas. Ganglion impar neurolysis has been reported in the palliative treatment for malignant pain.[14,16]

Limitations of the Current Technique

Multiple approaches have been described for ganglion impar block. The most widely used approach is the transsacrococcygeal approach with fluoroscopy by introducing the needle through the SCJ.[17,18]

Impacted stool or gas in the rectum can easily obscure the SCJ in the anteroposterior fluoroscopy view. Also a calcified sacrococcygeal disk will make it difficult to identify the SCJ even in the lateral fluoroscopy view.

With fluoroscopy, the needle may get stuck in the SCJ, however under US guidance, we can easily penetrate the SCJ by changing the needle's direction to match the angulation of the SCJ.[19]

Literature Review on Ultrasound-Guided Ganglion Impar Block

The classic transanococcygeal approach (curved needle placed through the anococcygeal ligament) was described with ultrasound guidance.[20] However, the authors prefer the transsacrococcygeal approach as it is more comfortable to the patient and it may avoid anal or rectal injuries.

Lin et al reported the safety of ultrasound-guided transsacrococcygeal approach in 15 patients.[19] The needle was accurately placed in all patients as confirmed with fluoroscopy. They reported that ultrasound was advantageous over fluoroscopy as the SCJ was easily identified in all 15 patients while it was difficult to visualize in 5 patients with fluoroscopy alone as the SCJ was obscured by rectal gas, impacted stool, or ossified sacrococcygeal disks.

Technique of Ultrasound-Guided Ganglion Impar Block

With the patient in the prone position, the sacral hiatus is palpated and a linear high-frequency transducer (or curved low-frequency transducer in obese patients) is placed transversely in the midline to obtain a transverse view of the sacral hiatus as described above in caudal block (Figure. 13.1). The transducer is then rotated 90° to obtain a longitudinal view of the sacral hiatus and the coccyx (Figure 13.5). The first cleft caudal to the sacral hiatus is the SCJ.

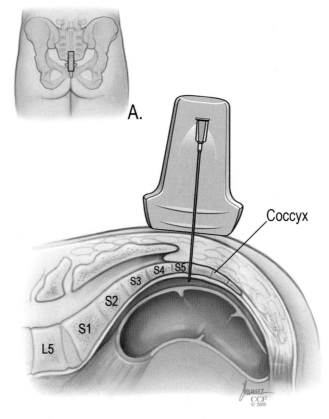

Figure 13.5. The placement of the ultrasound probe over the sacrococcygeal joint (SCJ) to obtain a longitudinal scan is shown. Reprinted with permission, Cleveland Clinic Center for Medical Art & Photography© 2008–2010. All rights reserved.

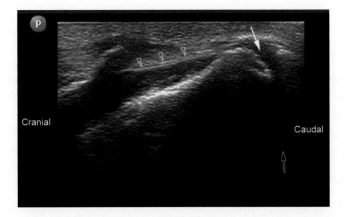

Figure 13.6. Long-axis sonogram showing the SCJ (*solid arrow*) and the sacrococcygeal ligament (*arrow heads*). Notice that the rectum (*hollow arrow*) can be insonated through the sacrococcygeal cleft. Reprinted with permission from Ohio Pain and Headache Institute.

After local anesthesia infiltration of the skin and subcutaneous tissue, a 22–25-gauge needle is then advanced into the SCJ under real-time ultrasonography. We use an out-of-plane approach while adjusting the needle's path to match the angulation of the SCJ cleft to allow for a traumatic needle insertion (Figure 13.6). The needle is advanced slightly through the SCJ cleft, and usually loss of resistance is felt indicating placement of the needle tip anterior to the ventral sacrococcygeal ligament. Lateral fluoroscopy may be obtained to confirm the depth of the needle and to monitor the spread of the injectate.

Limitations of the Ultrasound-Guided Technique

Ultrasound cannot accurately monitor the needle depth or the spread of the injectate because of the sacral and coccygeal bony artifacts. Ultrasound can be helpful when fluoroscopy is not available or insufficient in identifying the SCJ. We recommend using lateral fluoroscopic view to monitor the depth of the needle especially with neurolytic injections.[19]

Ultrasound-Guided Sacroiliac Joint Injection

Anatomy

The sacroiliac joint (SIJ) is a true diarthrodial joint with the articular surfaces of the sacrum and ilium separated by a joint space enclosed in a fibrous capsule.[21] It bears characteristics of a synovial joint, especially in the superoanterior and inferior aspects of the joint. The superoposterior joint surface lacks a joint capsule and contains the interosseous ligament. The anterior joint capsule gives origin to the anterior sacroiliac ligament. The posterior aspect also contains the posterior sacroiliac, sacrotuberous, and sacrospinous ligaments that stabilize the joint. With increasing age, degenerative changes occur with narrowing of the synovial cleft inferiorly and subsequent fibrous ankylosis.[22,23]

The muscular and fascial support of the SIJ is derived from the gluteus maximus and medius, the erector spinae, latissimus dorsi and thoracolumbar fascia, the biceps femoris, piriformis and the oblique muscles, and the transversus abdominis. The gluteus maximus, biceps, and piriformis attach to the sacrotuberous ligament while the thoracodorsal fascia connects to the remaining muscle groups. The anteroposterior and superoinferior wedge-shaped sacrum (forming a keystone configuration) and this extensive muscular support account for reduced mobility but high stability of the SIJ.[22-25] The posterior SIJ is predominantly innervated by lateral branches of the L4-S2 nerve roots with contributions from S3 and the superior gluteal nerve. The anterior SIJ innervation is from the L2-S2 segments.[26,27] The synovial capsule and ligaments contain free nerve endings as well as mechanoreceptors that transmit proprioceptive and pain sensation from the joint.[23]

Indications for SIJ Injection

Diagnostic SIJ injection: To identify pain stemming from the SIJ. Most provocative tests for diagnosing SIJ pain are not definitive and SIJ injections remain the gold standard. There are also no imaging studies that consistently provide findings to diagnose SIJ as the source of pain.

Therapeutic SIJ injection: After failure of conservative treatment including anti-inflammatory medications and physical therapy.

Literature Review on Ultrasound-Guided SIJ Injection

Pekkafahli et al[28] studied the feasibility of ultrasound-guided SIJ injections and reported a 76.7% overall success rate ($N = 60$), with a steep learning curve. The success rate improved from 60% with the first 30 injections to 93.5% in the next 30 injections. Klauser et al[29] assessed the feasibility of ultrasound-guided SIJ injection in ten human cadavers bilaterally at two different puncture sites. Upper level was defined at the level of the first posterior sacral foramen and the lower level at the level of the second posterior sacral foramen. Then they attempted the injection in ten patients with unilateral sacroiliitis. Computed tomography confirmed correct intra-articular needle placement in cadavers by showing the tip of the needle in the joint and intra-articular diffusion of contrast media in 80% of cases (upper level 70%; lower level 90%). In patients, 100% of US-guided injections were successful (eight lower levels, two upper levels).

Technique of Ultrasound-Guided SIJ Injection

The patient is placed in the prone position with a pillow underneath the abdomen to minimize lumbar lordosis. Usually a low-frequency curvilinear transducer is used, especially in obese patients to increase penetration. The transducer is placed transversely over the lower part of the sacrum (at the level of the sacral hiatus) and the lateral edge of the sacrum is identified. Then the transducer is moved laterally and cephalad till the bony contour of the ileum is clearly identified (Figure 13.7). The cleft seen between the medial border of the ileum and the lateral sacral edge represents the SI joint and the inferior most point is targeted.[30] A 22-gauge needle is then inserted at the medial end of the transducer and advanced laterally under direct vision in-plane with the ultrasound beam till it is seen entering the joint (Figure 13.8).

Limitations of Ultrasound-Guided SIJ Injection

The potential for periarticular rather than intra-articular injection may be increased compared to fluoroscopic or CT-guided SIJ injections as one can reliably obtain an arthrogram with contrast agent injection in most cases with the latter technique. Also, ultrasound is not very reliable in detecting intravascular injection while performing SIJ injections (Figure 13.9).

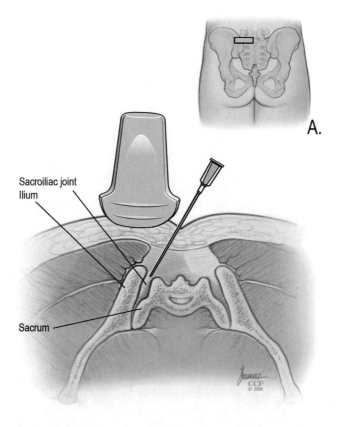

Figure 13.7. The placement of the ultrasound probe over the sacroiliac joint (SIJ) to obtain a short axis view is shown. Reprinted with permission, Cleveland Clinic Center for Medical Art & Photography© 2008–2010. All rights reserved.v

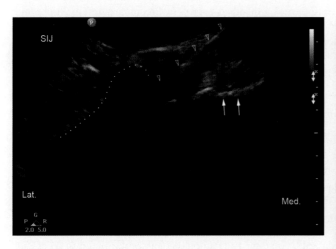

Figure 13.8. Short-axis sonogram showing the needle (in plane) inside the SIJ (*arrow heads*). The *dotted lines* outline the bony surface of the ilium and the *arrows* point at the dorsal surface of the sacrum. Reprinted with permission, Cleveland Clinic Center for Medical Art & Photography© 2008–2010. All rights reserved.

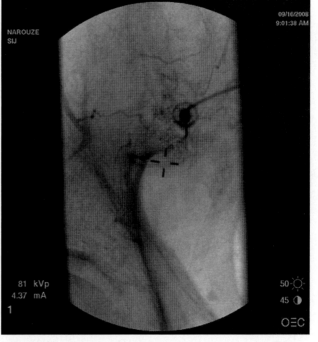

Figure 13.9. AP x-ray showing intravascular spread of the contrast agent during SIJ injection. Reprinted with permission from Ohio Pain and Headache Institute.

References

1. Senoglu N, Senoglu M, Oksuz H, et al. Landmarks of the sacral hiatus for caudal epidural block: an anatomical study. *Br J Anaesth*. 2005;95(5):692–695.

2. Hession WG, Stanczak JD, Davis KW, Choi JJ. Epidural steroid injections. *Semin Roentgenol*. 2004;39(1):7–23.

3. Parkin IG, Harrison GR. The topographical anatomy of the lumbar epidural space. *J Anat*. 1985;141:211–217.

4. Sekiguchi M, Yabuki S, Satoh K, Kikuchi S. An anatomic study of the sacral hiatus: a basis for successful caudal epidural block. *Clin J Pain*. 2004;20(1):51–54.

5. White AH, Derby R, Wynne G. Epidural injections for the diagnosis and treatment of low-back pain. *Spine*. 1980;5:78–86.

6. Stitz MY, Sommer HM. Accuracy of blind versus fluoroscopically guided caudal epidural injection. *Spine*. 1999;24:1371–1376.

7. Renfrew DL, Moore TE, Kathol MH, el-Khoury GY, Lemke JH, Walker CW. Correct placement of epidural steroid injections: fluoroscopic guidance and contrast administration. *AJNR Am J Neuroradiol*. 1991;12:1003–1007.

8. Furman MB, O'Brien EM, Zgleszewski TM. Incidence of intravascular penetration in transforaminal lumbosacral epidural steroid injections. *Spine*. 2000;25:2628–2632.

9. Bogduk N, Cherry D. Epidural corticosteroid agents for sciatica. *Med J Aust*. 1985;143:402–406.

10. Yoon JS, Sim KH, Kim SJ, Kim WS, Koh SB, Kim BJ. The feasibility of color Doppler ultrasonography for caudal epidural steroid injection. *Pain*. 2005;118:210–214.

11. Klocke R, Jenkinson T, Glew D. Sonographically guided caudal epidural steroid injections. *J Ultrasound Med*. 2003;22:1229–1232.

12. Chen CP, Tang SF, Hsu TC, et al. Ultrasound guidance in caudal epidural needle placement. *Anesthesiology*. 2004;101:181–184.

13. Raghunathan K, Schwartz D, Connelly NR. Determining the accuracy of caudal needle placement in children: a comparison of the swoosh test and ultrasonography. *Paediatr Anaesth*. 2008;18:606–612.

14. Waldman SD. Hypogastric plexus block and impar ganglion block. In: Waldman SD, ed. *Pain Management*. Philadelphia, PA: Saunders/Elsevier; 2007:1354–1357.

15. Reig E, Abejon D, del Pozo C, Insausti J, Contreras R. Thermocoagulation of the ganglion impar or ganglion of Walther: description of a modified approach. Preliminary results in chronic, nononcological pain. *Pain Pract*. 2005;5:103–110.

16. de Leon-Casasola OA. Critical evaluation of chemical neurolysis of the sympathetic axis for cancer pain. *Cancer Control*. 2000;7(2):142–148.

17. Wemm K Jr, Saberski L. Modified approach to block the ganglion impar (ganglion of Walther). *Reg Anesth*. 1995;20:544–545.

18. Toshniwal GR, Dureja GP, Prashanth SM. Transsacrococcygeal approach to ganglion impar block for management of chronic perineal pain: a prospective observational study. *Pain Physician*. 2007;10:661–666.

19. Lin CS, Cheng JK, Hsu YW, et al. Ultrasound-guided ganglion impar block: a technical report. *Pain Med*. 2010;11:390–394.

20. Gupta D, Jain R, Mishra S, Kumar S, Thulkar S, Bhatnagar S. Ultrasonography reinvents the originally described technique for ganglion impar neurolysis in perianal cancer pain. *Anesth Analg*. 2008;107(4):1390–1392.

21. Forst SL, Wheeler MT, Fortin JD, Vilensky JA. The sacroiliac joint: anatomy, physiology and clinical significance. *Pain Physician*. 2006;9:61–67.

22. Calvillo O, Skaribas I, Turnipseed J. Anatomy and pathophysiology of the sacroiliac joint. *Curr Rev Pain*. 2000;4:356–361.

23. Dreyfuss P, Dreyer SJ, Cole A, Mayo K. Sacroiliac joint pain. *J Am Acad Orthop Surg*. 2004;12: 255–265.

24. Foley BS, Buschbacher RM. Sacroiliac joint pain: anatomy, biomechanics, diagnosis, and treatment. *Am J Phys Med Rehabil*. 2006;85:997–1006.

25. Tuite MJ. Facet joint and sacroiliac joint injection. *Semin Roentgenol*. 2004;39:37–51.

26. Ikeda R. Innervation of the sacroiliac joint. Macroscopical and histological studies. *Nippon Ika Daigaku Zasshi*. 1991;58:587–596.

27. Grob KR, Neuhuber WL, Kissling RO. Innervation of the sacroiliac joint of the human. *Z Rheumatol*. 1995;54:117–122.

28. Pekkafahli MZ, Kiralp MZ, Ba ekim CC, et al. Sacroiliac joint injections performed with sonographic guidance. *J Ultrasound Med.* 2003;22:553–559.
29. Klauser A, De Zordo T, Feuchtner G, et al. Feasibility of ultrasound-guided sacroiliac joint injection considering sonoanatomic landmarks at two different levels in cadavers and patients. *Arthritis Rheum.* 2008;59:1618–1624.
30. Harmon D, O'Sullivan M. Ultrasound-guided sacroiliac joint injection technique. *Pain Physician.* 2008;11:543–547.

III

Ultrasound-Guided Abdominal and Pelvic Blocks

14

Ultrasound-Guided Transversus Abdominis Plane (TAP) Block

Samer N. Narouze

Introduction

The transversus abdominis plane (TAP) block is used to produce a dermatomal sensory block of the lower thoracic and upper lumbar afferents. With ultrasound imaging, the muscle layers are visible from the rectus medially through the aponeurotic area at the edge of the rectus to the three distinct layers of external, internal oblique, and transversus abdominis in the lateral abdominal wall. Installation of local anesthetics in this plane anesthetizes the anterior abdominal wall on this side. This block can be used as a diagnostic tool or as a therapeutic modality via a continuous indwelling catheter for postoperative lower abdominal pain or chronic pain syndromes arising from the anterior abdominal wall.

S.N. Narouze (✉)
Center for Pain Medicine, Summa Western Reserve Hospitals,
1900 23rd Street, Cuyahoga Falls, OH 44223, USA
e-mail: narouzs@hotmail.com

S.N. Narouze (ed.), *Atlas of Ultrasound-Guided Procedures in Interventional Pain Management*,
DOI 10.1007/978-1-4419-1681-5_14, © Springer Science+Business Media, LLC 2011

TAP block is a new technique for peripheral nerve blockade of the thoraco-lumbar nerves supplying the anterior abdominal wall and had been investigated for different applications for perioperative pain management following abdominal surgeries. The introduction of ultrasound-guided regional anesthesia allows the successful installation of local anesthetics around the anterior branches of the thoraco-lumbar ventral rami blocking somatic sensations from the anterior abdominal wall. Single injection as well as continuous infusions can be used for the treatment of chronic pain syndromes following lower abdominal open and laparoscopic surgeries.[1]

Abdominal pain is one of the most frequent complaints to a primary care physician, accounting for nearly 2.5 million office visits per year and in up to 50% of patients, no identifiable cause can be found.[2]

Somatosensory pain (abdominal wall pain) can be sometimes confused with the visceral pain origin and a differential epidural block is often performed to help differentiate between the two types of pain.[3] However, the interpretation of the differential epidural test sometimes is very confusing. It is time-consuming (takes few hours) and it carries the limitations and disadvantages of neuroaxial blocks. The author found that TAP block is very valuable in diagnosing pain stemming from the abdominal wall and thus help differentiate between somatosensory (abdominal wall) vs. visceral origin of pain.[1]

Anatomy

The abdominal wall consists of three muscle layers, the external oblique, the internal oblique, and the transversus abdominis and their associated fascial sheaths. These muscles are mainly innervated via the ipsilateral ventral rami of T7-L1 thoraco-lumbar nerves. After emerging through the intervertebral foramina, they follow a curvilinear course forward in the intercostal spaces toward the midline of the body. Along this course, they enter a fascial plane between the transversus abdominis and the internal oblique muscles what is known as the TAP accompanied by blood vessels. This neurovascular plan continues as far as the semilunar line. At the lateral border of the rectus abdominis muscle, the external oblique and the anterior lamella of the internal oblique aponeuroses pass anterior to the muscle forming the anterior rectus sheath. The aponeuroses from the posterior lamella of the internal oblique muscle and the transversus abdominis muscle pass posterior to the rectus muscle forming the posterior layer of the sheath. At this point, the ventral rami of the thoracic spinal nerves are located between the posterior border of the rectus muscle and the posterior rectus sheath. They run medially within the sheath before perforating the muscle anteriorly forming the anterior cutaneous branches.[4]

The anterior ramus of the 10th thoracic nerve reaches the skin at the level of the umbilicus, and the 12th thoracic nerve innervates the skin of the hypogastrium. The iliohypogastric and ilioinguinal nerves follow a similar course; however, they pierce the internal oblique muscle at different levels near the anterior superior iliac spine to supply the inguinal region (for more details, please refer to Chapter 16).

The Classic Approach

The TAP block was first described by Rafi and McDonell as a blind "double-pop" technique using a blunt needle introduced through the external and internal oblique muscles and fascia at the ilio-lumbar triangle of Petit.[5,6] This triangle is bounded posteriorly by the latissimus dorsi muscle and anteriorly by the external oblique, with the iliac crest forming the base of the triangle. The introduction of ultrasound allows modification of this technique and the TAP can be accessed anywhere between the iliac crest and costal margin behind the anterior axillary line. A higher subcostal approach may block the upper thoraco-lumbar nerves more effectively than a lower approach immediately above the iliac crest.[7]

Ultrasound-Guided Technique

The patient is positioned in the lateral decubitus position with the side to be blocked upward. A wedge can be placed underneath the patient in order to stretch the flank on the upper side. A high frequency or lower frequency transducers may be used according to body habitus. Preprocedural scanning of the anterior abdominal wall along the midaxillary line is recommended to decide the best view of the three muscle layers. Care should be taken that scanning more medially may only show two layers of muscles since the external oblique muscle forms an aponeurosis that joins the rectus sheath. From superficial to deep the following structures are recognized: skin and subcutaneous fat, external oblique, internal oblique, and transversus abdominis muscles with their investing fascia (Figures 14.1 and 14.2). Deeper to the transversus abdominis and its fascia, there is a fatty layer of preperitoneal

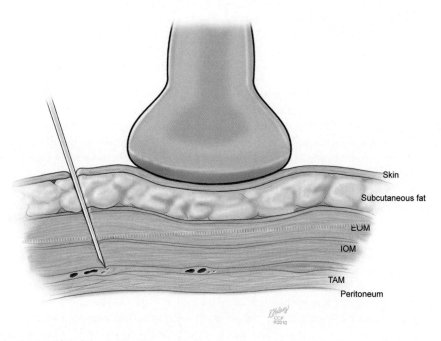

Figure 14.1. The abdominal wall muscles and the ultrasound transducer in place for performing TAP block is shown.

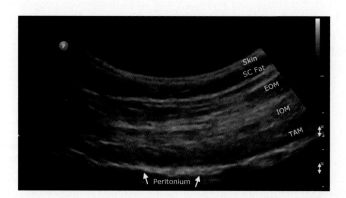

Figure 14.2. Preinjection short axis sonogram showing the abdominal wall muscle layers. *EOM* external oblique muscle, *IOM* internal oblique muscle, *TAM* transversus abdominis muscle. (Reprinted with permission from Ohio Pain and Headache Institute).

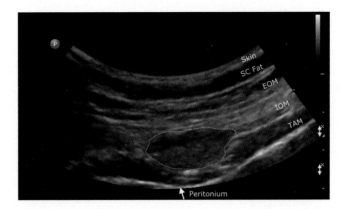

Figure 14.3. Postinjection short axis sonogram showing the spread of the injectate in the plane between the internal oblique muscle (IOM) and the transversus abdominis muscle (TAM). Note that the TAM and the peritoneum were pushed away by the injectate. (Reprinted with permission from Ohio Pain and Headache Institute).

fat separating it from the peritoneum and the bowels, which are often identified by its peristaltic movements. With ultrasound, the fascial layers appear as hyperechoic layers (whiter than the surrounding structures), and the muscles are identified by their relative hypoechoic structure with multiple striations. The neural structures are usually difficult to identify; however, scanning immediately cephalad to the ASIS can identify the iliohypogastric and ilioinguinal nerves (for more details, please refer to Chap. 21.)

The needle is inserted in-plane (parallel to the ultrasound beam) from the posterolateral side of the probe and is advanced in a medial and anterior direction. In order to have a clear picture of the needle, it is preferable to introduce it 1–2 in. far from the probe to avoid a steep introductory angle that can be unfavorable for the reflection of the ultrasound beam. The needle is advanced through the different layers with a tactile feeling of a "pop" when crossing each fascial layer. Gentle tapping on the needle can help identifying the tip advancing under ultrasound. Alternatively, the appropriate plane can be confirmed by injection of few millimeters of saline or local anesthetics (hydrolocalization). Correct placement is identified by the solution separating the internal oblique muscle superficially from the transversus abdominis muscle deep (Figure 14.3). Care should be taken to identify the injection along the appropriate plane vs. intramuscular injection, which leads to swelling of the muscles instead of separation.

It is important to use a blunt-tip needle for the TAP block to appreciate the tactile feedbacks when crossing different layers and to minimize the chances of peritoneal and bowel perforation. For single shot block, a blunt 22 G needle can be used while a Tuohy needle is used for continuous catheter technique. When a catheter is required, the space is dissected using 10 ml of saline followed by catheter insertion for about 5 cm beyond the tip of the needle.

Summary

Ultrasound-guided TAP block is a novel block with multiple applications for pain control following various lower abdominal surgeries. It produces a unilateral analgesia between the coastal margin and the inguinal ligament. It may also have applications in the diagnosis and management of chronic abdominal pain syndromes. Ultrasound-guided iliohypogastric and ilioinguinal nerve blocks are essentially a TAP block performed near the level of ASIS.

REFERENCES

1. Soliman LM, Narouze S. Ultrasound-guided transversus abdominis plane block for the management of abdominal pain: an alternative to differential epidural block. *Tech Reg Anesth Pain Manag.* 2009;13(3):117–120.
2. Klinkman MS. Episodes of care for abdominal pain in a primary care practice. *Arch Fam Med.* 1996;5:279–285.
3. Conwell DL, Vargo JJ, Zuccaro G, et al. Role of differential neuroaxial blockade in the evaluation and management of pain in chronic pancreatitis. *Am J Gastroenterol.* 2001;96:431-436.
4. Rozen WM, Tran TM, Ashton MW, Barrington MJ, Ivanusic JJ, Taylor GI. Refining the course of the thoracolumbar nerves: a new understanding of the innervation of the anterior abdominal wall. *Clin Anat.* 2008;21(4):325–333.
5. Rafi AN. Abdominal field block: a new approach via the lumbar triangle. *Anaesthesia.* 2001;56:1024–1026.
6. McDonnell JG, O'Donnell BD, Curley G, et al. The analgesic efficacy of the transversus abdominis plane block after abdominal surgery: a prospective randomized controlled trial. *Anesth Analg.* 2007;104:193–197.
7. Hebbard P. Subcostal transversus abdominis plane block under ultrasound guidance. *Anesth Analg.* 2008;106:674–675.

15

Ultrasound-Guided Celiac Plexus Block and Neurolysis

Samer N. Narouze and Hannes Gruber

Introduction

Celiac plexus block has been used in various upper abdominal malignant and nonmalignant pain syndromes with variable success. Pain signals stemming from visceral structures that are innervated by the celiac plexus can be interrupted by blocking the celiac plexus or the splanchnic nerves. These structures include the pancreas, liver, gallbladder, mesentery, omentum, and gastrointestinal tract from the lower esophagus to the transverse colon.

The most common application of neurolytic celiac plexus block is upper abdominal malignancy, especially pancreatic cancer; this was first described by Kappis in 1914.[1]

H. Gruber (✉)
Department of Radiology, Innsbruck Medical University,
TILAK, Anichstrasse 35, Innsbruck 6020, Austria
e-mail: hannes.gruber@i-med.ac.at

S.N. Narouze (ed.), *Atlas of Ultrasound-Guided Procedures in Interventional Pain Management*,
DOI 10.1007/978-1-4419-1681-5_15, © Springer Science+Business Media, LLC 2011

Anatomy of the Celiac Plexus

The celiac plexus is a dense network of autonomic nerves that lies anterior to the aorta and the crus of the diaphragm at L1 level. The plexus extends for few centimeters in front of the aorta surrounding the celiac trunk and the superior mesenteric artery (SMA).

Fibers within the plexus arise from efferent sympathetic preganglionic nerves (greater splanchnic nerve T5–T9, lesser splanchnic nerve T10–T11, least splanchnic nerve T12), parasympathetic preganglionic nerves (vagus, posterior trunk), sensory nerves from the phrenic and vagus nerves, and sympathetic postganglionic fibers. Afferent nociception fibers from the abdominal viscera pass diffusely through the celiac plexus and accompany the sympathetic fibers.

Three pairs of ganglia exist within the plexus; these include the celiac ganglia, the superior mesenteric ganglia, and the aortic renal ganglia (Figure 15.1). Postganglionic sympathetic nerves from these ganglia accompany blood vessels to the upper abdominal visceral structures. These fibers may play an important role in sympathetically mediated pain syndromes.[2]

Current Techniques for Celiac Plexus Block

There are two basic methods of performing CPB, which are different depending on the final needle placement relative to the diaphragm: retrocrural or anterocrural. The retrocrural technique also referred to as the deep splanchnic nerve block is considered the classic approach. This technique results in the spread of injectate cephalad and posterior to the diaphragmatic crura (Figure 15.2). On the other hand, the anterocrural technique typically involves the insertion of the needle from a posterior approach to a final position anterior to the aorta at the level of the celiac plexus.

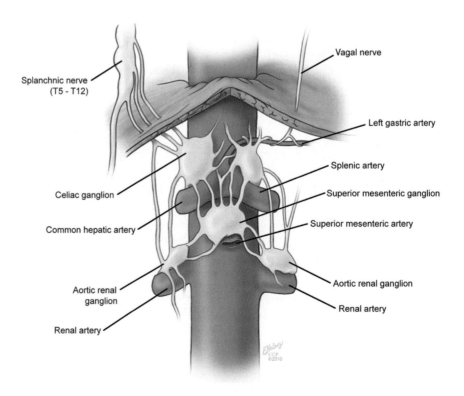

Figure 15.1. Celiac plexus anatomy. AP view. Reprinted with permission, Cleveland Clinic Center for Medical Art & Photography© 2010. All rights reserved.

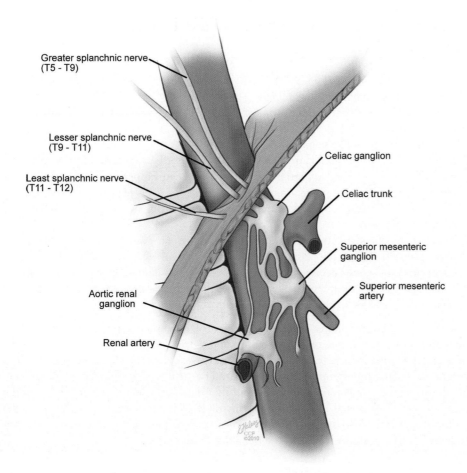

Figure 15.2. Celiac plexus anatomy. Lateral view showing the celiac plexus, the diaphragm, and the splanchnic nerves. Reprinted with permission, Cleveland Clinic Center for Medical Art & Photography© 2010. All rights reserved.

1. *Retrocrural approach or "classic" celiac plexus block (deep splanchnic block)*: This is commonly performed with fluoroscopy or CT guidance at L1 level in the prone position.[3] However, the classic technique of Kappis was performed with surface land marks in the lateral decubitus position.[1]
2. *Transcrural approach or "true" celiac plexus block*: The needle is advanced through the diaphragmatic crura and the tip is positioned on each side of the anterior aspect of the aorta with CT guidance.[4] Or the needle is advanced through the aorta with fluoroscopic guidance "transaortic approach."[5]
3. Anterocrural approach or true "anterior" approach. This was described initially using anatomical landmarks,[6] then later with CT[7] and ultrasound guidance.[8]

The Anterior Percutaneous Approach

Wendling reported the first anterior percutaneous approach to the splanchnic nerves.[6] A thin needle is inserted through the abdominal wall just below, and slightly to the left, of the xiphoid process. The needle is inserted perpendicular to the skin and advanced through the left lobe of the liver and the lesser omentum (occasionally bowel) toward the T12 vertebral body.

Interest in this technique has been revived with the introductions of the CT-guided[7] and US-guided approaches.[8]

Advantages of US-Guided Anterior Approach

1. It is the true anterocrural approach. The needle tip location is anterior to the aorta at the exact position of the celiac plexus.
2. More suitable for patients who cannot lie prone because of the abdominal pain or other reasons.
3. No radiation exposure compared to fluoroscopy or CT.
4. More suitable for terminal cancer patients that cannot be transferred to the radiology suite. The US machine is portable and the block can be performed, with adequate monitoring, in a regular procedure room.
5. Avoid injury to nerve roots and neuroaxial structures during needle placement with the posterior approach.
6. The authors believe that the most important advantage of the anterior approach is decreasing or even eliminating the potential risk of paraplegia with neurolytic celiac plexus block. Paraplegia and serious neurologic morbidity have been reported after celiac neurolysis.[9] Paraplegia now has been reported with essentially every posterior approach to celiac and splanchnic nerve technique except blockade by the anterior percutaneous approach.[2]

The most accepted postulated mechanism of neurologic injury is spinal cord ischemia or infarction as a consequence of disruption of small nutrient vessels by spasm, direct injury, or accidental intravascular injection.[2,10] Adamkiewicz's arteries, the largest spinal cord ventral radicular arteries, supply the lower ventral two thirds of the spinal cord. After leaving the aorta, they run laterally, about 80% of the time on the left, and typically reach the cord between T8 through L4, making it vulnerable to injury during celiac block by the posterior approach. Also the posterior retrocrural approach may allow the neurolytic agent to spread or leak posteriorly toward the neuroaxial structures.

Limitations of US-Guided Anterior Approach

1. Technically challenging in obese patients.
2. Patients with large pancreatic tumors or intra-abdominal masses anterior to the plexus will distort the anatomy and will make it very challenging to identify the aorta and the celiac trunk.
3. If the mass anterior to the plexus is vascular (by a prior CT or MRI) or as identified by ultrasound examination, the anterior approach should be abounded.

Sonoanatomy of the Epigastrium and Relevant Structures

The celiac plexus is a conglomerate of tiny nerve fibers and autonomic ganglia which form a rather heterogeneous tissue, that is – to date – not visualized clearly by high-resolution ultrasound. One should be familiar with the relevant sonoanatomy in order to safely and accurately perform the procedure. One landmark is the abdominal aorta, which is usually well visualized by ultrasound (best use 2–5 MHz broadband probes) in the median epigastrium as tubular pulsating more or less anechoic structure (Figure 15.3a, b). The US probe has to be tilted upward to meet the aorta as it enters the abdomen, where it is bordered by the muscular arcade of the diaphragm (Figure 15.4a, b). The first artery that arises from the aorta is the celiac trunk (CT), which provides arterial supply to the liver, stomach, spleen, and the pancreatic head. It is the "ultimate landmark" for the celiac plexus. As the celiac trunk exits the aorta, it presents as a typical ram-horn-like symmetric bifurcation (Figure 15.5a, b).

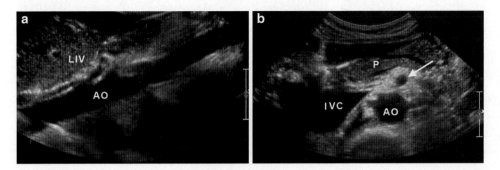

Figure 15.3. (a) Sagittal scan showing the epigastric segment of the aorta (AO) which is covered by liver tissue (LIV) anteriorly. (b) Axial scan showing the epigastric aorta (AO) as an anechoic disk neighbored by the anechoic cross section of the inferior vena cava (IVC) and covered by the pancreas (P). The *arrow* is pointing at the superior mesenteric artery (SMA).

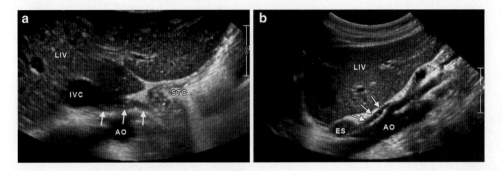

Figure 15.4. (a) Axial scan showing the muscular arcade of the aortic hiatus of the diaphragm (*three arrows*) which borders the aorta in the inferior vena cava (IVC), liver (LIV), and stomach (STO). (b) Corresponding sagittal scan showing the aorta (AO) with the first exiting arterial branches which are partially covered by the muscular arcade of the aortic hiatus (*arrows*). *ES* esophagus.

The second artery arising from the aorta is the SMA, which provides arterial supply to the proximal parts of the bowel – in combination with the CT – the pancreatic head, and the duodenum. The origins of the CT and the SMA are very close to each other that may provoke a wrong allocation in the axial scan. That is why we also perform a sagittal (longitudinal) scan to accurately identify both arteries (Figure 15.6a, b). In some rather rare cases, a common trunk for the CT and SMA is found and it serves as the unique landmark for the celiac plexus. The next artery after the SMA is the left renal artery (Figure 15.7).

So the area of the celiac plexus is broadly bordered by several organs (Figure 15.8a, b): by the left lobe of the liver, which is rather covering the scene to the ventral right; by the stomach, which frames the area to the ventral left up to its transition to the distal esophagus; and by the pancreas, which is more or less riding on the lienal vein. The cranial boundary is the diaphragm with its exiting aorta (muscular arcade of the aortic hiatus) and the esophagus (esophageal foramen). Inferiorly, the celiac plexus continues with the renal plexus around the origin of the renal arteries.

Percutaneous Ultrasound-Guided Celiac Plexus Block Technique

The patient is in the supine position and the ultrasound transducer is positioned over the epigastrium, just caudal to the xiphoid process (Figure 15.9). A scout scanning is performed so the operator will be familiar with the relevant anatomy especially in malignant cases where the anatomy may be distorted and accordingly plan on the safest and shortest path

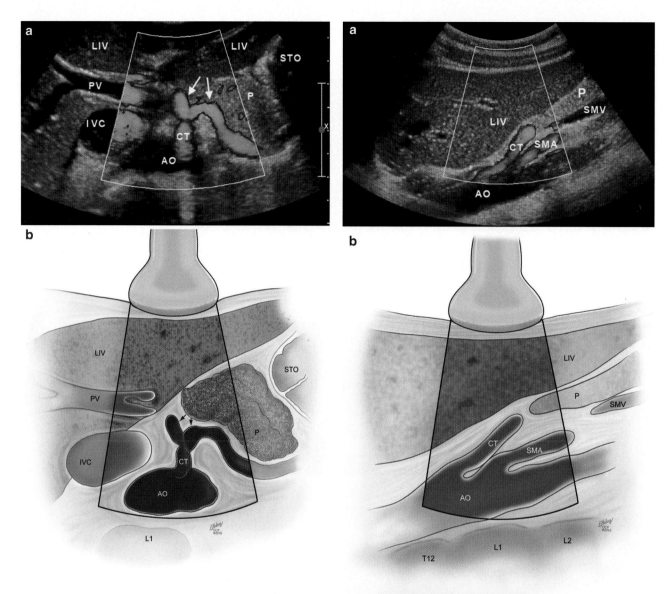

Figure 15.5. Axial scan with duplex mode (**a**) and corresponding illustration (**b**) showing the typical ram-horn-like appearance of the celiac trunk (CT). *AO* aorta, *IVC* inferior vena cava, *LIV* liver, *PV* portal vein, *P* pancreas, *STO* stomach. Reprinted with permission, Cleveland Clinic Center for Medical Art & Photography© 2010. All rights reserved.

Figure 15.6. Saggital scan with duplex mode (**a**) and corresponding illustration (**b**) showing the aorta (AO) with the both first arterial branches: the celiac trunk (CT) and the superior mesenteric artery (SMA). *LIV* liver, *P* pancreas, *SMV* superior mesenteric vein. Reprinted with permission, Cleveland Clinic Center for Medical Art & Photography© 2010. All rights reserved.

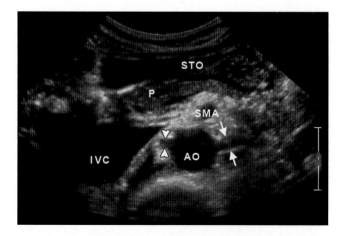

Figure 15.7. Axial scan more caudally showing the aorta (AO) and with the left renal artery (*arrows*) and the right renal artery (*arrowheads*). *IVC* inferior vena cava, *P* pancreas, *STO* stomach, *SMA* superior mesenteric artery.

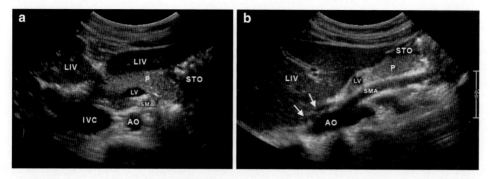

Figure 15.8. (a) Axial scan showing the left and right liver lobes separated by the echoic falciform ligament (LIV), the pancreas body (P), the stomach at the left (STO). The lienal vein entering the portal confluens (LV). *SMA* superior mesenteric artery, *IVC* inferior vena cava, *AO* Aorta. (b) Corresponding sagittal scan showing the structures of interest. The aorta (AO) with the exiting superior mesenteric artery (SMA), and the liver (LIV). The pancreas (P) covered by the distal parts of the stomach (STO). The proximal part of the lienal vein (LV) is depicted as well as the muscular arcade of the aortic hiatus (*arrows*).

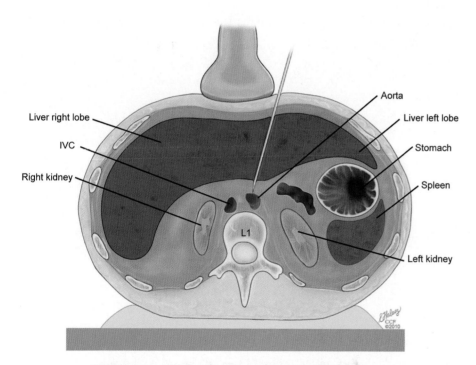

Figure 15.9. Short axis illustration showing the position of the US transducer and the needle to perform celiac plexus block. Reprinted with permission, Cleveland Clinic Center for Medical Art & Photography© 2010. All rights reserved.

for the needle (usually out-of-plane). We obtain both short-axis and long-axis views to correctly identify the celiac trunk (CT) and the SMA (see above). A 20- or 22-gauge needle is then introduced under direct vision in the short axis or the long axis. We prefer to advance the needle from the lateral side of the transducer (short-axis view) to lie just cephalad to the origin of the CT and not between the CT and SMA, to avoid injury to those vessels or their branches. The injection is carried out with real-time sonography after negative aspiration and negative test dose as ultrasound is not accurate in recognizing intravascular injections at such depth.

REFERENCES

1. Kappis M. Erfahrungen mit lokalanasthesie bei bauchoperationen. *Verh Dtsch Ges Chir*. 1914;43: 87–89.
2. Raj P. Celiac plexus/splanchnic nerve blocks. *Tech Reg Anesth Pain Manag*. 2001;5:102–115.
3. Moore DC, Bush WH, Burnett LL. Celiac plexus block: a roentgenographic, anatomic study of technique and spread of solution inpatients and corpses. *Anesth Analg*. 1981;60:369–379.
4. Singler RC. An improved technique for alcohol neurolysis of the celiac plexus. *Anesthesiology*. 1982;56:137–141.
5. Ischia S, Ischia A, Polati E, et al. Three posterior percutaneous celiac plexus block techniques. A prospective randomized study in 61 patients with pancreatic cancer pain. *Anesthesiology*. 1992;76:534–540.
6. Wendling H. Ausschaltung der nervi splanchnici durch leitungsanasthesie bei magenoperationen und anderen eingriffen in der oberen bauchhohle. *Brun's Beitr z Klin Chir*. 1918;110:517–550.
7. Matamala AM, Lopez FV, Martinez LI. The percutaneous approach to the celiac plexus using CT guidance. *Pain*. 1988;34:285–288.
8. Matamala AM, Lopez FV, Sanchez JLA, Bach LD. Percutaneous anterior approach to the celiac plexus using ultrasound. *Br J Anaesth*. 1989;62:637–640.
9. Cheshire WP, Santos CC, Massey EW, et al. Spinal cord infarction: etiology and outcome. *Neurology*. 1996;47:321–330.
10. Brown DL, Wright RM. Precautions against injection in the spinal artery during coeliac plexus block. *Anesthesia*. 1990;45:247–248.

16

Ultrasound-Guided Blocks for Pelvic Pain

Chin-Wern Chan and Philip W.H. Peng

P.W.H. Peng (✉)
Department of Anesthesia, University of Toronto, Toronto Western Hospital,
McL 2-405, 399 Bathurst Street, Toronto, ON, Canada M5T2S8
e-mail: Philip.Peng@uhn.on.ca

S.N. Narouze (ed.), *Atlas of Ultrasound-Guided Procedures in Interventional Pain Management*,
DOI 10.1007/978-1-4419-1681-5_16, © Springer Science+Business Media, LLC 2011

Introduction

Chronic pelvic pain (CPP) is defined as noncylic pain of at least 6 months duration, severe enough to cause disability or seek medical attention, occurring in locations such as the pelvis, anterior abdominal wall at or below the umbilicus, lower back, or buttocks.[1] The pathophysiology of CPP is complex. The pain generator may include the viscera (e.g., bladder, bowel), neuromuscular system (e.g., pudendal neuralgia, piriformis syndrome), or the gynecological system (e.g., endometriosis). Pathophysiological processes, both peripherally and centrally combined with psychological factors most likely contribute to the clinical picture.[2] Therefore, a multidisciplinary approach to management is recommended.[2] As part of this management plan, neural blockade and injection of muscles within the pelvis play both a diagnostic and therapeutic role.[2]

The technique of neural blockade has changed considerably in the past several decades. In the past, clinicians were not able to reliably visualize nerves. The methods of choice in the past were either landmark-based (blind) or equipment-guided techniques. The latter are indirect methods providing surrogate markers (such as bony landmarks for the nerve in fluoroscopy) or electrophysiological changes (such as nerve stimulation or electromyography). Both of them have intrinsic limitations in precisely locating a soft tissue structure. The introduction and increasing use of ultrasound to assist in needle placement and injection have provided the pain clinician with many benefits compared to previous modalities. Among the advantages of ultrasound are improved visualization of the nerve and surrounding vascular, bony, muscular, and visceral structures, more precise deposition of medication in the vicinity of the nerve of interest, real-time guidance on needle advancement, thereby improving target and reducing inadvertent damage to surrounding neurovascular structures, and the ability to better identify intravascular and intraneuronal injection.[3] Furthermore, the relatively easy access, portability, and lack of radiation exposure make ultrasonography an attractive imaging modality for the interventional pain physician.[4-8]

This chapter concentrates on anatomy, sonoanatomy, and ultrasound-guided techniques for needle placement of the following structures associated with CPP: (1) ilioinguinal, iliohypogastric, and genitofemoral nerves; (2) piriformis muscle; and (3) pudendal nerve.

Ilioinguinal, Iliohypogastric, and Genitofemoral Nerves

The ilioinguinal (II), iliohypogastric (IH), and genitofemoral (GF) nerves are known as the "border nerves," providing sensory innervation to the skin lying between the thigh and abdomen.[9] Due to their location and variable course, these nerves are susceptible to injury in surgical procedures involving the lower abdomen. Injury to the II and IH nerves is a known risk in open appendectomy incisions, postinguinal herniorrhaphy, low-transverse incisions (e.g., Pfannenstiel incision), and during trocar insertion for laparoscopic surgery of the abdomen and pelvis.[10-14] There are multiple mechanisms by which these nerves may be injured. Direct nerve trauma with or without neuroma formation, compression of the nerve with scar tissue or hematoma, and suturing of the nerve into fascial closure or mesh incorporation are several possible mechanisms.[15,16]

Patients presenting with pain secondary to irritation of these nerves usually complain of groin pain which may radiate to the scrotum or testicle in males, the labia majora in women, and the medial aspect of the thigh.[5] One review has identified chronic pain after inguinal repair to be as high as 54%.[17] Furthermore, one third of these patients report moderate to unbearable pain.[17] Blockade of the II and IH nerves are often performed to provide intra and postoperative analgesia for hernia repair.[18] In addition, blockade of these nerves serves a diagnostic and therapeutic purpose in patients complaining of chronic pain in this nerve distribution.[5,6,8]

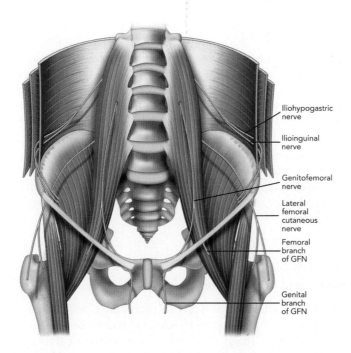

Figure 16.1. The pathway of ilioinguinal, iliohypogastric, and genitofemoral nerve (GFN) is shown. Reproduced with permission from USRA (www.usra.ca).

Anatomy

The II and IH nerves originate from the ventral rami of L1 with contributing filaments from T12.[9,19] The IH nerve emerges along the upper lateral border of psoas major (Figure 16.1). The nerve then crosses quadratus lumborum inferolaterally traveling to the iliac crest.[9] At a point midway between the iliac crest and 12th rib, the nerve pierces the transversus abdominis muscle superior to the anterior superior iliac spine (ASIS).[19] The IH nerve then runs inferomedially, piercing the internal oblique muscle above the ASIS.[19] From this point, the nerve runs between the internal and external oblique muscles, piercing the external oblique aponeurosis approximately 1 in. above the superficial inguinal ring.[9] As the nerve courses between the abdominal oblique muscles, it divides into lateral and anterior cutaneous branches.[12] The lateral cutaneous branch provides sensory innervations to the skin of the gluteal region.[19] The anterior cutaneous branch supplies the skin over the hypogastric region, including the skin over the lower region of the rectus abdominis muscle.[19] The II nerve emerges along the lateral border of psoas major, inferior to the IH nerve (Figure 16.1).[19] The II runs parallel and below the IH nerve. In contrast to the IH nerve, the ilioinguinal nerve pierces the internal oblique at its lower border, and then passes between the crura of the superficial inguinal ring, anterior to the spermatic cord.[9,19] The nerve provides sensory fibers to the skin over the root of penis and scrotum (mons pubis and labium majus) and superomedial thigh region.[19]

It should be noted from observation of the course of the nerves from imaging and cadaver studies, the most consistent area (90%) both II and IH nerves are found is at the point midway between the iliac crest and 12th rib, where the nerves are located between the TA and IO muscles.[19,20]

The GF nerve arises from the L1 and L2 nerve roots.[9] The nerve travels anteriorly, passing through the psoas muscle at the level of the third and fourth lumbar vertebrae.[9] It then runs on the ventral surface of the muscle, under the peritoneum and behind the ureter.[21] The nerve divides into the genital and femoral branches above the level of the inguinal ligament (Figure 16.1).[21] This point of division is variable. The genital branch passes through the deep inguinal ring providing motor innervation to the cremaster muscle and sensory fibers to the scrotum.[9,21] The course of this nerve in relation to the spermatic cord in the inguinal canal is varied, with ventral, dorsal, inferior locations[9,22] or as part of the cremaster muscle.[21] In females, the genital branch runs with the round ligament supplying mons pubis and labium majus.[9] The femoral branch follows the external iliac artery, passing through fascia lata providing sensory innervations to the skin of the femoral triangle.[9]

Success, consistency, and reliability in blockade of the border nerves with blind techniques have been poor.[23,24] This is likely due to the high degree of anatomic variability in not only the course of the nerves but also their branching patterns, areas of penetration of the fascial layers, and dominance patterns.[8] The above description of the II and IH nerve anatomy may only be consistent in 41.8% of patients.[25] Furthermore, the sites at which the II and IH nerves pierce the abdominal wall muscle layers are significantly variable.[14] However, by far the most consistent location of the II and IH nerves is lateral and superior to the ASIS where the nerves are found between the transversus abdominis and internal oblique muscular layers.[5,6,8,19]

Literature Review on the Injection Techniques for Ilioinguinal, Iliohypogastric, and Genitofemoral Nerve Block

A number of injection techniques for II and IH nerves have been described and virtually all are landmark-based.[26–28] Unfortunately, all these techniques suggest a needle entry anterior to the ASIS (Figure 16.2), where the anatomy of these nerves is highly variable. Thus, the failure rates with those techniques range between 10% and 45%.[18,23,24,29] Furthermore, the misguided needle may result in femoral nerve blockade[30] and bowel perforation and pelvic hematoma.[31–33]

There are two key elements contributing to the improvement in success rate. One is to perform the injection cephalad and posterior to the ASIS, where both the II and IH nerves (>90%) can be consistently found between the TA muscles at this point.[19] The

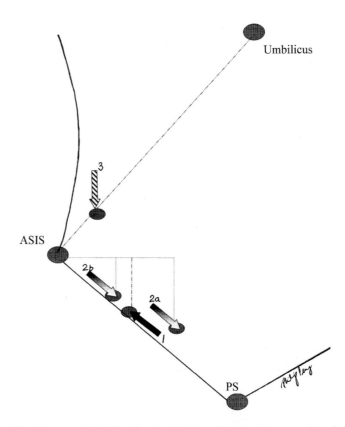

Figure 16.2. The three methods (four landmarks) described for ilioinguinal and iliohypogastric nerves injection are given in references[26–28]. *PS* pubic symphysis, *ASIS* anterior superior iliac spine. Reproduced with permission from American Society of Interventional Pain Physician.

other, is the use of ultrasound for the guidance of injection. Techniques utilizing ultrasound to inject the II and IH nerves have been published.[5,8,34,35] The accuracy of ultrasound guidance has been validated in a cadaver study with the injection site superior to ASIS and the block success rate was 95%.[34] The success of using ultrasound to guide II and IH nerve blockade has been replicated in the clinical setting. Based on visualization of the abdominal muscles, fascial planes, and the deep circumflex iliac artery, the authors were able to demonstrate a clinically successful block in all their cases based on sensory loss corresponding to the II and IH nerves following injection.[35,36] The ease and importance of identifying the abdominal muscle planes before attempting to visualize the nerves have been supported by a study assessing the training of anesthesiologists with little experience in using ultrasound to assist in needle placement.[37]

Neural blockade of the GF nerve is not commonly performed. Review of the literature yields that techniques described in the past were blind and rely on the pubic tubercle, inguinal ligament, inguinal crease, and femoral artery as landmarks.[38,39] One of the blind methods involves infiltration of 10 ml local anesthetic immediately lateral to the pubic tubercle, caudad to the inguinal ligament.[40] In another method, a needle is inserted into the inguinal canal to block the genital branch.[39] The latter method can only be reliably performed during surgery.[39] The blind techniques described are essentially infiltration techniques and rely on high volumes of local anesthetic for consistent results.[40]

Ultrasound-guided blockade of the genital branch of the GF nerve has been described in several review articles.[5,6,8] The genital nerve is difficult to visualize and blockade is achieved by identification of the inguinal canal.[5,6,8] In males, the GF nerve may travel within or outside the spermatic cord. Thus, the local anesthetic and steroid are deposited both outside and within the spermatic cord.[5,6,8]

Ultrasound-Guided Technique of Ilioinguinal, Iliohypogastric, and Genitofemoral Nerve

Ilioinguinal and Iliohypogastric Nerves

When performing II and IH nerve blockade under ultrasound guidance, it is important to clearly identify the abdominal wall muscle layers: EO, IO, and TA. The patient is placed in the supine position. Both nerves are relatively superficial, thus a high-frequency (6–13 MHz) linear probe will provide optimal visualization. The recommended area for initial scanning is posterior and superior to the ASIS. The probe should be placed perpendicular to the direction of the II and IH nerves (which is usually parallel to the inguinal ligament) with the lateral edge on top of the iliac crest (Figure 16.3). At this position, the iliac crest will appear as a hyperechoic structure adjacent to which will appear the three muscular layers of the abdominal wall (Figure 16.4). Below the TA, peristaltic movements of the bowel may be detected. The probe may need to be tilted either caudad or cephalad to optimize the image. Once the muscular layers are identified, the II and IH nerves will be found in the split fascial plane between the IO and TA muscle layers. Both nerves should be within 1.5 cm of the iliac crest at this site, with the II nerve closer to the iliac crest.[34] The nerves are usually in close proximity to each other[25] and located on the "upsloping" split fascia close to the iliac crest. In some cases, the nerves may run approximately 1 cm apart.[8] The deep circumflex iliac artery which is close to the two nerves in the same fascial layer can be revealed with the use of color Doppler (Figure 16.4). A neural structure within the fascial split may also be seen medial and on the flat part of the IO and TA muscle junction. This is the subcostal nerve and if mistaken for the II and IH nerve, the nerve blockade will result in aberrant distribution of anesthesia.

Once satisfied with visualization of the nerves, a 22-guage spinal needle is advanced to the nerves under real-time guidance. Either an out-of-plane or in-plane technique may be used although an in-plane technique is favored by the authors. The needle is advanced so the tip lies in the split fascial plane between the IO and TA muscles and adjacent to the II and IH nerves (Figure 16.4). At this point, hydrodissection with normal saline can

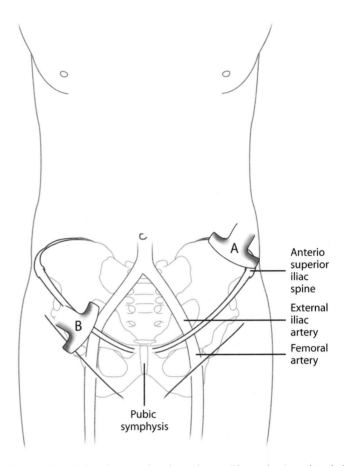

Anterio
superior
iliac
spine

External
iliac
artery

Femoral
artery

Pubic
symphysis

Figure 16.3. The position of the ultrasound probe is shown. The probe A is placed above and posterior to the anterior superior iliac spine and is in the short axis of the course of ilioinguinal nerve. The probe B is placed in the inguinal line in long axis of femoral and external iliac artery. Reproduced with permission from USRA (www.usra.ca).

confirm adequate position of the needle tip and spread within the fascial plane. In some cases, the nerves may be difficult to visualize. In this situation, injectate may be deposited in the fascial plane between the TA and IO muscles, ensuring satisfactory medial and lateral spread.[36] The injectate usually consists of 6–8 ml of local anesthetic (bupivacaine 0.5%) and steroid (depo-medrol 40 mg). The desired result is observation of spread of the solution in the split fascial plane to surround both nerves.

Genital Branch of Genitofemoral Nerve

The genital branch of the GF nerve cannot be visualized directly. The major structure that is sought on scanning is the inguinal canal and its content (spermatic cord in males or the round ligament in females).

The patient is positioned supine and a linear US probe with high frequency (6–13 MHz) is used. Initially, the probe is placed in the transverse plane below the inguinal ligament. In this plane, the femoral artery is identified and positioned in the middle of the screen. The probe is then rotated so that the artery lies in the long axis (Figure 16.3). The ultrasound probe is then moved cranially to trace the femoral artery until it dives deep into the abdomen to become the external iliac artery (Figure 16.5). At this point, an oval or circular structure may be seen superficial to the femoral artery. This structure is the inguinal canal and contains the spermatic cord in men and the round ligament in women. The probe may be moved slightly medial to trace the spermatic cord or round ligament. In males, arterial pulsations may be visible within the spermatic cord. These pulsations rep-

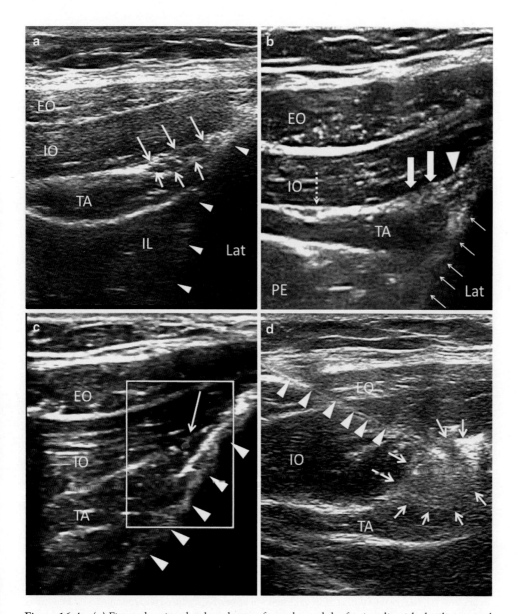

Figure 16.4. (a) Figure showing the three layers of muscles and the fascia split with the ilioinguinal and iliohypogastric nerves inside. *Solid triangles* outline the iliac crest. (**b**) Similar view as (**a**). *Solid arrows* show the ilioinguinal nerve (lateral) and iliohypogastric nerve (medial). *Solid triangle* shows the deep circumflex iliac artery. *Dashed line arrows* point to the fascia split with subcostal nerve (T12). Usually the fascia split for ilioinguinal and iliohypogastric nerves appears adjacent to the iliac crest. When it appears far away from the iliac crest like the one in this figure, one should suspect subcostal nerve. *Solid line arrows* outline the iliac crest. (**c**) Similar view as (**b**) with color Doppler. The deep circumflex iliac artery is shown in *red color*. *Line arrows* outline the iliac crest. (**d**) Figure showing the needle (outlined by *solid triangle*) inserted with in-plane technique and the *line arrows* outline the spread of the local anesthetic and steroid solution. *EO* external oblique muscle, *IO* internal oblique muscle, *TA* transverse abdominis muscle, *IL* iliacus, *PE* peritoneum, *LAT* lateral. Reproduced with permission from USRA (www.usra.ca).

resent the testicular artery and artery to the vas deferens. This may be confirmed by the use of color Doppler. The blood vessels may be made more prominent by asking the patient to perform a Valsalva maneuver, which increases blood flow through the pampiniform plexus. In addition to the arteries, a thin tubular structure within the spermatic cord may also be visible, which is the vas deferens. In females, the round ligament can be difficult to visualize and the target is the inguinal canal.

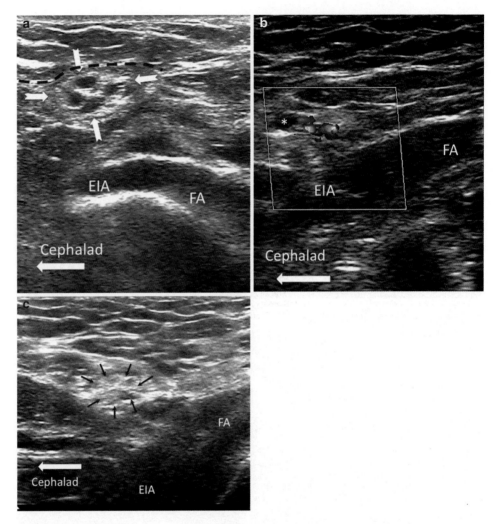

Figure 16.5. (a) Long-axis view of the femoral and external iliac artery showing the cross section of spermatic cord (outlined by *solid arrows*) in a male patient. The *red dashed line* outlines the deep abdominal fascia. (b) Similar view as (a) with color Doppler showing the vessels inside the spermatic cord. (c) Similar view as (a) but in a female patient showing the round ligament of uterus (outlined by *line arrows*). *EIA* external iliac artery, *FA* femoral artery. Reproduced with permission from USRA (www.usra.ca).

An out-of-plane technique is used to guide needle placement. The needle is inserted on the lateral aspect of the probe. The needle is directed to pierce the deep abdominal fascia and into the inguinal canal (Figure 16.5). Once the needle has pierced the fascia, hydrodissection with normal saline confirms spread within the inguinal canal. A volume of 4 ml of solution is deposited within the inguinal canal but outside the spermatic cord with another 4 ml deposited inside the spermatic cord. The reason for dividing the injection is due to the anatomic variability of the genital branch. The local anesthetic solution should not contain epinephrine as there is a risk of vasoconstriction of the testicular artery. In addition to local anesthetic, steroids may be added for cases with chronic pain. In females, 8 ml of the solution will be deposited into the inguinal canal.

Piriformis Syndrome

Piriformis syndrome is an uncommon cause of pain occurring in the back, buttock, or hip.[41–44] Typically, pain is felt in the region of the sacroiliac joint, greater sciatic notch, and piriformis muscle with radiation down the lower limb similar to sciatica.[45] The pain is exacerbated by walking, stooping, or lifting.[46] On physical examination, there may be gluteal atrophy and tenderness on palpation, pain on stretching of the piriformis muscle, and a positive Lasegue sign.[45,46] Often, it is a diagnosis of exclusion with clinical assessment and investigations necessary to rule out pathology of the lumbar spine, hips, and sacroiliac joint.[46,47]

Often, piriformis syndrome will improve with a conservative regimen of physical therapy and simple analgesic pharmacotherapy. For those patients not responding, more interventional therapy may be required in the form of muscle injections or surgery.[48] The piriformis muscle may be injected with local anesthetic and steroid[49] which will also aid in diagnosis if therapeutically successful. Furthermore, botulinum toxin has been injected into the piriformis muscle with evidence of longer periods of analgesia.[50,51] In those cases, in which there is failure to improve after three injections, surgical release of the piriformis muscle should be considered.[41]

Anatomy

The origin of the piriformis muscle is via fleshy digitations on the ventral surface of the S2 to S4 vertebrae (Figure 16.6).[44] Running laterally anterior to the sacroiliac joint, the piriformis muscle exits the pelvis through the greater sciatic foramen.[45] At this point, the muscle becomes tendinous inserting into the upper border of the greater trochanter as a round tendon.[47] The piriformis functions as an external rotator of the lower limb in the erect position, an abductor when supine, and a weak hip flexor when walking.[47]

All neurovascular structures exiting the pelvis to the buttock pass through the greater sciatic foramen.[47] The superior gluteal nerve and artery pass superior to the piriformis.[47] Inferior to the piriformis lie the inferior gluteal artery and nerve, the internal pudendal

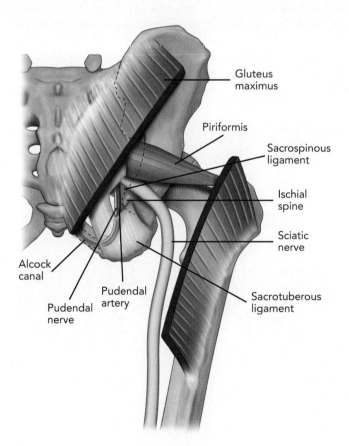

Figure 16.6. Posterior view of pelvis showing the pudendal neurovascular bundle and piriformis muscle. The gluteus maximus muscle was cut to show the deeper structures. Note that the pudendal nerve and artery run in the interligamentous plane between the sacrospinous and sacrotuberous ligament and subsequently into the Alcock's canal. Reproduced with permission from USRA (www.usra.ca).

artery, the pudendal nerve, nerve to obturator internus, posterior femoral cutaneous nerve, nerve to quadratus lumborum, and the sciatic nerve.[47] The anatomical relationship between the piriformis muscle and sciatic nerve is variable. Most commonly (78–84%), the sciatic nerve passes below the piriformis muscle.[52,53] Less frequently (12–21%), the nerve is divided, passing through and below the muscle.[53] Less common variations are the divided nerve passing through and above the piriformis; the divided nerve passing above and below the muscle; undivided nerve passing above piriformis; or undivided nerve passing through the muscle.[52,53] The close relationship of the piriformis muscle to the sciatic nerve explains why patients experiencing piriformis syndrome may also experience symptoms of sciatic nerve irritation.[43]

Literature Review on Piriformis Muscle Injections

There have been reports of different techniques utilized to inject the piriformis muscle, including fluoroscopy,[49] CT,[54] and MRI[55] to assist with accurate needle placement within the muscle. Electrophysiologic guidance has been used alone and in conjunction with the above modalities.[51,56,57] Irrespective of whether EMG guidance is used, fluoroscopically guided piriformis muscle injections depend on the presence of a characteristic intrapiriformis contrast pattern to confirm needle placement within the piriformis muscle (Figure 16.7),[49] which has been shown to be unreliable.[58] A validation study with cadavers suggested that the fluoroscopically guided contrast-controlled injection was only accurate in guiding an intrapiriformis injection in 30% of the injections.[58] In cases where the needle was incorrectly placed, the usual final position of the needle was within the gluteus maximus muscle, which overlies piriformis.

In contrast, ultrasound is seen as an attractive imaging technique as it provides visualization of the soft tissue and neurovascular structures, and allows real-time imaging of needle insertion toward the target.[59] Multiple reports of ultrasound-guided piriformis muscle injection have been published with similar techniques described.[4,5,58,60,61] The accuracy of needle placement with ultrasound was recently validated in a cadaveric study suggesting an accuracy of 95%.[58]

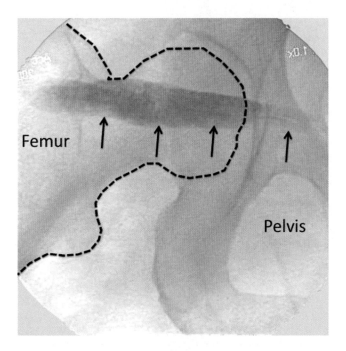

Figure 16.7. Radiographic contrast (indicated by *line arrows*) outlining the piriformis muscle. Reproduced with permission from USRA (www.usra.ca).

Ultrasound-Guided Technique for Piriformis Muscle Injection

The patient is placed in the prone position. A low-frequency (2–5 Hz) curvilinear probe is held in the transverse plane and initially positioned over the posterior superior iliac spine (PSIS). The transducer is then moved laterally to visualize the ilium, which will be identifiable as a hyperechoic line descending diagonally across the screen from the superomedial to inferolateral corners (Figure 16.8). Once the ilium is visualized, the probe

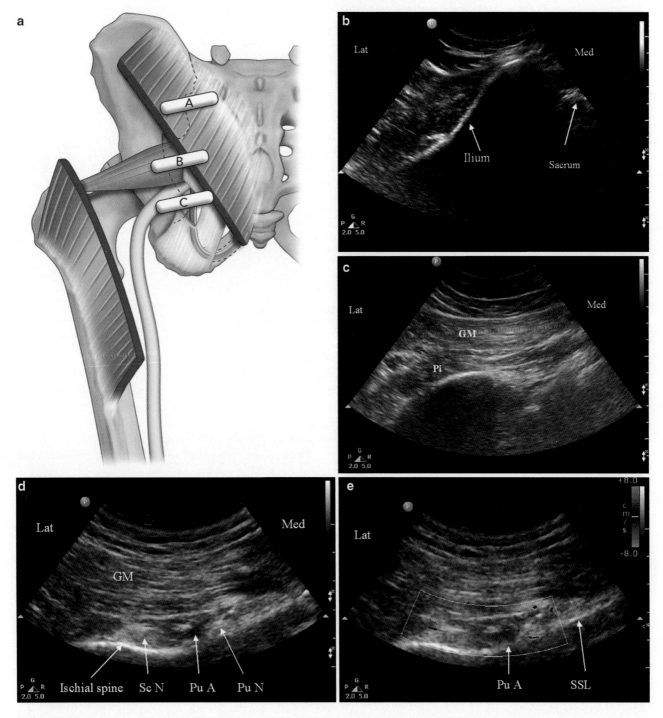

Figure 16.8. Ultrasonographic scan of the piriformis muscle and the pudendal nerve. (**a**) Three different positions of ultrasound probe. Reproduced with permission from USRA (www.usra.ca). (**b**) Ultrasound image at probe position A. (**c**) Ultrasound image at probe position B. (**d**) Ultrasound image at probe position C. (**e**) Color Doppler to show pudendal artery. *Pu A* pudendal artery, *Pu N* pudendal nerve, *SSL* sacrospinous ligament, *Sc N* sciatic nerve, *GM* gluteus maximus muscle. (**b–e**) From Rofaeel et al.[7] Reproduced with permission from Lippincott Williams & Wilkins.

is orientated in the direction of the piriformis muscle and moved in a caudad direction until the sciatic notch is found (Figure 16.8). At the sciatic notch level, the hyperechoic shadow of the bone will disappear from the medial aspect and two muscle layers will be visible: the gluteus maximus and the piriformis (Figure 16.8). Confirmation of the piriformis muscle can be made by having an assistant rotating the hip externally and internally with the knee flexed. This movement will demonstrate side to side gliding of the piriformis muscle on ultrasound. It is important to identify the sciatic notch, as failure to do so may lead the practitioner to mistakenly identify one of the other external hip rotators (e.g., the gemelli muscles) as piriformis.

Due to the depth of the muscle, a 22-guage, 120 mm nerve stimulating needle is used. The authors recommend the concomitant use of a nerve stimulator to avoid unintentional injection of the sciatic nerve, as the passage of the sciatic nerve in this territory is variable as described above. In addition, the use of a nerve stimulator also allows identification of the needle tip within the piriformis muscle by the visualization of piriformis muscle twitches on the monitor.

An in-plane technique is used with the needle being inserted on the medial aspect of the probe and passing laterally into the muscle belly of the piriformis in the sciatic notch. If intramuscular injection is the objective, the needle should be slowly advanced further until strong contractions of the piriformis muscle are evident on the monitor. A small volume of normal saline (0.5 ml) may be injected to confirm position within the muscle. Once satisfied with needle position, a small volume (1–2 ml) of medication (either a mixture of 1 ml of 0.5% bupivacaine and 40 mg depo-medrol or 50 units of Botulinum toxin A diluted in 1 ml of normal saline) may be injected into the muscle.

Pudendal Neuralgia

The pudendal nerve supplies the anterior and posterior urogenital areas (clitoris, penis, vulva, and perianal area).[62-64] Pudendal neuralgia refers to CPP where pain is experienced in these regions innervated by the pudendal nerve.[62] Typically, the pain is exacerbated by sitting and may be reduced by lying on the nonpainful side, standing, and sitting on a toilet seat.[65] On physical examination, there may be evidence of hypoesthesia, hyperalgesia, or allodynia in the perineal area.[65] The pain may be reproduced or exaggerated when pressure is applied against the ischial spine during a vaginal or rectal examination. Pudendal nerve block is an important tool in the diagnosis of this condition.[66]

Often the cause of the symptoms in patients suffering from pudendal neuralgia will not be readily identifiable. However, bicycle riding,[67] vaginal delivery,[68,69] countertraction devices in orthopedic surgery,[70,71] pelvic trauma,[70] and intensive athletic activity[72] are recognized risk factors in the development of pudendal neuralgia. There are two anatomical regions in which the pudendal nerve is susceptible to entrapment along its path: (1) the interligamentous plane, which lies between the sacrotuberous and sacrospinous ligaments at the level of the ischial spine[73]; (2) Alcock's canal.[74]

Anatomy

The pudendal nerve contains both motor and sensory fibers.[75] Relative to the major nerves of the extremities, the pudendal nerve is thin (0.6–6.8 mm) and is situated deep within the body, surrounded by fatty tissue.[76] The nerve arises from the anterior rami of the second, third, and fourth sacral nerves (S2, S3, and S4)[75] and passes through the greater sciatic notch.[76] Once out of the pelvis, the pudendal nerve travels ventrally in the interligamentous plane between the sacrospinous and sacrotuberous ligament at the level of the ischial spine (Figure 16.6).[62,77] At this level, 30–40% of pudendal nerves will be two- or three-trunked.[62,78,79] Within the interligamentous plane, the pudendal artery is located lateral to the pudendal nerve in the vast majority of cases (90%).[76] This region is of clinical importance as the nerve may be compressed between the sacrospinous and sacrotuberous ligaments.[73] Furthermore, elongation of the ischial spine due to repetitive muscular forces represents a potential source of microtrauma affecting the pudendal nerve.[72]

Following its passage between the two ligaments, the pudendal nerve swings anteriorly to enter the pelvis through the Alcock's canal of the lateral ischiorectal fossa.[78–80] Alcock's canal is a fascial sheath formed by the duplication of the obturator internus muscle, underlying the plane of levator ani.[78] At this site, the pudendal nerve is also susceptible to entrapment either by the fascia of the obturator internus or by the falciform process of the sacrotuberous ligament.[74]

As the pudendal nerve travels through the ischiorectal fossa, it gives off three terminal branches: the dorsal nerve of the penis, inferior rectal nerve, and the perineal nerve. The dorsal nerve of the penis runs lateral to the dorsal artery and deep dorsal vein of the penis, terminating in the glans penis.[77,81,82] The course of the nerve under the subpubic arch makes it susceptible to compression by the saddle nose of a bicycle.[83] The inferior rectal nerve supplies the external anal sphincter.[77,81,82] The remaining portion of the pudendal nerve trunk becomes the perineal nerve which continues to supply sensation of the skin of the penis (clitoris), perianal area, and the posterior surface of the scrotum or labia majora.[82] The perineal nerve also provides motor supply to the deep muscles of the urogenital triangle.[81,82]

Literature Review on the Pudendal Nerve Injections

There are two anatomical regions at which blockade of the pudendal nerve may be performed: the interligamentous plane[73] and Alcock's canal.[74]

The pudendal nerve has been blocked by various routes in the literature. These include the transvaginal[84], transperineal,[85,86] and transgluteal approaches.[87] The transgluteal approach is popular allowing blockade at the ischial spine and Alcock's canal. Traditionally, fluoroscopy has been used to guide needle placement, using the ischial spine as a surrogate landmark.[62] The needle is placed medial to the ischial spine which corresponds to the course of the pudendal nerve at this level.[87,88] The major limitation of fluoroscopy is that it cannot accurately demonstrate the interligamentous plane.[5,8] At the level of the ischial spine, the pudendal artery lies between the pudendal nerve and the pudendal artery in the majority of cases (76–100%).[7,76] Therefore, injectate may not spread to the pudendal nerve using this landmark. In addition, the potential proximity of the sciatic nerve at this level makes it susceptible to the anesthetic if spread of the injectate is not visualized in real time. Furthermore, the depth for needle insertion cannot be assessed with fluoroscopy.

Both ultrasound and computed tomography (CT) scan are ideal for visualizing the interligamentous plane as they identify all the important landmarks: ischial spine, sacrotuberous ligament, sacrospinous ligament, pudendal artery, and the pudendal nerve.[8] Furthermore, it also allows visualization of the sciatic nerve and other vascular structures, so more selective needle placement and blockade can occur. Ultrasound has the advantage of avoiding exposing the patient to radiation and is more accessible to clinicians. While early reports only described ultrasound visualization of the pudendal nerve,[76,89] the actual technique of blockade has been reported in greater detail recently.[5,7,8] A consistent feature of published techniques on ultrasound-guided pudendal nerve blockade is identifying the ischial spine and its medial aspect which contains the sacrotuberous and sacrospinous ligaments, internal pudendal artery, and pudendal nerve.[5–8]

At the level of Alcock's canal, ultrasound cannot accurately identify or guide needle placement. CT guidance is the only form of imaging which can accurately guide the needle into the canal.[90]

Ultrasound-Guided Technique for Pudendal Nerve Injection

Pudendal nerve blockade at the level of the ischial spine with ultrasound guidance is performed via the transgluteal approach with the patient in the prone position. The aim of scanning is to identify the ischial spine and therefore reliably identify the interligamentous plane which will appear on its medial aspect. A curvilinear probe (2–5 Hz) is recommended for scanning due to the depth of the nerve. Scanning begins with the probe held in the transverse plane over the PSIS, a technique similar to that of scanning the piriformis muscle (Figure 16.8). The probe is then moved caudad until the piriformis muscle is identified as described above for the piriformis muscle injection. At this level the ischium can be identified as a curved hyperechoic line. The probe is then moved further caudad to identify the ischial spine. The following four features will help to identify the level of the ischial spine (Figure 16.8):

> The ischial spine will appear as a straight hyperechoic line as opposed to the ischium which is a curved hyperechoic line.
>
> The sacrospinous ligament will be visualized as a hyperechoic line lying medial and in contact with the ischial spine. The sacrospinous ligament, however, does not cast an anechoic shadow deep to its image, as opposed to that casted by bone structures.
>
> The piriformis muscle will disappear. Deep to the gluteus maximus lies the sacrotuberous ligament. Although it is difficult to differentiate between this ligament and the fascial plane of the gluteus maximus, the sacrotuberous ligament can be felt easily as the needle is advancing through this thick ligament.
>
> The internal pudendal artery can be seen, usually situated on the medial portion of the ischial spine. This can be confirmed with color Doppler.

The pudendal nerve will lie medial to the pudendal artery at this level. However, due to the depth and the small diameter of the nerve it may be difficult to visualize. On dynamic scan, the sciatic nerve and inferior gluteal artery can be seen lateral to the ischial spine tip. Visualization of these structures is important because if these are mistaken for the internal pudendal artery, sciatic nerve blockade will result.

Once satisfied with the identification of the ischial spine, pudendal artery, and the interligamentous plane, a 22-guage, 120 mm insulated peripheral nerve stimulating needle is inserted from the medial aspect of the probe. The target is for the needle tip to be situated between the sacrotuberous ligament and sacrospinous ligament. Due to the depth of the pudendal nerve, it is helpful to insert the needle several centimetres medial to the medial edge of the probe to reduce the steepness of the needle path and therefore assist in visualization of the needle tip as it passes to the target site. The needle is advanced so that it will pass through the sacrotuberous ligament, on the medial side of the pudendal artery. As the needle is passing through the sacrotuberous ligament, increased resistance will be felt. Once the needle is through, the resistance will diminish. A small volume of normal saline is injected to confirm position within the interligamentous plane. The pudendal nerve itself will be difficult to visualize due to a combination of its depth,[7,76] small diameter,[62,76,79] and possibility of anatomical division into two or three trunks.[62,78,79]

If hydrodissection confirms adequate spread within the interligamentous plane and no intravascular spread, a mixture of local anesthetic and steroid may be injected. In the author's experience, a mixture of 4 ml of 0.5% bupivacaine and 40 mg of steroid (depo-medrol) is commonly injected and clinical signs of pudendal nerve blockade are present shortly after. During injection, the clinician should ensure that there is a spread of the injectate medial to the pudendal artery and that the injectate does not pass too far laterally past the artery. Excessive lateral spread may result in inadvertent sciatic nerve blockade. It is recommended that the patient is assessed for signs of successful blockade following the procedure. This may be achieved simply by assessing sensation to pin prick and alcohol swab in the perineal area ipsilateral to site of blockade. Successful blockade will result in reduced sensation to both stimuli in this region.

Conclusion

Ultrasound is a valuable tool for imaging peripheral structures, guiding needle advancement, and confirming the spread of injectate around the target tissue, all without exposing healthcare providers and patients to the risks of radiation. In patients with CPP, the target structures for the interventional procedures can be well visualized with the use of ultrasound. Most of the ultrasound-guided interventional procedures in CPP have been validated and thus allow the accurate performance of these procedures.

References

1. American College of Obstetricians and Gynecologists. Chronic pelvic pain: ACOG practice bulletin no. 51. *Obstet Gynecol.* 2004;103:589–605.
2. Fall M, Baranowski AP, Elniel S, et al. EAU guidelines on chronic pelvic pain. *Eur Urol.* 2010;57:35–48.
3. Chan VWS. *A Practical Guide to Ultrasound Imaging for Regional Anesthesia.* 2nd ed. Toronto, ON: Toronto Printing; 2009.
4. Smith J, Hurdle M-F, Locketz AJ, Wisniewski SJ. Ultrasound-guided piriformis injection: technique description and verification. *Arch Phys Med Rehabil.* 2006;87(12):1664–1667.
5. Peng PWH, Tumber PS. Ultrasound-guided interventional procedures for patients with chronic pelvic pain – a description of techniques and review of the literature. *Pain Physician.* 2008;11: 215–224.
6. Bellingham GA, Peng PWH. Ultrasound-guided interventional procedures for chronic pelvic pain. *Tech Reg Anesth Pain Manag.* 2009;13:171–178.
7. Rofaeel A, Peng P, Louis I, et al. Feasibility of real-time ultrasound for pudendal nerve block in patients with chronic perineal pain. *Reg Anesth Pain Med.* 2008;33(2):139–145.
8. Peng P, Narouze S. Ultrasound-guided interventional procedures in pain medicine: a review of anatomy, sonoanatomy, and procedures. Part I nonaxial structures. *Reg Anesth Pain Med.* 2009;34(5):458–474.
9. Rab M, Ebmer J, Dellon AL. Anatomic variability of the ilioinguinal and genitofemoral nerve: implications for the treatment of groin pain. *Plast Reconstr Surg.* 2001;108(6):1618–1623.
10. Cardosi RJ, Cox CS, Hoffman MS. Postoperative neuropathies after major pelvic surgery. *Obstet Gynecol.* 2002;100(2):240–244.
11. Luijendijk RW, Jekel J, Storm RK, et al. The low transverse Pfannenstiel incision and the prevalence of incisional hernia and nerve entrapment. *Ann Surg.* 1997;225(14):365–369.
12. Choi PD, Nath R, Mackinnon SE. Iatrogenic injury to the ilioinguinal and iliohypogastric nerves in the groin: case report, diagnosis, and management. *Ann Plast Surg.* 1996;37(1):60–65.
13. Sippo WC, Burghardt A, Gomez AC. Nerve entrapment after Pfannenstiel incision. *Am J Obstet Gynecol.* 1987;157(2):420–421.
14. Whiteside JL, Barber MD, Walters MD, Falcone T. Anatomy of the ilioinguinal and iliohypogastric nerves in relation to trocar placement and low transverse incisions. *Am J Obstet Gynecol.* 2003;189(16):1574–1578.
15. Grosz CR. Iliohypogastric nerve injury. *Am J Surg.* 1981;142(5):628.
16. Lantis JC II, Schwaitzberg SD. Tack entrapment of the ilioinguinal nerve during laparoscopic hernia repair. *J Laparoendosc Adv Surg Tech A.* 1999;9(3):285–289.
17. Poobalan AS, Bruce J, Smith EC, King PM, Krukowski ZH, Chambers WA. A review of chronic pain after inguinal herniorrhaphy. *Clin J Pain.* 2003;19(1):48–54.
18. Lim SL, Ng Sb A, Tan GM. Ilioinguinal and iliohypogastric nerve block revisited: single shot versus double shot technique for hernia repair in children. *Paediatr Anaesth.* 2002;12(3):255–260.
19. Mandelkow H, Loeweneck H. The iliohypogastric and ilioinguinal nerves. Distribution in the abdominal wall, danger areas in surgical incisions in the inguinal and pubic regions and reflected visceral pain in their dermatomes. *Surg Radiol Anat.* 1988;10(2):145–149.
20. Jamieson RW, Swigart LL, Anson BJ. Points of parietal perforation of the ilioinguinal and iliohypogastric nerves in relation to optimal sites for local anaesthesia. *Q Bull Northwest Univ Med Sch.* 1952;26(1):22–26.
21. Liu WC, Chen TH, Shyu JF, et al. Applied anatomy of the genital branch of the genitofemoral nerve in open inguinal herniorrhaphy. *Eur J Surg.* 2002;168(3):145–149.

22. Ducic I, Dellon AL. Testicular pain after inguinal hernia repair: an approach to resection of the genital branch of genitofemoral nerve. *J Am Coll Surg.* 2004;198(2):181–184.
23. Thibaut D, de la Cuadra-Fontaine JC, Bravo MP, et al. Ilioinguinal/iliohypogastric blocks: where is the anesthetic injected? *Anesth Analg.* 2008;107(2):728–729.
24. Weintraud M, Marhofer P, Bosenberg A, et al. Ilioinguinal/iliohypogastric blocks in children: where do we administer the local anesthetic without direct visualization. *Anesth Analg.* 2008;106(1):89–93.
25. al-Dabbagh AK. Anatomical variations of the inguinal nerves and risks of injury in 110 hernia repairs. *Surg Radiol Anat.* 2002;24(2):102–107.
26. Brown DL. *Atlas of Regional Anesthesia.* Philadelphia, PA: WB Saunders; 1999.
27. Waldman SD. *Atlas of Interventional Pain Management.* Philadelphia, PA: Saunders; 2004.
28. Katz J. *Atlas of Regional Anesthesia.* Norwalk, CT: Appleton-Century-Crofts; 1985.
29. van Schoor AN, Boon JM, Bosenberg AT, Abrahams PH, Meiring JH. Anatomical considerations of the pediatric ilioinguinal/iliohypogastric nerve block. *Paediatr Anaesth.* 2005;15(5): 371–377.
30. Lipp AK, Woodcock J, Hensman B, Wilkinson K. Leg weakness is a complication of ilio-inguinal nerve block in children. *Br J Anaesth.* 2004;92(2):273–274.
31. Johr M, Sossai R. Colonic puncture during ilioinguinal nerve block in a child. *Anesth Analg.* 1999;88(5):1051–1052.
32. Amory C, Mariscal A, Guyot E, Chauvet P, Leon A, Poli-Merol ML. Is ilioinguinal/iliohypogastric nerve block always totally safe in children? *Paediatr Anaesth.* 2003;13(2):164–166.
33. Vaisman J. Pelvic hematoma after an ilioinguinal nerve block for orchialgia. *Anesth Analg.* 2001;92(4):1048–1049.
34. Eichenberger U, Greher M, Kirchmair L, Curatolo M, Morigg B. Ultrasound-guided blocks of the ilioinguinal and iliohypogastric nerve: accuracy of a selective new technique confirmed by anatomical dissection. *Br J Anaesth.* 2006;97(2):238–243.
35. Gofeld M, Christakis M. Sonographically guided ilioinguinal nerve block. *J Ultrasound Med.* 2006;25(12):1571–1575.
36. Hu P, Harmon D, Frizelle H. Ultrasound-guided blocks of the ilioinguinal/iliohypogastric nerve block: a pilot study. *Ir J Med Sci.* 2007;176(2):111–115.
37. Ford S, Dosani M, Robinson AJ, et al. Defining the reliability of sonoanatomy identification by novices in ultrasound-guided pediatric ilioinguinal and iliohypogastric nerve blockade. *Anesth Analg.* 2009;109(6):1793–1798.
38. Broadman L. Ilioinguinal, iliohypogastric, and genitofemoral nerves. In: Gay SG, ed. *Regional Anesthesia. An Atlas of Anatomy and Techniques.* St Louis, MA: Mosby; 1996:247–254.
39. Conn D, Nicholls B. Regional anaesthesia. In: Wilson IH, Allman KG, eds. *Oxford Handbook of Anaesthesia.* 2nd ed. New York: Oxford University Press; 2006:1055–1104.
40. NYSORA. *Genitofemoral Nerve Block.* <http://nysora.com/peripheral_nerve_blocks/classic_block_techniques/3081-genitofemoral>; 2009. Accessed 11.12.09.
41. Parziale JR, Hudgins TH, Fishman LM. The piriformis syndrome. *Am J Orthop.* 1996;25(12): 819–893.
42. Barton PM. Piriformis syndrome: a rational approach to management. *Pain.* 1991;47(3):345–352.
43. Durrani Z, Winnie AP. Piriformis muscle syndrome: an underdiagnosed cause of sciatica. *J Pain Symptom Manage.* 1991;6(6):374–379.
44. Hallin RP. Sciatic pain and the piriformis muscle. *Postgrad Med.* 1983;74(2):69–72.
45. Benzon HT, Katz JA, Enzon HA, Iqbal MS. Piriformis syndrome anatomic considerations, a new injection technique, and a review of the literature. *Anesthesiology.* 2003;98(6):1442–1448.
46. Robinson D. Piriformis syndrome in relations to sciatic pain. *Am J Surg.* 1947;73:335–358.
47. Papadopoulos EC, Khan SN. Piriformis syndrome and low back pain: a new classification and review of the literature. *Orthop Clin North Am.* 2004;35(1):65–71.
48. Benson ER, Schutzer SF. Posttraumatic piriformis syndrome: diagnosis and results of operative treatment. *J Bone Joint Surg Am.* 1999;81(7):941–949.
49. Fishman S, Caneris O, Bandman T, Audette J, Borsook D. Injection of the piriformis muscle by fluoroscopic and electromyographic guidance. *Reg Anesth Pain Med.* 1998;23(6):554–559.
50. Lang AM. Botulinum toxin type B in piriformis syndrome. *Am J Phys Med Rehabil.* 2004;83(3):198–202.
51. Fishman L, Konnoth C, Rozner B. Botulinum neurotoxin type B and physical therapy in the treatment of piriformis syndrome: a dose finding study. *Am J Phys Med Rehabil.* 2004;83(1):42–50.
52. Pecina M. Contribution to the etiological explanation of the piriformis syndrome. *Acta Anat.* 1979;105(2):181–187.

53. Beason LE, Anson BJ. The relation of the sciatic nerve and its subdivisions to the piriformis muscle. *Anat Rec.* 1937;70:1–5.

54. Fanucci E, Masala S, Sodani G, et al. CT-guided injection of botulinic toxin for percutaneous therapy of piriformis muscle syndrome with preliminary MRI results about denervative process. *Eur Radiol.* 2001;11(12):2543–2548.

55. Filler A, Haynes J, Jordan S, et al. Sciatic pain of non-disc origin and piriformis syndrome: diagnosis by magnetic resonance neurography and interventional magnetic resonance imaging with outcome of resulting treatment. *J Neurosurg Spine.* 2005;2(2):99–115.

56. Fishman LM, Dombi GW, Michaelson C, et al. Piriformis syndrome: diagnosis, treatment, and outcome – a 10 year study. *Arch Phys Med Rehabil.* 2002;83(3):295–301.

57. Fishman LM, Andersen C, Rosner B. Botox and physical therapy in the treatment of piriformis syndrome. *Am J Phys Med Rehabil.* 2002;81(12):936–942.

58. Finoff JT, Hurdle MFB, Smith J. Accuracy of ultrasound-guided versus fluoroscopically guided contrast controlled piriformis injections. A cadaveric study. *J Ultrasound Med.* 2008;27(8): 1157–1163.

59. Koski JM. Ultrasound-guided injections in rheumatology. *J Rheumatol.* 2000;27(9):2131–2138.

60. Broadhurst NA, Simmons ND, Bond MJ. Piriformis syndrome: correlation of muscle morphology with symptoms and signs. *Arch Phys Med Rehabil.* 2004;85(12):2036–2039.

61. Huerto AP, Yeo SN, Ho KY. Piriformis muscle injection using ultrasonography and motor stimulation – report of a technique. *Pain Physician.* 2007;10(5):687–690.

62. Robert R, Prat-Pradal D, Labat JJ, et al. Anatomic basis of chronic perineal pain: role of the pudendal nerve. *Surg Radiol Anat.* 1998;20(2):93–98.

63. Benson JT, Griffis K. Pudendal neuralgia, a severe pain syndrome. *Am J Obstet Gynecol.* 2005;192(5):1663–1668.

64. Amarenco G, Kerdraon J, Bouju P, et al. Treatments of perineal neuralgia caused by involvement of the pudendal nerve. *Rev Neurol.* 1997;153(5):331–334.

65. Peng PWH, Antolak SJ Jr, Gordon AS. Pudendal neuralgia. In: Pukall C, Goldstein GI, Goldstein A, eds. *Female Sexual Pain Disorders.* 1st ed. Hoboken, NJ: Wiley-Blackwell; 2009:112–118.

66. Labat JJ, Riant T, Robert R, et al. Diagnostic criteria for pudendal neuralgia by pudendal nerve entrapment (Nantes criteria). *Neurourol Urodyn.* 2008;27(4):306–310.

67. Leibovitch I, Mor Y. The vicious cycling: bicycling related urogenital disorders. *Eur Urol.* 2005;47(3):277–287.

68. Allen RE, Hosker GL, Smith AR, Warrell DW. Pelvic floor damage and childbirth: a neurophysiological study. *Br J Obstet Gynaecol.* 1990;97(9):770–779.

69. Lien KC, Morgan DM, Delancey JO, Ashton-Miller JA. Pudendal nerve stretch during vaginal birth: a 3D computer simulation. *Am J Obstet Gynecol.* 2005;192(5):1669–1676.

70. Soulie M, Vazzoler N, Seguin P, Chiron P, Plante P. Urological consequences of pudendal nerve trauma during orthopedic surgery: review and practical advice. *Prog Urol.* 2002;12(3):504–509.

71. Amarenco G, Ismael SS, Bayle B, Denys P, Kerdraon J. Electrophysiological analysis of pudendal neuropathy following traction. *Muscle Nerve.* 2001;24(1):116–119.

72. Antolak S, Hough D, Pawlina W, Spinner RJ. Anatomical basis of chronic pelvic pain syndrome: the ischial spine and pudendal nerve entrapment. *Med Hypotheses.* 2002;59(3):349–353.

73. Labat JJ, Robert R, Bensignor M, Buzelin JM. Neuralgia of the pudendal nerve. Anatomo-clinical considerations and therapeutical approach. *J Urol (Paris).* 1990;96(5):329–344.

74. Amarenco G, Lancoe Y, Ghnassia RT, Goudal H, Pernigot M. Alcock's canal syndrome and perineal neuralgia. *Rev Neurol (Paris).* 1988;144(8–9):523–526.

75. Juenemann K-P, Lue TF, Scmidt RA, Tanagho EA. Clinical significance of sacral and pudendal nerve anatomy. *J Urol.* 1988;139(1):74–80.

76. Gruber H, Kovacs P, Piegger J, Brenner E. New, simple, ultrasound-guided infiltration of the pudendal nerve: topographic basics. *Dis Colon Rectum.* 2001;44(9):1376–1380.

77. Mahakkanukrauh P, Surin P, Vaidhayakarn P. Anatomical study of the pudendal nerve adjacent to the sacrospinous ligament. *Clin Anat.* 2005;18(3):200–205.

78. Shafik A, Doss SH. Pudendal canal: surgical anatomy and clinical implications. *Am Surg.* 1999;65(2):176–180.

79. O'Bichere A, Green C, Phillips RK. New, simple approach for maximal pudendal nerve exposure: anomalies and prospects for functional reconstruction. *Dis Colon Rectum.* 2000;43(7):956–960.

80. Thompson JR, Gibbs S, Genadry R, Burros L, Lambrou N, Buller JL. Anatomy of pelvic arteries adjacent to the sacrospinous ligament: importance of the coccygeal branch of the inferior gluteal artery. *Obstet Gynecol.* 1999;94(6):973–977.

81. Shafik A, el-Sherif M, Youssef A, Olfat ES. Surgical anatomy of the pudendal nerve and its clinical implications. *Clin Anat.* 1995;8(2):110–115.
82. Schraffordt SE, Tjandra JJ, Eizenberg N, Dwyer PL. Anatomy of the pudendal nerve and its terminal branches: a cadaver study. *ANZ J Surg.* 2004;74(1–2):23–26.
83. Sedy J, Nanka O, Belisova M, Walro JM, Jarolim L. Sulcus nervi dorsalis penis/clitoridis: anatomic structure and clinical significance. *Eur Urol.* 2006;50(5):1079–1085.
84. Bowes WA. Clinical aspects of normal and abnormal labour. In: Resnick R, Creasy RK, eds. *Maternal-Fetal Medicine: Principles and Practice.* 2nd ed. Philadelphia, PA: WB Saunders; 1989:510–546.
85. Naja Z, Ziade MF, Lonnqvist PA. Nerve stimulator-guided pudendal nerve block decreases posthemorrhoidectomy pain. *Can J Anaesth.* 2005;52(1):62–68.
86. Imbelloni LE, Viera EM, Gouveia MA, Netinho JG, Spirandelli LD, Cordeiro JA. Pudendal block with bupivacaine for postoperative pain relief. *Dis Colon Rectum.* 2007;50(10):1656–1661.
87. Prat-Pradal D, Metge L, Gagnard-Landra C, Mares P, Dauzat M, Godlewski G. Anatomical basis of transgluteal pudendal nerve block. *Surg Radiol Anat.* 2009;31(4):289–293.
88. Choi SS, Lee PB, Kim YC, Kim HJ, Lee SC. C-arm guided pudendal nerve block: a new technique. *Int J Clin Pract.* 2006;60(5):553–556.
89. Kovacs P, Gruber H, Piegger J, Bodner G. New, simple, ultrasound-guided infiltration of the pudendal nerve: ultrasonographic technique. *Dis Colon Rectum.* 2001;44(9):1381–1385.
90. Hough DM, Wittenberg KH, Pawlina W, et al. Chronic perineal pain caused by pudendal nerve entrapment: anatomy and CT-guided perineural injection technique. *AJR Am J Roentgenol.* 2003;181(2):561–567.

IV

Ultrasound-Guided Peripheral Nerve Blocks and Continuous Catheters

17

Ultrasound-Guided Nerve Blocks of the Upper Extremity

Anahi Perlas, Sheila Riazi, and Cyrus C.H. Tse

A. Perlas (✉)
Department of Anesthesia, University of Toronto, Toronto Western Hospital,
399 Bathurst Street, MP 2-405, Toronto, ON, Canada M5T 2S8
e-mail: anahi.perlas@uhn.on.ca

S.N. Narouze (ed.), *Atlas of Ultrasound-Guided Procedures in Interventional Pain Management*,
DOI 10.1007/978-1-4419-1681-5_17, © Springer Science+Business Media, LLC 2011

Introduction

Traditional peripheral nerve block techniques are performed without image guidance and are based on the identification of surface anatomical landmarks. Anatomical variations among individuals, the small size of target neural structures, and proximity to blood vessels, the lung, and other vital structures make these techniques often difficult, of varying success, and sometimes associated with serious complications.

Ultrasonography is the first imaging modality to be broadly used in regional anesthesia practice. Ultrasound (US) provides real-time imaging that can help define individual regional anatomy, guide needle advancement with precision, and ensure adequate local anesthetic spread, potentially optimizing nerve block efficacy and safety. The brachial plexus and its branches are particularly amenable to sonographic examination given their superficial location. The small distances from the skin make it possible to image these nerves with high-frequency (10–15 MHz) linear probes, which provide high-resolution images.

Brachial Plexus Anatomy

Thorough knowledge of brachial plexus anatomy is required to facilitate the technical aspects of block placement and to optimize patient-specific block selection.

The brachial plexus originates from the ventral primary rami of spinal nerves C5–T1 and extends from the neck to the apex of the axilla (Figure 17.1). Variable contributions may also come from the fourth cervical (C4) and the second thoracic (T2) nerves. The C5 and C6 rami typically unite near the medial border of the middle scalene muscle to form the superior trunk of the plexus; the C7 ramus becomes the middle trunk; and the C8 and T1 rami unite to form the inferior trunk. The C7 transverse process lacks an anterior tubercle, which facilitates the ultrasonographic identification of the C7 nerve root.[1] The roots and trunks pass through the interscalene groove, a palpable surface anatomic landmark between the anterior and middle scalene muscles. The three trunks undergo primary anatomic separation into anterior (flexor) and posterior (extensor) divisions at the lateral border of the first rib. The anterior divisions of the superior and middle trunks form the lateral cord of the plexus, the posterior divisions of all three trunks form the posterior cord, and

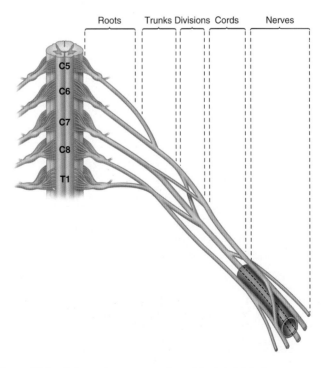

Figure 17.1. Schematic representation of the brachial plexus structures.

the anterior division of the inferior trunk forms the medial cord. The three cords divide and give rise to the terminal branches of the plexus, with each cord possessing two major terminal branches and a variable number of minor intermediary branches. The lateral cord contributes the musculocutaneous nerve and the lateral component of the median nerve. The posterior cord generally supplies the dorsal aspect of the upper extremity via the radial and axillary nerves. The medial cord contributes the ulnar nerve and the medial component of the median nerve. Important intermediary branches of the medial cord include the medial antebrachial cutaneous nerve and the medial cutaneous nerve, which joins with the smaller intercostobrachial nerve (T2) to innervate the skin over the medial aspect of the arm.[2,3]

The brachial plexus provides sensory and motor innervation to the upper limb. In addition, the lateral pectoral nerve (C5–7) and the medial pectoral nerve (C8, T1), which are branches of the brachial plexus, supply the pectoral muscles; the long thoracic nerve (C5–7) supplies the serratus anterior muscle; the thoracodorsal nerve (C6–8) supplies the latissimus dorsi muscle; and the suprascapular nerve supplies the supraspinatus and infraspinatus muscles.

Interscalene Block

Anatomy

The roots of the brachial plexus are found in the interscalene groove (defined by the anterior and middle scalene muscles) deep to the sternocleidomastoid muscle.

Indication

Interscalene block remains the brachial plexus approach of choice to provide anesthesia or analgesia for shoulder surgery as it targets the proximal roots of the plexus (C4–C7). Local anesthetic spread after interscalene administration extends from the distal roots/proximal trunks and follows a distribution to the upper dermatomes of the brachial plexus that consistently includes the (nonbrachial plexus) supraclavicular nerve (C3–C4), which supplies sensory innervation to the cape of the shoulder.[4] The more distal roots of the plexus (C8–T1) are usually spared by this approach.[5]

Procedure

The patient is positioned supine with the head turned 45° to the contralateral side. A transverse image of the plexus roots in the interscalene area is obtained on the lateral aspect of the neck in an axial oblique plane (Figure 17.2). The anterior and middle scalene muscles define the interscalene groove, located deep to the sternocleidomastoid muscle lateral to the carotid artery and internal jugular vein.[6] The nerve roots appear hypoechoic, with a round or oval cross section. The roots are often best imaged at the C6 or C7 level. The C6 vertebra may be identified as the most caudad cervical vertebra with a transverse process that has both anterior and posterior tubercles. The anterior tubercle of C6 (Chassaignac's tubercle) is the most prominent of all cervical vertebrae. Scanning more caudally, C7 has only a posterior tubercle. The vertebral artery and vein may be seen adjacent to the vertebral transverse process distal to C6, deep to the interscalene space (approximately within 1 cm). One of the most common side effects of interscalene block is secondary phrenic nerve palsy and transient hemidiaphragmatic paresis. This is usually asymptomatic in otherwise healthy patients but may be poorly tolerated in patients with limited respiratory reserve, which makes it contraindicated in patients with significant underlying respiratory disease.[7] Recent data suggest that ultrasound-guided interscalene block may provide adequate postoperative analgesia with only 5 ml of local anesthetic, and this is associated with a lower incidence and lower severity of hemidiaphragmatic paresis than 20 ml of the same local anesthetic solution.[8]

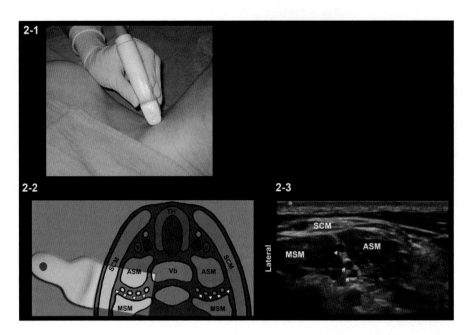

Figure 17.2. Interscalene approach to brachial plexus block. (1) Ultrasound probe placement. (2) Illustration showing the anatomical structures within the ultrasound transducer range. (3) Ultrasound view of interscalene area. MSM middle scalene muscle, ASM anterior scalene muscle, SCM sternocleidomastoid muscle, Vb vertebral body, Tr trachea, TH thyroid gland, A carotid artery, V internal jugular vein, *arrow heads* brachial plexus.

Unintentional epidural or spinal anesthesia and spinal cord injury are very rare complications of interscalene block. Recent data suggest that ultrasound guidance reduces the number of needle passes required to perform interscalene block and that more consistent anesthesia of the lower trunk is possible with ultrasound-guided techniques.[9,10]

Supraclavicular Block

Anatomy

In the supraclavicular area, the brachial plexus presents most compactly, at the level of trunks (superior, middle, and lower) and/or their respective anterior and posterior divisions, and this may explain its traditional reputation for a short latency and complete, reliable anesthesia.[11] The brachial plexus is located lateral and posterior to the subclavian artery as they both cross over the first rib and under the clavicle toward the axilla.

Indication

The supraclavicular approach to the brachial plexus is indicated for surgeries of the arm, forearm, or hand.

Procedure

With the patient in the supine position and the head turned 45° contralaterally, a transverse view of the subclavian artery and the brachial plexus may be obtained by scanning

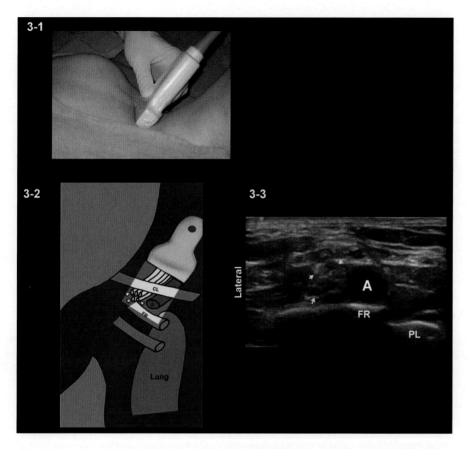

Figure 17.3. Supraclavicular approach to brachial plexus block. (1) Ultrasound probe placement. (2) Illustration showing the anatomical structures within the ultrasound transducer range. (3) Ultrasound view of supraclavicular area. *CL* clavicle, *FR* first rib, *PL* pleura, *A* subclavian artery, *arrow heads* brachial plexus.

over the supraclavicular fossa in a coronal oblique plane (Figure 17.3). The plexus appears most commonly as a group of several neural structures in this area, having been compared to a "bunch of grapes." The subclavian artery ascends from the mediastinum and moves laterally over the pleural surface on the dome of the lung. It is in this area, medial to the first rib that the brachial plexus becomes close to the subclavian artery, located posterolateral to it. It is critical for the safe performance of supraclavicular block and the prevention of pneumothorax to properly recognize the sonoanatomy of the above structures. Although both rib and pleural surface appear as hyperechoic linear surfaces on ultrasound imaging, a number of characteristics can help differentiate one from the other. A dark "anechoic" area underlies the first rib, while the area under the pleura often presents a "shimmering" quality, with occasional comet tail's signs.[12] In addition, the pleural surface moves both with normal respiration and with subclavian artery pulsation, while the rib presents no appreciable movement in response to normal respiration or arterial pulsation. Once the desired location is chosen, a needle is advanced usually in-plane in either a medial-to-lateral or lateral-to-medial orientation. Local anesthetic needs to be delivered within the plexus compartment ensuring spread to all the brachial plexus components. In order to anesthetize the lower trunk, which is required for distal limb surgeries, it has been suggested that it is best to deposit most of the local anesthetic bolus immediately above the first rib and next to the subclavian artery.[13]

The risk of pneumothorax has made the supraclavicular block an "unpopular" one for several decades. The advent of real-time ultrasound guidance has renewed interest in this particular block. The ability to consistently image the first rib and the pleura clearly and maintain the needle tip away from the latter may potentially help perform this block safely while minimizing this risk, although no comparative studies have been done. In a case series of 510 consecutive cases of ultrasound-guided supraclavicular block, complications listed were symptomatic hemidiaphragmatic paresis (1%), Horner syndrome (1%), unintended vascular puncture (0.4%), and transient sensory deficit (0.4%).[12] In contrast to the contention that UGRA facilitates blockade with smaller volumes of local anesthetic, the minimum volume required for UGRA supraclavicular blockade in 50% of patients is 23 ml, which is similar to recommended volumes for traditional nerve localization techniques.[14] Concomitant use of nerve stimulation does not seem to improve the efficacy of ultrasound-guided brachial plexus block.[15]

Infraclavicular Block

Anatomy

In the infraclavicular area, the cords of the brachial plexus are located posterior to pectoralis major and minor muscles, around the second part of the axillary artery. The lateral cord of the plexus lies superior and lateral, the posterior cord lies posterior, and the medial cord lies posterior and medial to the axillary artery. It typically represents the deepest of all supraclavicular locations (approximately 4–6 cm from the skin).[16]

Indication

This approach to the brachial plexus has similar indications to the supraclavicular block.[17]

Procedure

Both linear and curved probes may be used to image the plexus in this area near the coracoid process in a parasagittal plane.[18] In children or slim adults, a 10-MHz probe may be used.[19] However, for many adults a probe of lower resolution may be needed (4–7 MHz, for example) to obtain the required image penetration (up to 5–6 cm). With the patient positioned supine and the arm on the side, or abducted 90°, the axillary artery and vein can be readily identified in a transverse view scanning in a parasagittal plane (Figure 17.4). The three adjacent brachial plexus cords appear hyperechoic with the lateral cord most commonly superior (9–12 o'clock position), the medial cord inferior (3–6 o'clock position), and the posterior cord posterior (6–9 o'clock position), to the artery.[20] Abducting the arm 110° and externally rotating the shoulder moves the plexus away from the thorax and closer to the surface of the skin often improving identification of the cords.[21] A block needle is usually inserted in plane with the ultrasound beam (parasagittal plane) in a cephalo-to-caudad orientation. Medial needle orientation toward the chest wall needs to be avoided, as pneumothorax remains a risk with this approach as well.[22] Local anesthetic spread in a "U" shape posterior to the artery provides consistent anesthesia to the three cords.[23,24] Preliminary data suggest that low-dose ultrasound-guided infraclavicular blocks (16 ± 2 ml) can be performed without compromise to block success or onset time.[25]

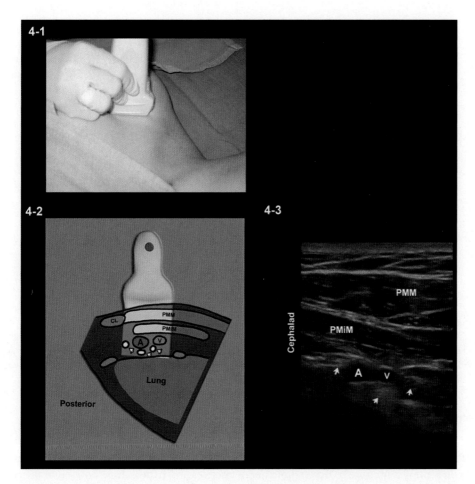

Figure 17.4. Infraclavicular approach to brachial plexus block. (1) Ultrasound probe placement. (2) Illustration showing the anatomical structures within the ultrasound transducer range. (3) Ultrasound view of infraclavicular area. *PMM* pectoralis major muscle, *PMiM* pectoralis minor muscle, *CL* clavicle, *A* axillary artery, *V* axillary vein, *arrowheads* brachial plexus.

Axillary Block

Anatomy

The axillary approach to the brachial plexus targets the terminal branches of the plexus, which include the median, ulnar, radial, and musculocutaneous nerves. The musculocutaneous nerve often departs from the lateral cord in the proximal axilla and is commonly spared by the axillary approach, unless specifically targeted.

Indication

Axillary brachial plexus block is usually indicated for distal upper limb surgery (hand and wrist).

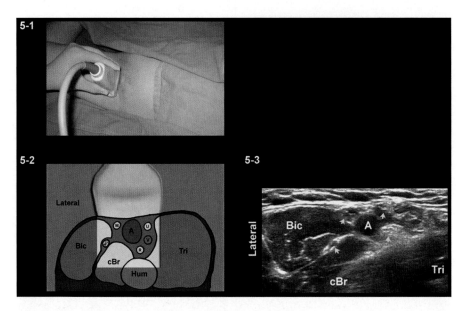

Figure 17.5. Axillary approach to brachial plexus block. (1) Ultrasound probe placement. (2) Illustration showing the anatomical structures within the ultrasound transducer range. (3) Ultrasound view of axillary area. *Bic* biceps muscle, *cBr* coracobrachialis muscle, *Hum* humerus, *Tri* triceps muscle, A axillary artery, V axillary vein, MC musculocutaneous nerve, M median nerve, U ulnar nerve, R radial nerve, *arrow heads* brachial plexus.

Procedure

The transducer is placed along the axillary crease, perpendicular to the long axis of the arm. Nerves in the axilla have mixed echogenicity and a "honeycomb" appearance (representing a mixture of hypoechoic nerve fascicles and hyperechoic nonneural fibers). The median, ulnar, and radial nerves are usually located in close proximity to the axillary artery between the anterior (biceps and coracobrachialis) and posterior (triceps) muscle compartments (Figure 17.5).[26] The median nerve is commonly found anteromedial to the artery, the ulnar nerve medial to the artery, and the radial nerve posteromedial to it. The musculocutaneous nerve often branches off more proximally, and may be located in a plane between the biceps and coracobrachialis muscles.[27] Separate blockade of each individual nerve is recommended to ensure complete anesthesia. Similarly to other brachial plexus approaches, because of the superficial location of all terminal nerves, it is useful to use a needle-in-plane approach. Ultrasound guidance has been associated with higher block success rates and lower volumes of local anesthetic solution required compared to nonimage-guided techniques.[28,29]

Distal Peripheral Nerves in the Upper Extremity

Blocking individual nerves in the distal arm or forearm may be useful as supplemental blocks if a single nerve territory is "missed" with a plexus approach. Scanning along the upper extremity, these peripheral nerves may be followed and blocked in many locations along their course. Five milliliters of local anesthetic solution is generally sufficient to block any of the terminal nerves individually. We herein suggest some frequently used locations in the arm.

Median nerve can be located just proximal to the elbow crease, medial to the brachial artery (Figure 17.6).

The radial nerve can be located in the lateral aspect of the distal part of the arm, deep to the brachialis and brachioradialis muscles and superficial to the humerus (Figure 17.7).

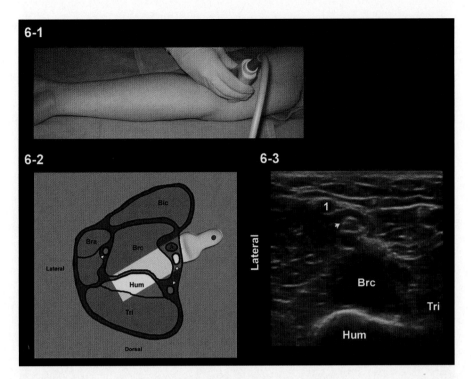

Figure 17.6. Median nerve block in distal arm. (1) Ultrasound probe placement. (2) Illustration showing the anatomical structures within the ultrasound transducer range. (3) Ultrasound view of median nerve in distal arm. *Bic* biceps muscle, *Bra* brachioradialis muscle, *Brc* brachialis muscle, *Hum* humerus, *Tri* triceps muscle, *A* brachial artery, *arrow head* within the ultrasound transducer range; median nerve.

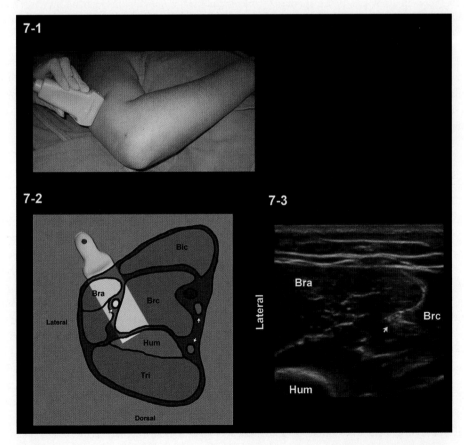

Figure 17.7. Radial nerve block in distal arm. (1) Ultrasound probe placement. (2) Illustration showing the anatomical structures within the ultrasound transducer range. (3) Ultrasound view of radial nerve in distal arm. *Bic* biceps muscle, *Bra* brachioradialis muscle, *Brc* brachialis muscle, *Hum* humerus, *Tri* triceps muscle, *A* brachial artery, *arrow head* within the ultrasound transducer range; radial nerve.

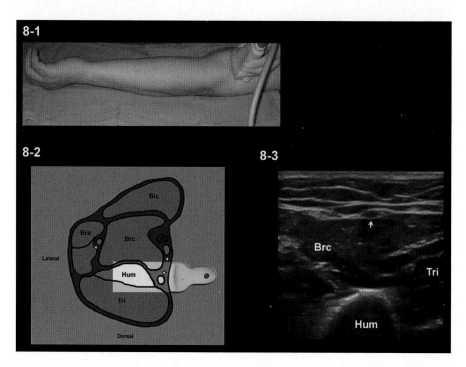

Figure 17.8. Ulnar nerve block in distal arm. (1) Ultrasound probe placement. (2) Illustration showing the anatomical structures within the ultrasound transducer range. (3) Ultrasound view of ulnar nerve in distal arm. *Bic* biceps muscle, *Bra* brachioradialis muscle, *Brc* brachialis muscle, *Hum* humerus, *Tri* triceps muscle, *A* brachial artery, *arrow head* within the ultrasound transducer range; ulnar nerve.

The ulnar nerve is superficially located in the arm. Blockade of the ulnar nerve at the elbow (ulnar groove) is traditionally discouraged as the nerve is circumscribed by rigid structures (bones and ligaments) and there is the potential for entrapment. However, it may be safely blocked proximal to the ulnar groove (Figure 17.8).

Summary

In this chapter, we have discussed some common approaches of ultrasound-guided blocks of the brachial plexus and its terminal nerves. Ultrasound-guided regional anesthesia is a rapidly evolving field. Recent advances in ultrasound technology have enhanced the resolution of portable equipment and improved the image quality of neural structures and the regional anatomy relevant to peripheral nerve blockade. The ability to image the anatomy in real time, guide a block needle under image, and tailor local anesthetic spread is a unique advantage of ultrasound imaging vs. traditional landmark-based techniques. Much research is currently underway to study if these potential advantages result in greater efficacy and improved safety.

REFERENCES

1. Martinoli C, Bianchi S, Santacroca E, Pugliese F, Graif M, Derchi LE. Brachial plexus sonography: a technique for assessing the root level. *AJR Am J Roentgenol.* 2002;179:699–702.
2. Gray's Anatomy. The Anatomical Basis of Clinical Practice. 39th ed. In: Standring S, ed. Edinburgh: Elsevier Churchill Livingstone; 2005.
3. Neal JM, Gerancher JC, Hebl JR, et al. Upper extremity regional anesthesia: essentials of our current understanding. *Reg Anesth Pain Med.* 2009;34:134–170.

4. Urmey WF, Grossi P, Sharrock NE, Stanton J, Gloeggler PJ. Digital pressure during interscalene block is clinically ineffective in preventing anesthetic spread to the cervical plexus. *Anesth Analg.* 1996;83:366–370.

5. Lanz E, Theiss D, Jankovic D. The extent of blockade following various techniques of brachial plexus block. *Anesth Analg.* 1983;62:55–58.

6. Chan VWS. Applying ultrasound imaging to interscalene brachial plexus block. *Reg Anesth Pain Med.* 2003;28(4):340–343.

7. Urmey WF, Talts KH, Sharrock NE. One hundred percent incidence of hemidiaphragmatic paresis associated with interscalene brachial plexus anesthesia as diagnosed by ultrasonography. *Anesth Analg.* 1991;72:498–503.

8. Riazi S, Carmichael N, Awad I, Holtby RM, McCartney CJL. Effect of local anesthetic volume (20 vs 5 ml) on the efficacy and respiratory consequences of ultrasound-guided interscalene brachial plexus block. *Br J Anaesth.* 2008;101:549–556.

9. Kapral S, Greher M, Huber G, et al. Ultrasonographic guidance improves the success rate of interscalene brachial plexus blockade. *Reg Anesth Pain Med.* 2008;33:253–258.

10. Liu SS, Zayas VM, Gordon MA, et al. A prospective, randomized, controlled trial comparing ultrasound versus nerve stimulator guidance for interscalene block for ambulatory shoulder surgery for postoperative neurological symptoms. *Anesth Analg.* 2009;109:265–271.

11. Brown DL, Cahill DR, Bridenbaugh LD. Supraclavicular nerve block: anatomic analysis of a method to prevent pneumothorax. *Anesth Analg.* 1993;76:530–534.

12. Perlas A, Lobo G, Lo N, Brull R, Chan V, Karkhanis R. Ultrasound-guided supraclavicular block. Outcome of 510 consecutive cases. *Reg Anesth Pain Med.* 2009;34:171–176.

13. Soares LG, Brull R, Lai J, Chan VW. Eight ball, corner pocket: the optimal needle position for ultrasound-guided supraclavicular block. *Reg Anesth Pain Med.* 2007;32:94–95.

14. Duggan E, El Beheiry H, Perlas A, et al. Minimum effective volume of local anesthetic for ultrasound-guided supraclavicular brachial plexus block. *Reg Anesth Pain Med.* 2009;34:215–218.

15. Beach ML, Sites BD, Gallagher JD. Use of a nerve stimulator does not improve the efficacy of ultrasound-guided supraclavicular block. *J Clin Anesth.* 2006;18:580–584.

16. Sauter AR, Smith HJ, Stubhaug A, Dodgson MS, Klaastad O. Use of magnetic resonance imaging to define the anatomical location closest to all three cords of the infraclavicular brachial plexus. *Anesth Analg.* 2006;103:1574–1576.

17. Arcand G, Williams S, Chouinard P, et al. Ultrasound guided infraclavicular versus supraclavicular block. *Anesth Analg.* 2005;101:886–890.

18. Sandhu NS, Manne JS, Medabalmi PK, Capan LM. Sonographically guided infraclavicular brachial plexus block in adults: a retrospective analysis of 1146 cases. *J Ultrasound Med.* 2006;25:1555–1561.

19. Marhofer P, Sitzwohl C, Greher M, Kapral S. Ultrasound guidance for infraclavicular brachial plexus anesthesia in children. *Anesthesia.* 2004;59:642–646.

20. Porter J, Mc Cartney C, Chan V. Needle placement and injection posterior to the axillary artery may predict successful infraclavicular brachial plexus block: a report of three cases. *Can J Anaesth.* 2005;52:69–73.

21. Bigeleisen P, Wilson M. A comparison of two techniques for ultrasound guided infraclavicular block. *Br J Anaesth.* 2006;96:502–507.

22. Koscielniak-Nielsen ZJ, Rasmussen H, Hesselbjerg L. Pneumothorax after an ultrasound guided lateral sagittal infraclavicular block. *Acta Anaesthesiol Scand.* 2008;52:1176–1177.

23. Tran DQ, Charghi R, Finlayson RJ. The "double bubble" sign for successful infraclavicular brachial plexus blockade. *Anesth Analg.* 2006;103:1048–1049.

24. Bloc S, Garnier T, komly B, et al. Spread of injectate associated with radial or median nerve-type motor response during infraclavicular brachial plexus block: an ultrasound evaluation. *Reg Anesth Pain Med.* 2007;32:130–135.

25. Sandhu NS, Bahniwal CS, Capan LM. Feasibility of an infraclavicular block with a reduced volume of lidocaine with sonographic guidance. *J Ultrasound Med.* 2006;25(1):51–56.

26. Retzl G, Kapral S, Greher M, et al. Ultrasonographic findings of the axillary part of the brachial plexus. *Anesth Analg.* 2001;92:1271–1275.

27. Spence B, Sites B, Beach M. Ultrasound-guided musculocutaneous nerve block: a description of a novel technique. *Reg Anesth Pain Med.* 2005;30(2):198–201.

28. Lo N, Brull R, Perlas A, et al. Evolution of ultrasound guided axillary brachial plexus blockade: retrospective analysis of 662 blocks. *Can J Anaesth.* 2008;55:408–413.

29. O'Donnell BD, Iohom G. An estimation of the minimum effective anesthetic volume of 2% lidocaine in ultrasound-guided axillary brachial plexus block. *Anesthesiology.* 2009;111:25–29.

18

Ultrasound-Guided Nerve Blocks of the Lower Limb

Haresh Mulchandani, Imad T. Awad, and Colin J.L. McCartney

C.J.L. McCartney (✉)
Department of Anesthesia, Sunnybrook Health Sciences Center, University of Toronto,
2075 Bayview Avenue, Toronto, ON, Canada M4N 3M5
e-mail: cjlmccartney@sympatico.ca

S.N. Narouze (ed.), *Atlas of Ultrasound-Guided Procedures in Interventional Pain Management*,
DOI 10.1007/978-1-4419-1681-5_18, © Springer Science+Business Media, LLC 2011

General Considerations

Ultrasound imaging has transformed the practice of regional anesthesia in the last 6 years by providing direct visualization of needle tip as it approaches the desired nerves and real-time control of the spread of local anesthetics.[1,2] The use of ultrasound imaging has also been expanding in the field of chronic pain management recently with the availability of smaller, less expensive, and more portable machines. Compared with the traditional fluoroscopy, ultrasound imaging overheads are lower as it does not require an x-ray compatible suite and protective clothing and has no radiation hazards to patients and staff. It does though have its limitations, possessing only a narrow imaging window, which is very sensitive to the probe's position and direction.[3]

The ultrasound device used ideally possesses a high-frequency (7–12 MHz) linear array probe, suited for looking at superficial structures (up to an approximate depth of 50 mm), and a low-frequency (2–5 MHz) curved array probe, which provides better tissue penetration and a wider field of view (but at the expense of resolution) (Figure 18.1). Appropriate covering or sheathing of the ultrasound probe is required to maintain sterility of the procedure and to protect the US probe itself and prevent the possibility of any cross infection between patients.

When using the ultrasound machine to assist with blocks, the operator should assume the most ergonomic positioning of their equipment, and themselves (Figure 18.2). The ultrasound machine is commonly placed on the opposite side to where the block is to be performed. Where possible the operator should be seated and the height of the patient's stretcher should be adjusted accordingly. When holding the probe it is often helpful to steady its position by gripping it lower down and placing the operator's fingers against the patient's skin.[4] When scanning if possible the operator's arm should rest on the stretcher. All these things together help prevent operator fatigue and discomfort.

The lower limb peripheral nerve block techniques are discussed below, with those employed more frequently described first.

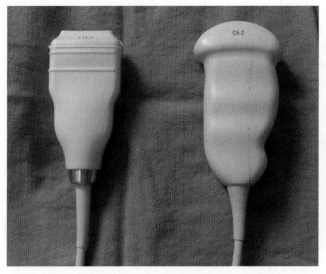

Figure 18.1. Linear probe (*left*), curvilinear probe (*right*).

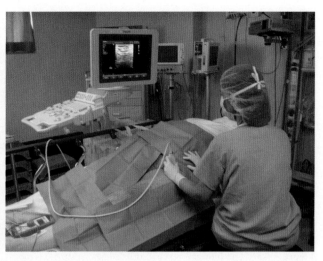

Figure 18.2. Proper positioning of operator using ultrasound machine.

Femoral Nerve Block

Clinical Application

The femoral nerve block provides analgesia and anesthesia to the anterior aspect of the thigh and knee, as well as the medial aspect of the calf and foot via the saphenous nerve. A single injection or continuous catheter technique can be used. When combined with a sciatic nerve block it provides complete anesthesia and analgesia below the knee joint. Studies have demonstrated that ultrasound guidance leads to faster and denser blocks, as well as a reduction in local anesthetic requirements, when compared to nerve stimulation guidance.[5,6]

Anatomy (Figures 18.3 and 18.4)

The femoral nerve arises from the lumbar plexus (L2, L3, and L4 spinal nerves) and travels through the body of the psoas muscle.[7] It lies deep to the fascia iliaca, which extends from the posterior and lateral walls of the pelvis and blends with the inguinal ligament, and superficial to the iliopsoas muscle. The femoral artery and vein lie anterior to the fascia iliaca. The vessels pass behind the inguinal ligament and become invested in the fascial sheath. Thus the femoral nerve, unlike the femoral vessels, does not lie within the fascial sheath, but lies posterior and lateral to it. The fascia lata overlies all three femoral structures: nerve, artery, and vein. Thus the femoral nerve is amenable to sonographic examination, given its superficial location and consistent position lateral to the femoral artery.

Preparation and Positioning

Noninvasive monitors are applied and intravenous access obtained. The patient is placed supine with the leg in the neutral position. Intravenous sedative agents and oxygen therapy are administered as required. In patients with high body mass index, it may be necessary to retract the lower abdomen to expose the inguinal crease. This may be performed by an assistant, or by using adhesive tape, going from the patient's abdominal wall to an anchoring structure such as the side arms of the stretcher. Skin disinfection is then performed and a sterile technique observed.

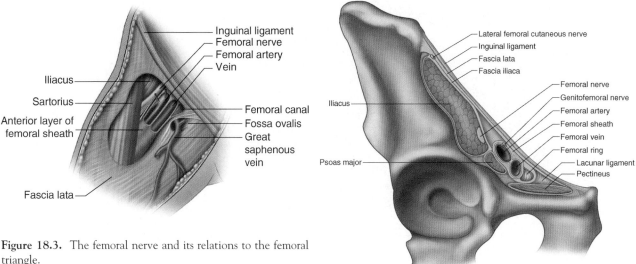

Figure 18.3. The femoral nerve and its relations to the femoral triangle.

Figure 18.4. The femoral nerve.

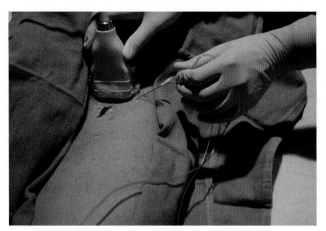

Figure 18.5. Femoral nerve block in-plane approach.

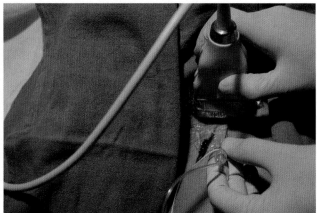

Figure 18.6. Femoral nerve block out-of-plane approach.

Ultrasound Technique

A high-frequency (7–12 MHz) linear ultrasound is placed along the inguinal crease. Either an in-plane or out-of-plane approach may be used, with the latter favored for placement of continuous femoral nerve catheters (Figures 18.5 and 8.6).

The ultrasound probe is placed to identify the femoral artery and then moved laterally, keeping the femoral artery visible on the medial aspect of the screen. It is often easier to see the femoral nerve when visualized more proximally beside the common femoral artery rather than distal to the branching of the profunda femoris artery. Thus, if two arteries are identified, scan more proximally until only one artery is visible. The femoral nerve appears as a hyperechoic flattened oval structure lateral to the femoral artery (Figure 18.7).

The femoral nerve is usually observed 1–2 cm lateral to the femoral artery. Once the femoral nerve has been identified lidocaine is infiltrated into the overlying skin and subcutaneous tissue. The distension of the subcutaneous tissues with infiltration of the lidocaine can be seen on the ultrasound image.

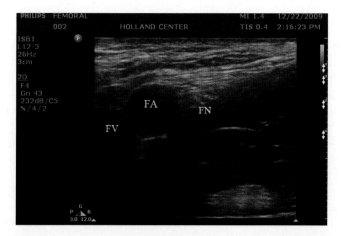

Figure 18.7. Transverse scan of inguinal region (*FN* femoral nerve, *FA* femoral artery, *FV* femoral vein).

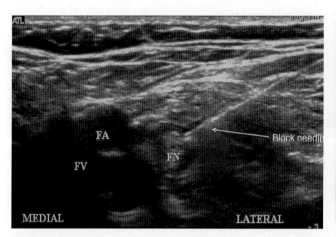

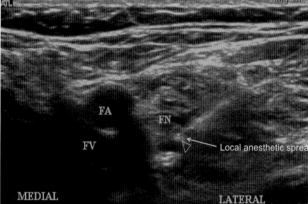

Figure 18.8. Femoral structures with block needle in-plane approach (*FN* femoral nerve, *FA* femoral artery, *FV* femoral vein).

Figure 18.9. Local anesthetic spread around femoral structures (*FN* femoral nerve, *FA* femoral artery, *FV* femoral vein).

Single-Injection Technique

A 20 ml syringe is attached to the 50-mm block needle and the needle is flushed with the local anesthetic solution contained therein. The block needle is inserted either in an in-plane or out-of-plane approach. Whether using an in-plane or out-of-plane approach, the needle tip should be constantly visualized with ultrasound. The advantage of the in-plane approach is that it is usually possible to visualize the whole shaft of the needle, whereas only the tip may be visible with an out-of-plane approach. The needle is aimed adjacent to the nerve. If nerve stimulation is used, quadriceps muscle contraction (patellar twitch) is sought. If the sartorius muscle contracts instead (inner thigh movement), then the needle needs to be redirected deeper and more laterally. After a negative aspiration test for blood, 20 ml of local anesthetic is injected in 5 ml increments. The spread of the local anesthetic can be visualized in real time as hypoechoic solution surrounding the femoral nerve, and the needle tip is repositioned if required to ensure appropriate spread. Using ultrasound guidance alone, it is possible to deliberately direct the needle a few centimeters lateral to the femoral vessels and nerve under the fascia iliaca. Figures 18.8 and 18.9 illustrate the image of the femoral nerve before and after the injection of local anesthetic around it. In the former, the femoral structures are identified with the block needle in place. The latter shows the spread of local anesthetic around the femoral nerve.

Continuous Catheter Technique

This is similar to the single-injection technique. In our center, an out-of-plane technique is used more commonly to enable the catheter to pass more easily along the longitudinal axis of the nerve. An in-plane technique may also be employed though. A 80-mm 17 G insulated needle with a 20-G catheter is used. If nerve stimulation is utilized, then it is attached to the catheter and not to the introducing needle. The catheter is placed within the introducer needle such that its tip is well within the introducer needle. This is to prevent any catheter tip damage as the introducer is positioned. Care must be taken to grip the catheter together with the introducer needle at its hub to prevent any unwanted migration of the catheter further into the introducer needle. An electrical circuit is still formed as current passes from the tip of the catheter to the tip of the introducer needle and into the patient. The introducer needle tip is visualized in the correct position by ultrasound, and the quadriceps contraction at a current of 0.3–0.5 mA if electrical stimulation is utilized. The needle may be repositioned at this point to a more horizontal position, to enable the threading of the catheter. The catheter is now advanced and electrical stimulation maintained (if used). Catheter insertion should be without resistance. If not, then the needle needs to be repositioned. The catheter is usually advanced further in the space as the introducer needle is removed, such that it is approximately 5 cm beyond where the tip of the introducer needle was placed (thus usually around 10 cm at the skin). The catheter's position is secured and dressings applied. Local anesthetic spread can be visualized as it surrounds the femoral nerve both in the transverse and longitudinal planes.

By applying the same basic principles outlined above continuous catheters may be inserted in nearly all lower limb blocks. The exceptions to this rule are the blocks where there is insufficient space in the subcutaneous tissues to permit the insertion of a catheter (for example, in ankle blocks).

Sciatic Nerve Block

Clinical Application

Blockage of the sciatic nerve results in anesthesia and analgesia of the posterior thigh and lower leg. When combined with a femoral or lumbar plexus block, it provides complete anesthesia of the leg below the knee.

Anatomy

The last two lumbar nerves (L4 and L5) merge with the anterior branch of the first sacral nerve to form the lumbosacral trunk. The sacral plexus is formed by the union of the lumbosacral trunk with the first three sacral nerves (Figure 18.10). The roots form on the anterior surface of the lateral sacrum and become the sciatic nerve on the ventral surface of the piriformis muscle. It exits the pelvis through the greater sciatic foramen below the piriformis muscle and descends between the greater trochanter of the femur and the ischial tuberosity between the piriformis and gluteus maximus, and then quadratus femoris and gluteus maximus. More distally it runs anterior to biceps femoris before entering the popliteal triangle. At a variable point before the lower third of the femur, it divides into the tibial and common peroneal nerves.

Preparation and Positioning

Noninvasive monitors are applied and intravenous access obtained. Intravenous sedative agents and oxygen therapy are administered. The patient needs to be in a lateral decubitus position with the side to be blocked uppermost. The knee is flexed and the foot positioned so that twitches of the foot are easily seen. The sciatic nerve lies within a palpable groove

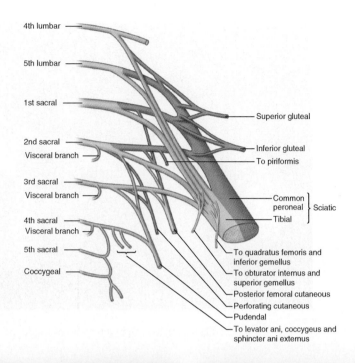

Figure 18.10. The sacral plexus.

4th lumbar

5th lumbar

1st sacral

Superior gluteal

2nd sacral
Visceral branch

Inferior gluteal
To piriformis

3rd sacral
Visceral branch

Common peroneal ⎱ Sciatic
Tibial

4th sacral
Visceral branch

5th sacral

To quadratus femoris and inferior gemellus
To obturator internus and superior gemellus

Coccygeal

Posterior femoral cutaneous
Perforating cutaneous
Pudendal
To levator ani, coccygeus and sphincter ani externus

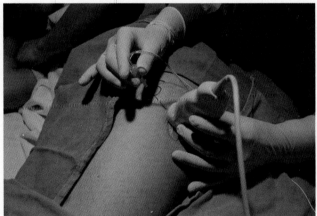

Figure 18.11. Sciatic nerve block in-plane approach.

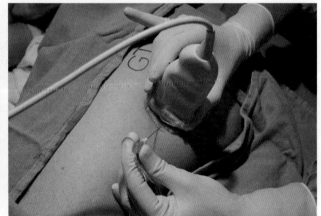

Figure 18.12. Sciatic nerve block out-of-plane approach.

which can be marked prior to using the ultrasound. Skin disinfection is then performed and a sterile technique observed.

Ultrasound Technique

The sciatic nerve is the largest peripheral nerve in the body, measuring more than 1 cm in width at its origin and approximately 2 cm at its greatest width. Multiple different approaches are described using surface landmarks, which are often difficult to palpate, together with topographical geometry to estimate the point of needle insertion. The sciatic nerve though is amenable to imaging with ultrasound, it is considered a technically challenging block due to the lack of any adjacent vascular structures and its deep location relative to skin. It can be approached with either an in-plane (Figure 18.11) or out-of-plane approach (Figure 18.12).

A low-frequency curved array probe (2–5 MHz) is preferred. The US probe is placed over the greater trochanter of the femur and its curvilinear bony shadow is delineated. The probe is moved medially to identify the curvilinear bony shadow of the ischial tuberosity. The sciatic nerve is visible in a sling between these two hyperechoic bony shadows (Figure 18.13). It usually appears as a wedge-shaped hyperechoic structure, that is easier to

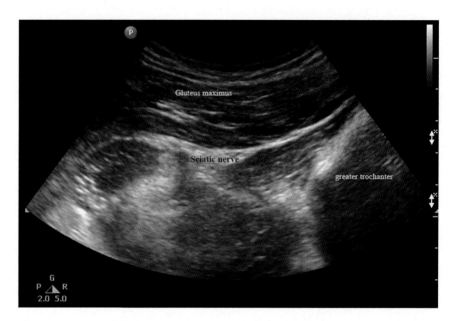

Figure 18.13. Transverse scan of sciatic nerve.

identify more proximally, and then followed down to the infragluteal region. It is often easier to identify it from its surrounding structures by decreasing the gain on the US machine. The depth of the sciatic nerve varies mainly with body habitus. In order to reach the target, the angle of approach of the needle is often close to perpendicular to the skin.[8] This makes visualization of the entire needle shaft using the in-plane approach more difficult. An out-of-plane approach is often used whereby only a cross-sectional view of the needle is visible. The skin is infiltrated with lidocaine at the point of insertion of the block needle. The needle tip is tracked at all times if possible. Imaging of the needle tip this deep can be problematic and its position is often inferred from the movement of the tissues around it, and by injections of small volumes of D5W, local anesthetic, or air. Electrical stimulation can be used to help confirm needle to nerve contact. It is useful to use the US to observe the pattern of local anesthetic spread around the sciatic nerve in real time. The aim is to reposition the needle tip if required to obtain circumferential spread around the nerve. However, be aware this is not always possible, as moving the needle around the nerve can be technically challenging.

Sciatic Nerve Blockade in the Popliteal Fossa

Clinical Application

Sciatic nerve blockade distally at the popliteal fossa is used for anesthesia and analgesia of the lower leg. As opposed to more proximal sciatic nerve block, popliteal fossa block anesthetizes the leg distal to the hamstrings muscles, allowing patients to retain knee flexion.

Anatomy

The sciatic nerve is a nerve bundle containing two separate nerve trunks, the tibial and common peroneal nerves. The sciatic nerve passes into the thigh and lies anterior to the hamstring muscles [semimembranosus, semitendinosus, and biceps femoris (long and short heads)], lateral to adductor magnus, and posterior and lateral to the popliteal artery and vein. At a variable level, usually between 30 and 120 mm above the popliteal crease, the sciatic nerve divides into the tibial (medial) and common peroneal (lateral) components.[9] The tibial nerve is the larger of the two divisions and descends vertically through the popliteal fossa, where distally it accompanies the popliteal vessels. Its terminal branches are the medial and lateral plantar nerves. The common peroneal nerve continues downward and descends along the head and neck of the fibula. Its superficial branches are the superficial and deep peroneal nerves. Since most foot and ankle surgical procedures involve both tibial and common peroneal components of the nerve, it is essential to anesthetize both nerve components. Blockade of the nerve before it divides therefore simplifies the technique.

Preparation and Positioning

Noninvasive monitors are applied and intravenous access obtained. The patient is placed prone. The foot on the side to be blocked is positioned so that any movement of the foot can be easily seen placed with the foot hanging off the end of the bed with a pillow under the ankle. Oxygen therapy and adequate intravenous sedation is administered. Skin disinfection is performed and a sterile technique observed. Once the block has been inserted the patient is moved supine for the operative procedure.

Ultrasound Technique

The advent of ultrasound-guided techniques allows the nerves to be followed to determine their exact level of division, removing the need to perform the procedure an arbitrary distance above the popliteal fossa. Thus an insertion point can be chosen which minimizes the distance to the nerve from skin. Both the in-plane and the out-of-plane approach may be used (Figures 18.14 and 18.15).

A high-frequency (7–12 MHz) linear array probe is appropriate for this block. Start with US probe in a transverse plane above the popliteal crease. The easiest method for finding the sciatic nerve is to follow the tibial nerve. Locate the popliteal artery at the popliteal crease. The tibial nerve will be found lateral and posterior to it as a hyperechoic structure. Follow this hyperechoic structure until it is joined further proximal in the popliteal fossa by the peroneal nerve. The sciatic nerve can also be found directly above the popliteal fossa by looking deep and medial to the biceps femoris and semitendinosus muscle and superficial and lateral to the popliteal artery (Figure 18.16).

It is often useful to angle the US probe caudally to enhance nerve visibility. If nerve visualization is difficult, get the patient to plantar flex and dorsiflex the foot. This causes the tibial and peroneal components to move during foot movement, called the "see saw" sign.

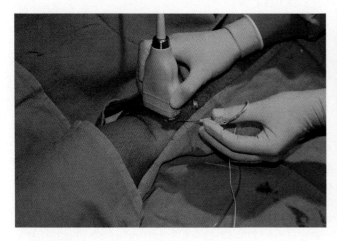

Figure 18.14. Popliteal nerve block in-plane approach.

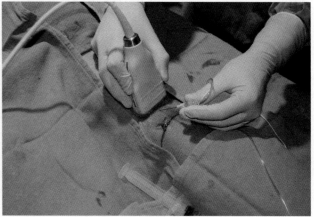

Figure 18.15. Popliteal nerve block out-of-plane approach.

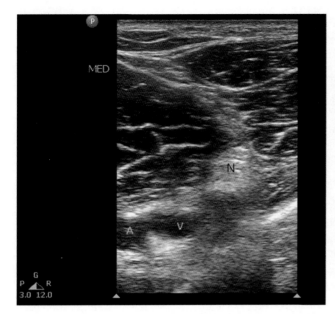

Figure 18.16. Transverse section of popliteal region showing popliteal nerve, vein, and artery.

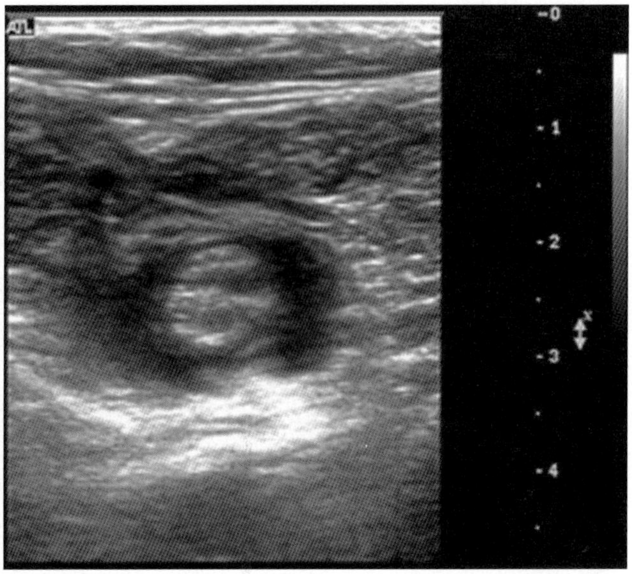

Figure 18.17. View of popliteal nerve after injection of local anesthetic.

Once the sciatic nerve has been identified in the popliteal fossa, the skin is infiltrated with lidocaine at the desired point of insertion of the block needle. The out-of-plane technique is commonly used, as it is simpler and less uncomfortable for the patient, but it does not allow visualization of the whole needle shaft.

The block needle is inserted and directed next to the sciatic nerve. Once the needle tip lies adjacent to the nerve, a muscle contraction can be elicited if preferred by slowly increasing the nerve stimulator current until a twitch is seen (commonly less than 0.5 mA). After negative aspiration for blood, local anesthetic is incrementally injected. It is important to examine the spread of local anesthetic and ensure that spread is seen encircling the nerve. Needle repositioning may be needed to ensure adequate spread on either side of the nerve (Figure 18.17).

Lumbar Plexus Block

Clinical Application

Lumbar plexus block (also frequently referred to as the psoas compartment block) leads to anesthesia and analgesia of the hip, knee, and anterior thigh regions. Combined with sciatic nerve blockade it provides anesthesia and analgesia for the whole leg.

Anatomy

The lumbar plexus is formed from the anterior divisions of L1, L2, L3, and part of L4 (Figure 18.18). The L1 root often receives a branch from T12. The lumbar plexus is situated most commonly in the posterior one third of the psoas major muscle, anterior to the transverse processes of the lumbar vertebrae. The major branches of the lumbar plexus are the genitofemoral nerve, lateral cutaneous femoral nerve of the thigh, femoral, and obturator nerves.

Figure 18.18. The lumbar plexus.

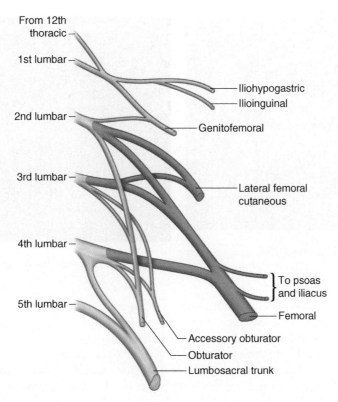

From 12th thoracic

1st lumbar

Iliohypogastric

Ilioinguinal

2nd lumbar

Genitofemoral

3rd lumbar

Lateral femoral cutaneous

4th lumbar

To psoas and iliacus

5th lumbar

Femoral

Accessory obturator

Obturator

Lumbosacral trunk

Preparation and Positioning

The patient is placed in the lateral decubitus position with the side to be blocked uppermost. The leg needs to be positioned such that contractions of the quadriceps muscle are visible. Noninvasive monitors are applied and intravenous access obtained. Intravenous sedative agents and oxygen therapy are administered as required. More sedation is usually required for lumbar plexus blocks compared to other techniques, as the block needle has to pass through multiple muscle planes. Skin disinfection is performed and a sterile technique observed.

Ultrasound Technique

Note this is considered as an advanced technique due to the depth of the target from the skin and the technical difficulty of using the ultrasound to perform real imaging as the block is performed.

The target is to place the needle in the paraspinal area at the level of L3/4. Ultrasound can be used both to confirm correct vertebral level and to guide needle tip under direct vision. A low-frequency (2–5 MHz) curved array probe is used. It is placed in a paramedian longitudinal position (Figure 18.19). Firm pressure is required to obtain good quality images. Identify the transverse processes at the L3/4 space by moving the US probe laterally from the spinous processes in the midline, staying in the longitudinal plane. Going from the midline and moving the probe laterally, the articular processes are seen, with the adjoining superior and inferior articular processes of the facets forming a continuous "sawtooth" hyperechoic line. As the probe is moved further laterally, the transverse processes are seen, with the psoas muscle lying between them. The image is of a "trident" (Figure 18.20) with the transverse processes causing bony shadows, and the psoas muscle lying in between.

At this point, the US probe is usually 3–5 cm off the midline. The lumbar plexus is not usually directly visualized, but lies within the posterior third of the psoas muscle (i.e., the closest third of the psoas muscle seen with the US probe). The distance from the skin to the psoas

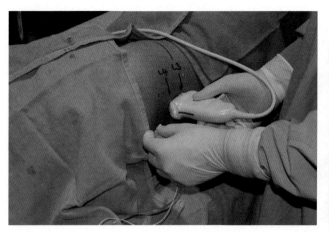

Figure 18.19. Positioning for ultrasound-guided lumbar plexus block.

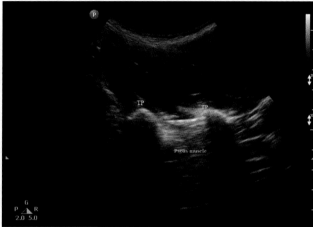

Figure 18.20. Paravertebral scan of L3–L4. *TP* transverse process.

muscle can be measured using the caliper function of the ultrasound machine. This gives an estimate of the depth of the lumbar plexus before needle insertion. Note that anterior to the psoas muscle (further away from the skin in this US view) lie the peritoneal cavity, the great vessels, and kidney. Thus care with needle tip placement should be maintained at all times.

The depth of the plexus is most often between 50 and 100 mm from the skin surface. An in-plane or an out-of-plane technique may be used. If an in-plane approach is used the usual direction for insertion is from caudad to cephalad. For the out-of-plane approach, the site for the block needle is on the medial side of the US probe (which is maintained in its longitudinal position). The needle needs to be placed at the center of the probe, directed slightly laterally such that in its path it comes directly under the US beam. Advancing the needle from a medial to a lateral direction is also preferred to avoid insertion into the dural cuff, which can extend laterally beyond the neural foramina. Lidocaine is infiltrated into the skin and subcutaneous tissue at the point where the block needle is to be inserted. The needle is observed in real time and targeted toward the posterior third of the psoas muscle bulk. Electrical stimulation is commonly used to confirm proximity to the lumbar plexus. The target is to elicit quadriceps muscle contraction. When satisfied with needle tip position, the local anesthetic is injected incrementally (with frequent aspiration to monitor for blood or CSF), and its spread observed, looking for fluid and tissue expansion in the psoas muscle bulk.

Obturator Nerve Block

Clinical Application

The obturator nerve sends articular branches to the hip and knee joints, and innervates a relatively small dermatome area on the medial aspect of the knee. The obturator nerve also supplies the adductor muscles on the medial aspect of the thigh. Blockade of the obturator nerve using the "3-in-1" technique is unreliable and ultrasonography offers again an excellent opportunity of direct visualization and subsequent effective blockade of that nerve.

Anatomy

The anterior divisions of L2-4 ventral rami form this nerve. It descends toward the pelvis from the medial border of the psoas major muscle and travels through the obturator canal. Once it emerges from the obturator canal, it enters the medial aspect of the thigh, and divides into anterior and posterior divisions that run anterior and posterior to the adductor brevis. The anterior division supplies the adductor brevis and longus, while the posterior division supplies the knee joint and adductor magnus.

Preparation and Positioning

Slight abduction of the hip and external rotation of the thigh help to open up the space. Noninvasive monitors are applied and intravenous access obtained. Intravenous sedative agents and oxygen therapy are administered as required. The groin is exposed on the side to be blocked. Skin disinfection is then performed and a sterile technique observed.

Ultrasound Technique

A high-frequency (7–12 MHz) linear array probe is appropriate for this block. Ultrasonography is performed just below the inguinal ligament to see the femoral artery and vein. The probe should be moved medially and slightly caudal maintaining its horizontal position. The obturator nerve lies between the pectineus, adductor longus, and short adductor brevis muscles. The anterior branch of the obturator nerve lies in a fascial layer between the pectineus, adductor longus, and adductor brevis muscles. The posterior branch lies between the adductor brevis and the adductor magnus muscles.

Going laterally the pectineus is identified and then the adductor muscles. The anterior branch of the obturator nerve can be found between the adductor longus and the (deeper) adductor brevis. The posterior branch is found between the adductor brevis and the (deeper) adductor magnus muscles. In both cases (anterior and posterior), the obturator nerve is often seen as a hyperechoic structure, although sometimes only the fascial planes can be distinguished (Figure 18.21).

An in-plane or an out-of-plane approach may be used. It is useful to obtain an ultrasound image where both branches are visible, and then choose a single needle insertion point from which both branches of the nerve may be blocked. The skin is infiltrated with lidocaine at this point. When the block needle tip is positioned at the correct site between the fascial planes, local anesthetic solution is injected. The local anesthetic should be observed to cause distension of the intermuscular fascial planes and surround the nerve (if visible).

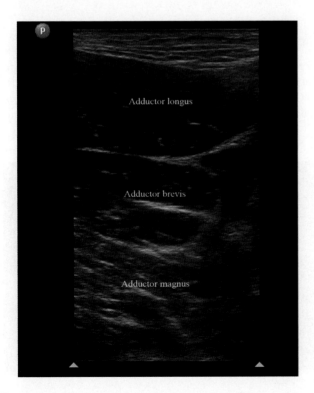

Figure 18.21. Transverse image of medial aspect of upper thigh showing adductor longus, brevis, and magnus muscles.

To aid localization of the obturator nerve, low-current nerve stimulation may be used to elicit adductor muscle contraction. It is possible to perform the block without the use of nerve stimulation, and also without exactly identifying the obturator nerve branches themselves.[10] The important steps when using ultrasound guidance are correct identification of the muscle layers, and deposition of the local anesthetic into the appropriate interfascial planes.

Lateral Femoral Cutaneous Nerve Block

Clinical Application

The lateral femoral cutaneous nerve (LFCN) provides sensory innervation to the lateral thigh. Blockade of the LFCN can be used for analgesia for femoral neck surgery in older patients. It can be used for the diagnosis and management of meralgia paresthetica, a chronic pain syndrome caused by entrapment of the nerve (frequently by adipose layers over the iliac crest).[11] The LFCN has a highly variable course, thus ultrasound guidance to block this nerve leads to a much higher success rate compared to blind approaches.[12]

Anatomy

The LFCN is a pure sensory nerve arising from the dorsal divisions of L2/3. After emerging from the lateral border of the psoas major muscle, it follows a highly variable path: it may pass inferior or superior to the anterior superior iliac spine (ASIS) (Figure 18.22). If it passes medial to the ASIS, it can be less than 1 cm or more than 7 cm away from it.[13] It is located between the fascia lata and iliaca. It passes under the inguinal ligament and crosses the lateral border of the sartorius muscle at a variable distance (between 2 and 11 cm) inferior to ASIS, where it divides into anterior and superior branches.

Preparation and Positioning

The patient is positioned supine with the leg in a neutral position. Noninvasive monitors are applied and intravenous access obtained. The groin is exposed and the ASIS marked. Intravenous sedative agents and oxygen therapy are administered as required. Skin disinfection is then performed over the ASIS/groin area and a sterile technique observed.

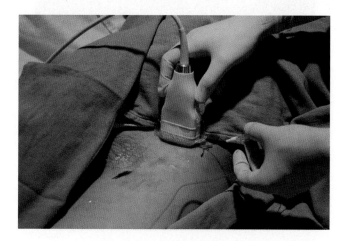

Figure 18.22. In-plane approach of blocking the lateral femoral cutaneous nerve of the thigh.

Ultrasound Technique

For this superficial technique, a 7–12 MHz high-frequency linear array probe is placed immediately medial to the ASIS along the inguinal ligament, with the lateral end of the probe on the ASIS. The ASIS casts a bony shadow on the US image. The US probe is moved medially and inferiorly from this point. An in-plane or out-of-plane approach may be used. The fascia lata, fascia iliaca, and sartorius muscle are identified. The nerve is identified as a small hypoechoic structure found between the fascias above the sartorius muscle. As it is a superficial structure an in-plane approach is used, with a shallow angle of approach. The skin is infiltrated with lidocaine and the block needle is inserted to reach the desired skin plane immediately medial and inferior to the ASIS. Using US guidance, the LFCN can be blocked with a much lower dose of local anesthetic, and blockage with as little as 0.3 ml of lidocaine has been reported in the literature.[14]

Saphenous Nerve Block

Clinical Application

The saphenous nerve is a sensory branch of the femoral nerve. It innervates the skin over the medial, anteromedial, and posteromedial aspect of the lower limb from above the knee to the foot. Thus blockade of the saphenous nerve produces anesthesia and analgesia of the anteromedial aspect of the lower leg, ankle, and foot, but without producing quadriceps muscle weakness. It is commonly used with a sciatic nerve block to provide complete anesthesia and analgesia of the lower leg. Its small size and lack of a motor component makes it difficult to localize with conventional nerve localization techniques, thus ultrasound increases the success rate of blocking this nerve.[15]

Anatomy

The saphenous nerve is a terminal branch of the femoral nerve, leaving the femoral canal proximally in the femoral triangle, descending within the adductor canal, and remaining deep to the sartorius muscle with the femoral artery (Figure 18.23). It is initially found

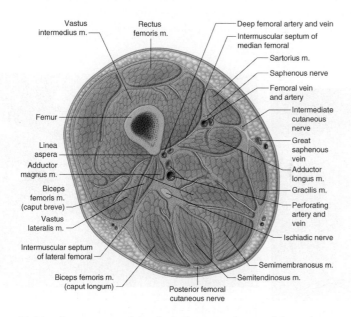

Figure 18.23. Cross section of the thigh showing position of the saphenous nerve.

lateral to the femoral artery, and then becomes more medial and superior to the vessel at the distal end of the adductor magnus muscle.[16] It is a sensory nerve, covering the medial aspect of the calf, ankle, foot, and great toe.

Preparation and Positioning

The patient is in a supine position, with the leg slightly externally rotated. Noninvasive monitors are applied and intravenous access obtained. Intravenous sedative agents and oxygen therapy are administered as required. The medial aspect of the thigh is exposed down to the knee. Skin disinfection is then performed here and a sterile technique observed.

Ultrasound Technique

In the mid to distal thigh, the saphenous nerve can be easily approached. The nerve can be blocked with an in-plane approach or an out-of-plane approach (Figures 18.24 and 18.25). A high-frequency (7–12 MHz) linear ultrasound is placed transverse to the longitudinal axis, and is used to scan the medial aspect of the thigh. The saphenous nerve is frequently difficult to visualize, but its relationship to the sartorius muscle and vessels is relatively constant. At the medial side of the mid thigh region (approximately 15 cm proximal to the patella), the sartorius muscle and femoral artery are identified. The saphenous nerve lies in a position below the sartorius muscle. Move the US probe in a caudal direction from this point along the long axis of the thigh until the femoral artery is seen "diving" deeper, toward the posterior aspect of the thigh where it becomes the popliteal artery. This area is the "adductor hiatus." From here move 2–3 cm proximally, to the distal adductor canal, and block the nerve at this level (Figure 18.26).

Note that the diameter of the saphenous nerve varies widely. The aim is to insert the needle deep to the sartorius and depositing the local anesthetic medial to the artery. More distally in the thigh, 5–7 cm proximal to the popliteal crease, the saphenous nerve is superficial to the descending branch of the femoral artery, deep to the sartorius muscle and posterior to the vastus medialis muscle.

More distally, the saphenous nerve pierces the fascia lata between the sartorius and gracilis tendons to join the subcutaneous saphenous vein. The saphenous nerve is posteromedial to the vein at the level of the tibial tuberosity, although it is difficult to visualize using ultrasound. Ultrasound-guided paravenous injection of local anesthetic using light pressure with a high-frequency linear transducer probe is easily performed at this level.

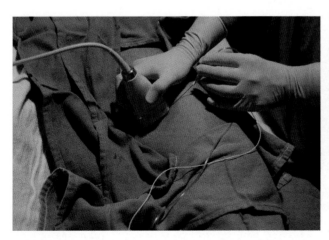

Figure 18.24. In-plane approach of blocking the saphenous nerve.

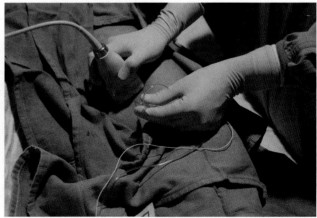

Figure 18.25. Out-of-plane approach of blocking the saphenous nerve.

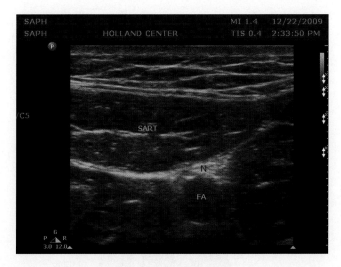

Figure 18.26. Transverse view showing saphenous nerve and sartorius muscle.

Ankle Block

Clinical Application

Ankle block can be used for anesthesia and analgesia of the foot. It can be used for diagnostic and therapeutic purposes with spastic talipes equinovarus and sympathetically mediated pain. It is useful for postoperative pain relief as it causes no motor blockade of the foot, thus patients can ambulate with crutches immediately after surgery, which facilitates faster discharge home.

Anatomy

Five peripheral nerves innervate the foot area (Figure 18.27):

– The saphenous nerve, a terminal branch of the femoral nerve, supplies the medial side of the foot. The remainder of the foot is innervated by branches of the sciatic nerve.
– The sural nerve innervates the lateral aspect of the foot. This is formed from the tibial and communicating superficial peroneal branches.
– The posterior tibial nerve supplies the deep plantar structures, the muscles, and the sole of the foot.
– The superficial peroneal nerve innervates the dorsal aspect of the foot.
– The deep peroneal nerve supplies the deep dorsal structures and the web space between the first and second toes.

The saphenous, superficial peroneal, and sural nerves lie subcutaneously at the level of the malleoli. The posterior tibial nerve and deep peroneal nerve lie deeper in the tissues, under the flexor retinaculum (for the tibial nerve) and the extensor retinaculum (for the deep peroneal nerve). The posterior tibial nerve passes with the posterior tibial artery posterior to the medial malleolus. The deep peroneal nerve passes lateral to the anterior tibial artery under the flexor retinaculum before emerging more superficially to travel with the dorsalis pedis artery on the dorsum of the foot.

The exact areas of the foot supplied by each nerve vary significantly in the population. Thus for surgical procedures that require a tourniquet, blockage of all five nerves is required.

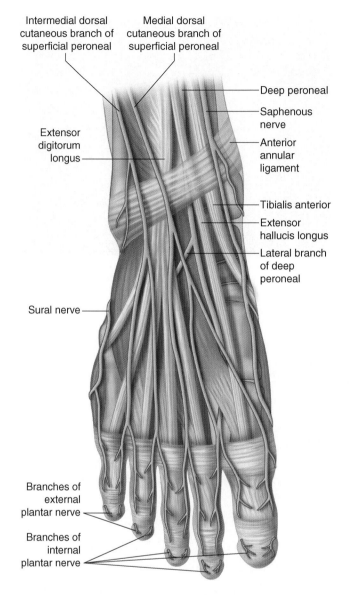

Figure 18.27. Nerve supply to the ankle.

Preparation and Positioning

The patient is placed supine. Noninvasive monitors are applied and intravenous access obtained. Intravenous sedative agents and oxygen therapy are administered as required. Elevate the foot with a pillow (or similar) such that the anterior and medial aspects of the ankle are accessible. Skin disinfection is then performed and a sterile technique observed.

Ultrasound Technique

Traditionally, blockade of the superficial peroneal, saphenous, and sural nerves is performed by infiltration subcutaneously without the use of ultrasound. This is performed by a circumferential subcutaneous injection of local anesthetic over the anterior aspect of the ankle, in a line just proximal to the malleoli. Ten to fifteen cubic meter of local anesthetic solution is sufficient. However, a newer technique describing the use of ultrasound to locate the sural nerve has been described in the literature. This was performed applying a tourniquet and looking 1 cm proximal to the lateral malleolus for the distended lesser saphenous vein.[17] No attempt is made to identify the sural nerve itself, and the local anesthetic is inserted using an out-of-plane approach to obtain circumferential perivascular spread (usually achieved with less than 5 cm³ of local anesthetic).

Ultrasound also facilitates blockade of the two deep nerves that supply the foot, namely the posterior tibial and deep peroneal nerves.

Posterior Tibial Nerve Block

A 7–12-MHz linear array US probe is used as the structures usually lie within 2–3 cm of the skin. If present on the US machine, the 10–15-MHz "hockey stick" US probe may also be used for this block. The probe is placed immediately superior and slightly posterior to the medial malleolus, in the transverse plane (Figures 18.28 and 18.29). The bony landmark of the medial malleolus is easily identified as a hyperechoic curvilinear shadow. The tibial arterial pulsation and the hyperechoic tibial nerve are seen posterior and superficial to the medial malleolus. The order of the structures seen going posteriorly from the medial malleolus is tendons, then artery, then nerve ("TAN").

Both an in-plane and an out-of-plane approach may be used. An in-plane approach is most often used, and nerve stimulation can be used to confirm position if required before insertion of local anesthetic. Ultrasound can be used to confirm circumferential spread of local anesthetic around the nerve, and using this method 5 cm³ of local anesthetic is sufficient.

Deep Peroneal Nerve Block

The deep peroneal nerve is not readily visualized using ultrasound. Thus its position is usually inferred by locating the dorsalis pedis artery. The US probe is placed on the dorsum of the foot at the intermalleolar line. The dorsalis pedis pulsation is identified and sometimes the deep peroneal is seen as a round hyperechoic structure lateral to the artery.

The dorsal foot is convex in shape and the nerve is in a superficial location, making it difficult to use the in-plane approach for this block. Thus the out-of-plane approach is commonly used for needle insertion. Once identified, 2–3 cm³ of local anesthetic is deposited around the deep peroneal nerve. If not seen, the local anesthetic can be deposited lateral to the dorsalis pedis artery.

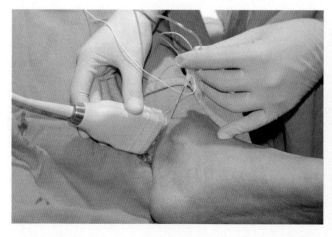 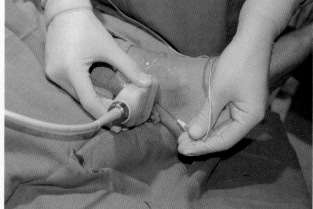

Figure 18.28. In-plane approach to block the posterior tibial nerve.   **Figure 18.29.** Out-of-plane approach to block posterior tibial nerve.

References

1. Liu SS, Ngeow JE, YaDeau JT. Ultrasound-guided regional anesthesia and analgesia: a qualitative systematic review. *Reg Anesth Pain Med.* 2009;34:47–59.
2. Marhofer P, Chan VW. Ultrasound-guided regional anesthesia: current concepts and future trends. *Anesth Analg.* 2007;104:1265–1269.
3. Gofeld M. Ultrasonography in pain medicine: a critical review. *Pain Pract.* 2008;8:226–240.
4. Chin KJ, Perlas A, Chan VW, Brull R. Needle visualization in ultrasound-guided regional anesthesia: challenges and solutions. *Reg Anesth Pain Med.* 2008;33:532–544.
5. Marhofer P, Schrogendorfer K, Koining H, et al. Ultrasonic guidance improves sensory block and onset time of three-in-one blocks. *Anesth Analg.* 1997;85:854–857.
6. Casati A, Baciarello M, Di Cianni S, et al. Effects of ultrasound guidance on the minimum effective anaesthetic volume required to block the femoral nerve. *Br J Anaesth.* 2007;98:823–827.
7. Awad IT, Duggan EM. Posterior lumbar plexus block: anatomy, approaches, and techniques. *Reg Anesth Pain Med.* 2005;30:143–149.
8. Chan VW, Abbas S, Brull R, et al. *Ultrasound Imaging for Regional Anesthesia.* 2nd ed. 2009.
9. Vloka JD, Hadzić A, April E, Thys DM. The division of the sciatic nerve in the popliteal fossa: anatomical implications for popliteal nerve blockade. *Anesth Analg.* 2001;92:215–217.
10. Sinha SK, Abrams JH, Houle TT, et al. Ultrasound-guided obturator nerve block: an interfacial injection approach without nerve stimulation. *Reg Anesth Pain Med.* 2009;34:261–264.
11. Harney D, Patijn J. Meralgia paresthetica: diagnosis and management strategies. *Pain Med.* 2007;8:669–677.
12. Ng I, Vaghadia H, Choi PT, et al. Ultrasound imaging accurately identifies the lateral femoral cutaneous nerve. *Anesth Analg.* 2008;107:1295–1302.
13. Grothaus MC, Holt M, Mekhail AO, et al. Lateral femoral cutaneous nerve: an anatomic study. *Clin Orthop Relat Res.* 2005;437:164–168.
14. Bodner G, Bernathova M, Galiano K, et al. Ultrasound of the lateral femoral cutaneous nerve: normal findings in a cadaver and in volunteers. *Reg Anesth Pain med.* 2009;34:265–268.
15. Manickam B, Perlas A, Duggan E, et al. Feasibility and efficacy of ultrasound-guided block of the saphenous nerve in the adductor canal. *Reg Anesth Pain Med.* 2009;34:578–580.
16. Tsui BCH, Ozelsel T. Ultrasound-guided transsartorial perifemoral artery approach for saphenous nerve block. *Reg Anesth Pain Med.* 2009;34:177–178.
17. Redborg KE, Sites BD, Chinn CD, et al. Ultrasound improves the success rate of a sural nerve block at the ankle. *Reg Anesth Pain Med.* 2009;34:24–28.

19

Ultrasound-Guided Continuous Peripheral Nerve Blocks

Edward R. Mariano and Brian M. Ilfeld

E.R. Mariano (✉)
Anesthesiology and Perioperative Care Service, Veterans Affairs Palo Alto Health Care System,
Stanford University School of Medicine, 3801 Miranda Avenue (112A), Palo Alto, CA 94304, USA
e-mail: emariano@stanford.edu

S.N. Narouze (ed.), *Atlas of Ultrasound-Guided Procedures in Interventional Pain Management*,
DOI 10.1007/978-1-4419-1681-5_19, © Springer Science+Business Media, LLC 2011

Introduction

Continuous peripheral nerve block (CPNB) catheters, also known as "perineural" catheters, extend the potential duration of anesthesia and analgesia provided by peripheral nerve block techniques. In the ambulatory setting, the use of CPNB has been shown to increase the quality of pain control experienced by patients at home as well as reduce the incidence of side effects produced by conventional opioid analgesics.[1-3] For hospitalized patients, CPNB techniques have similarly demonstrated postoperative analgesia efficacy following major surgery,[4-7] facilitating early rehabilitation,[4,8] and shortening the time to achieve hospital discharge criteria in arthroplasty patients.[6,7,9] In select patients, joint replacement with only overnight hospitalization and outpatient management of perineural infusions is feasible[10-12] and offers potential economic benefits.[13]

The use of electrical nerve stimulation guidance for CPNB performance, employing either stimulating or nonstimulating perineural catheters, is well established.[1,2,14-16] However, ultrasound guidance is emerging as a reliably effective and efficient technique for perineural catheter insertion.[17-23]

Applications

Ultrasound-guided CPNB techniques may be performed in a variety of locations: along the brachial plexus,[17,18,22-25] femoral nerve,[21,26,27] sciatic nerve,[19,22,27,28] paravertebral,[29] and ilioinguinal and iliohypogastric nerves.[30] Essentially, perineural catheters may be placed in the vicinity of nearly all peripheral nerves for continuous local anesthetic infusion using ultrasound guidance. To date, most published ultrasound-guided perineural catheter insertion techniques share a common step of injecting fluid via the placement needle around the target nerve under direct visualization, creating sufficient space for subsequent catheter insertion.[17,19-22] The specific techniques differ mainly in the choice of needle insertion site and trajectory relative to transducer position (in-plane vs. out-of-plane) and transducer orientation relative to the target nerve (short axis vs. long axis).[31,32]

Overview of Ultrasound-Guided Perineural Catheter Insertion

Nerve in Short Axis, Needle In-Plane Approach (Figure 19.1)

The imaging of target nerves in short axis (cross-sectional imaging) permits differentiation of neural tissue from surrounding anatomic structures such as muscle and adipose.[32] Insertion of a 17- or 18-gauge Touhy-tip needle and real-time guidance within the ultrasound beam (in-plane) allows the practitioner to visualize the entire length of the needle including the tip, thereby avoiding inadvertent intravascular or intraneural needle insertion during the CPNB procedure.[31] Fluid injected via the needle may be directed around the target nerve in a deliberate fashion prior to perineural catheter placement. A potential disadvantage of the in-plane needle guidance technique with short-axis imaging is the needle orientation perpendicular to the path of the target nerve, which may result in catheters being inserted beyond the nerve and misplacement of the subsequent local anesthetic infusion.[33] The use of a flexible epidural-type catheter may prevent catheter tip misplacement and may be more appropriate for in-plane ultrasound-guided CPNB techniques utilizing short axis imaging.[17,19,21]

Specific challenges in adopting the in-plane needle guidance approach include acceptance of "new" needle insertion sites that differ from traditional nerve stimulation techniques[19,21] and technical difficulty in visualizing the needle tip throughout the CPNB procedure.

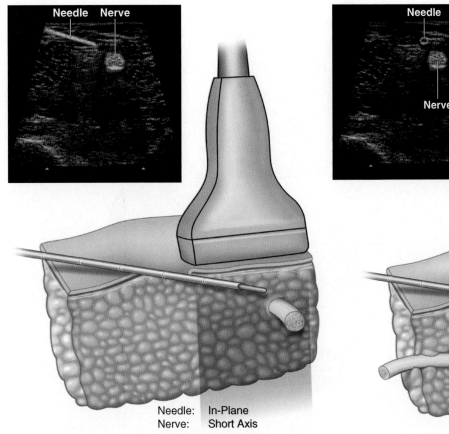

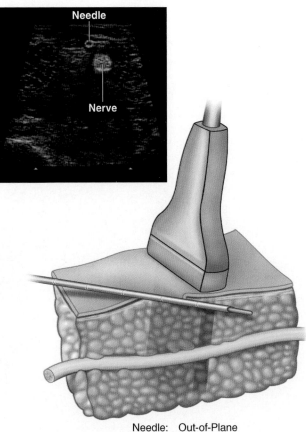

Figure 19.1. Short-axis imaging of the target nerve with needle advancement under in-plane ultrasound guidance. Adapted from: Regional Anesthesia and Pain Medicine, vol. 35, issue 2, pp. 123–126. Brian Ilfeld, Michael Fredrickson, and Edward Mariano. Ultrasound-Guided Perineural Catheter Insertion: Three Approaches but Few Illuminating Data. Copyright © 2010, American Society of Regional Anesthesia and Pain Medicine.

Figure 19.2. Short-axis imaging of the target nerve with the needle advancement under out-of-plane ultrasound guidance. Adapted from: Regional Anesthesia and Pain Medicine, vol. 35, issue 2, pp. 123–126. Brian Ilfeld, Michael Fredrickson, and Edward Mariano. Ultrasound-Guided Perineural Catheter Insertion: Three Approaches but Few Illuminating Data. Copyright © 2010, American Society of Regional Anesthesia and Pain Medicine.

Nerve in Short Axis, Needle Out-of-Plane (Figure 19.2)

In this approach, the target nerve is visualized in short axis, but the placement needle is inserted in approximately the same predicted sites recommended by nerve stimulation techniques, only guided by the ultrasound-guided nerve localization. Since the needle passes through the plane of the ultrasound beam, needle tip identification can be difficult or impossible.[32,34] However, practitioners have recommended the use of local tissue movement and intermittent injection of fluid via the placement needle to infer the position of the needle tip.[22,34] Once the placement needle is in proximity to the target nerve, the possible advantage of this technique over the in-plane approach is the potential to advance the perineural catheter nearly parallel to the path of the nerve. Additionally, the needle insertion sites involved are more familiar to practitioners who practice stimulation-guided regional anesthesia.

Nerve in Long Axis, Needle In-Plane

In theory, visualizing the target nerve in long axis while guiding the needle and perineural catheter in-plane should be the optimal approach. Unfortunately, imaging these structures within the same plane is challenging, to say the least, and limited to specific circumstances.[27] Anatomically, few nerves maintain a trajectory that is straight enough to permit long-axis imaging.[27,35] To date, this approach has not been described for brachial plexus perineural catheter insertion (Figure 19.3).

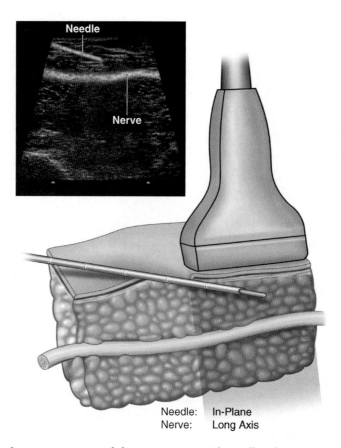

Figure 19.3. Long-axis imaging of the target nerve with needle advancement under in-plane ultrasound guidance. Adapted from: Regional Anesthesia and Pain Medicine, vol. 35, issue 2, pp. 123–126. Brian Ilfeld, Michael Fredrickson, and Edward Mariano. Ultrasound-Guided Perineural Catheter Insertion: Three Approaches but Few Illuminating Data. Copyright © 2010, American Society of Regional Anesthesia and Pain Medicine.

Preparation for Ultrasound-Guided Perineural Catheter Insertion

Sterile Technique

Prior to perineural catheter insertion, the planned procedural site should be shaved, if necessary, to accommodate catheter dressings. For all perineural catheter insertion procedures, sterile technique is recommended.[36] This includes skin preparation with chlorhexidine gluconate solution, a sterile fenestrated surgical drape, sterile equipment included protective ultrasound transducer sleeve, and conductive gel, sterile gloves, and surgical cap and mask.

Standard Perineural Catheter Equipment

Various needle and perineural catheter equipment sets have been presented. For practitioners employing a short-axis imaging and in-plane needle guidance technique, the nonstimulating flexible epidural-type catheter and Tuohy-tip placement needle are preferred.[17,19–21] Stimulating perineural catheters may also be used with ultrasound guidance.[18,23,25,28,33] Many other nonstimulating catheter and placement needle combinations have been employed for ultrasound-guided perineural catheter techniques.[22,34,37] An electrical nerve stimulator will also be required if using a combined technique of ultrasound guidance and electrical stimulation. Local anesthetic (e.g., 1% lidocaine) should also be included within the perineural catheter set for skin infiltration and injection within the subcutaneous and muscular tissue that comprise the trajectory of the placement needle.

Ultrasound-Guided Perineural Catheter Insertion Techniques for Common Surgical Procedures

Interscalene CPNB

Indications: Shoulder or proximal humerus surgery.

Transducer selection: High frequency, linear.

Preparation and equipment: As above.

Patient positioning: Supine, with the head turned away from the affected side[38] or lateral decubitus with the affected side nondependent.[18,25]

Technique: The ultrasound transducer should be placed at the level of the cricoid cartilage perpendicular to the skin with the anterior portion of the transducer over the clavicular head of the sternocleidomastoid (SCM) muscle (Figure 19.4a). After identifying the brachial plexus between the anterior and middle scalene muscles (Figure 19.4b), insert the placement needle either in a caudad direction out-of-plane[34,39] or a posterior-to-anterior direction in-plane[18,24,25] and advance the needle until the tip is in the proximity of the

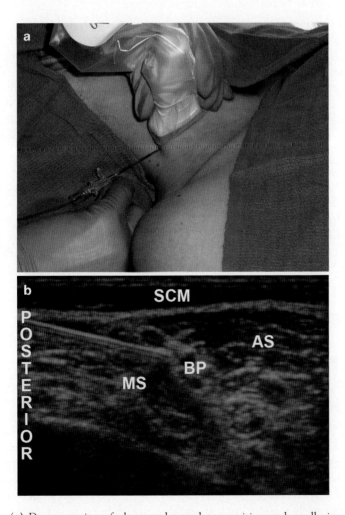

Figure 19.4. (a) Demonstration of ultrasound transducer position and needle insertion site for right interscalene brachial plexus perineural catheter insertion. The patient is positioned supine with the head turned away from the side to be blocked. (b) Sample image from ultrasound-guided interscalene brachial plexus perineural catheter insertion. *SCM* sternocleidomastoid muscle, *AS* anterior scalene muscle, *MS* middle scalene muscle, *BP* brachial plexus.

target nerve. Injectate solution (local anesthetic, saline, or dextrose-containing water) via the placement needle facilitates subsequent perineural catheter insertion. Catheter tip position may be inferred using electrical stimulation,[25] agitated injectate,[40] or air injected via the catheter.[41]

Pearls: Identify the SCM over the internal jugular vein, and follow the deep fascia of the SCM posteriorly. The adjacent muscles posterior and deep to the SCM are the scalene muscles. If the plane between the anterior and middle scalene muscles is not apparent, slide the transducer caudad until the separation of the two muscles can be visualized. When advancing the placement needle through the middle scalene muscle using an in-plane technique, direct the tip of the needle toward hyperechoic connective tissue or perineural fat rather than the hypoechoic neural structures to avoid inducing paresthesias.

Infraclavicular CPNB

Indications: Distal humerus, elbow, forearm, and hand surgery.

Transducer selection: low frequency, small curvilinear (preferred) or high frequency, linear.

Preparation and equipment: As above.

Patient positioning: Supine, with the affected arm abducted, if feasible, and head turned away from the side to be blocked.[17,20]

Technique: The ultrasound transducer is applied medial and caudad to the ipsilateral coracoid process and oriented in a parasagittal plane (Figure 19.5a). After identifying the brachial plexus cords around the axillary artery in short axis (Figure 19.5b), the placement needle is directed cephalad-to-caudad in-plane to permit needle tip visualization and avoid inadvertent vascular puncture.[17,20] Injectate solution can be distributed via the placement needle around each of the three cords separately[17] or as a single deposit posterior to the axillary artery[42] prior to perineural catheter insertion. A nonstimulating flexible epidural-type catheter[17,20] or stimulating catheter[23] should be placed posterior to the axillary artery.

Pearls: Although the infraclavicular CPNB can be placed with the arm in any position, abducting the arm at the shoulder facilitates cross-sectional imaging of the brachial plexus and vasculature and reduces the depth of these structures by stretching the pectoralis muscles and moving them further away from the chest wall. With a recent study demonstrating equal efficacy for single-injection and triple-injection techniques for infraclavicular CPNB,[42] a single-injection posterior to the axillary artery with subsequent perineural catheter insertion is recommended for procedures performed solely for postoperative pain. For perineural infusion settings, consider a higher basal rate of dilute local anesthetic solution (e.g., 0.2% ropivacaine) to maximize analgesia and minimize the incidence of an insensate extremity.[43]

Femoral CPNB

Indications: Thigh and knee surgery.

Transducer selection: High frequency, linear.

Preparation and equipment: As above.

Patient positioning: Supine, with the affected leg straight. The ultrasound transducer should be applied perpendicular to the skin at the level of the inguinal crease oriented parallel to the inguinal ligament and immediately lateral to the femoral artery pulse (Figure 19.6a). After identifying the femoral nerve below the fascia iliaca lateral to the femoral artery (Figure 19.6b), the placement needle may be inserted and directed cephalad out-of-plane,[22,26] lateral-to-medial in-plane,[21] or cephalad in-plane[27] until the tip is in proximity to the femoral nerve and the injectate solution can be deposited via the needle around the nerve. A perineural catheter can then be inserted through the placement needle.

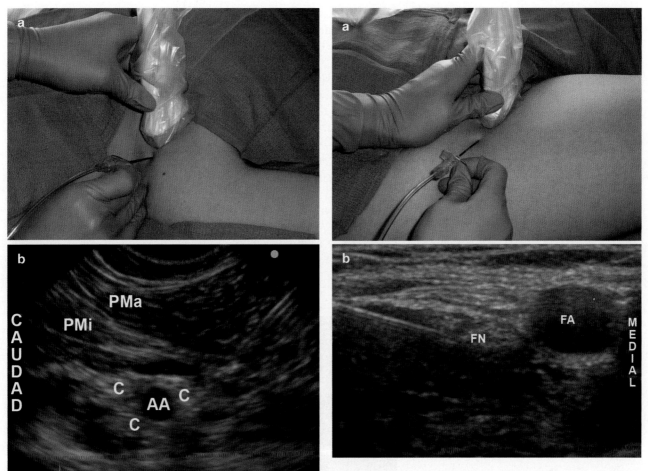

Figure 19.5. (a) Demonstration of ultrasound transducer position and needle insertion site for right infraclavicular brachial plexus perineural catheter insertion. The patient is positioned supine with the head turned away from the side to be blocked and the right arm abducted. (b) Sample image from ultrasound-guided infraclavicular brachial plexus perineural catheter insertion. *PMa* pectoralis major muscle, *PMi* pectoralis minor muscle, *AA* axillary artery, *C* brachial plexus cord.

Figure 19.6. (a) Demonstration of ultrasound transducer position and needle insertion site for right femoral perineural catheter insertion. The patient is positioned supine with the affected leg straight. (b) Sample image from ultrasound-guided femoral perineural catheter insertion. *FA* femoral artery, *FN* femoral nerve.

Pearls: Utilize color Doppler to aid in the identification of the femoral artery. If the profunda femoris artery is visualized, follow this branch cephalad until it joins the femoral artery. The femoral nerve will typically be at the same depth as the femoral artery. Identify the curved fascia iliaca over the iliacus muscle from lateral to medial. The femoral nerve is located where the fascia iliaca separates off of the iliacus muscle medially. Consider using a hydro-dissection technique after piercing the fascia iliaca to avoid inadvertently traumatizing the nerve. Perineural catheters placed for knee surgery should be placed along the lateral aspect of the femoral nerve,[44] and low basal infusions should be employed for ambulatory patients to minimize the risk of falls.[7]

Subgluteal Sciatic CPNB

Indications: Foot and ankle surgery.

Transducer selection: High frequency, linear or large low-frequency, curvilinear (preferred).

Preparation and equipment: As above.

Patient Positioning: Semi-prone (Sims position) with the knee on the affected side flexed and crossed over the dependent unaffected leg. Apply the ultrasound transducer in axial orientation perpendicular to the skin between the ischial tuberosity and greater trochanter of the femur (Figure 19.7a).[45,46] Identify the sciatic nerve medial to the femur and deep to the fascia of the gluteus maximus muscle (Figure 19.7b).[45] Insert the placement needle in a lateral-to-medial direction with in-plane guidance or in a cephalad direction with out-of-plane guidance.[28] When the needle tip is in proximity of the sciatic nerve, injectate solution is administered via the placement needle. Following confirmation of circumferential injectate spread around the sciatic nerve, the flexible epidural-type or styleted stimulating[28] perineural catheter can be inserted through the placement needle.

Pearls: The subgluteal approach can also be performed in the prone position, although the Sims position offers the advantage of stretching the gluteus muscles and reducing the depth from skin to target nerve. The sciatic nerve is reliably located between the femur and the ischial tuberosity. When subgluteal sciatic perineural catheters are used for postoperative analgesia in a basal-bolus infusion regimen, local anesthetic consumption can be expected to be lower than that of popliteal catheter infusions for similar surgical indications.[47]

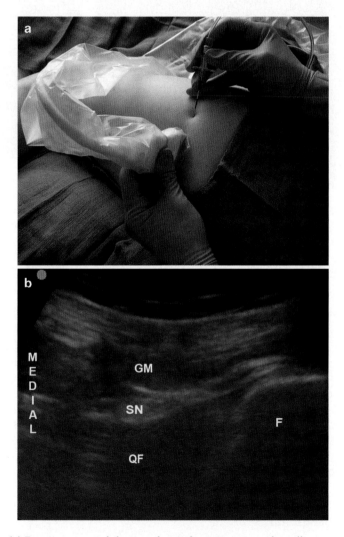

Figure 19.7. (a) Demonstration of ultrasound transducer position and needle insertion site for left subgluteal sciatic perineural catheter insertion. The patient is in Sims position with the right side dependent. (b) Sample image from ultrasound-guided subgluteal sciatic perineural catheter insertion. *GM* gluteus maximus muscle, *QF* quadrates femoris muscle, *F* femur, *SN* sciatic nerve.

Popliteal Sciatic CPNB

Indications: Foot and ankle surgery.

Transducer selection: high frequency, linear (preferred) or low frequency, curvilinear (obese patients).

Preparation and equipment: As above.

Patient Positioning: Prone with the ankle of the affected side supported by a pillow or towel. Apply the ultrasound transducer in axial orientation perpendicular to the skin at the level of the intertendinous junction (Figure 19.8a).[48] After identifying the sciatic nerve anterior and medial to the fascia of the biceps femoris muscle (Figure 19.8b), the placement needle

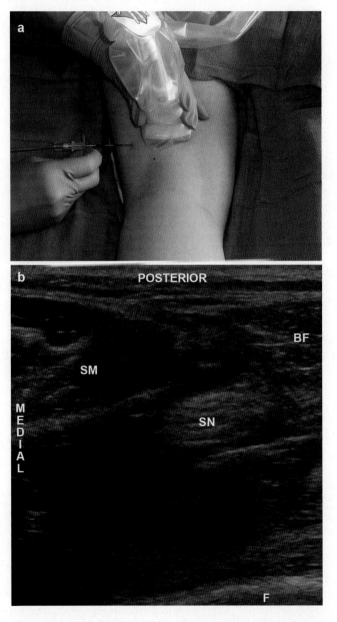

Figure 19.8. (a) Demonstration of ultrasound transducer position and needle insertion site for left popliteal sciatic perineural catheter insertion. The patient is positioned prone with the affected extremity slightly flexed at the knee. (b) Sample image from ultrasound-guided popliteal sciatic perineural catheter insertion. *SM* semimembranosus muscle, *BF* biceps femoris muscle, *F* femur, *SN* sciatic nerve.

may be inserted in a cephalad direction out-of-plane[22] or lateral-to-medial with in-plane guidance.[19] When the needle tip is in proximity of the sciatic nerve, injectate solution is administered via the placement needle. Following confirmation of circumferential injectate spread around the sciatic nerve, the flexible[19] or standard[22] epidural-type perineural catheter is deployed through the placement needle.

Pearls: The use of ultrasound guidance facilitates the performance of popliteal-sciatic CPNB in the supine and lateral positions as well. When searching for the nerve, first identify the surface of the femur as it serves as a lateral landmark and depth limit; the sciatic nerve will always be medial and posterior to the femur. Follow the biceps femoris muscle and investing fascia posteriorly and medially from the femur. The sciatic nerve is reliably located medial to the fascia of the biceps femoris muscle. For postoperative perineural infusion, avoid high basal rates of dilute local anesthetic to minimize the incidence of an insensate extremity.[49]

Tranversus Abdominis Plane CPNB

Indications: Abdominal wall surgery (e.g., inguinal and ventral hernia repairs or laparotomy).

Transducer selection: High frequency, linear or low frequency, curvilinear (obese patients).

Preparation and equipment: As above.

Patient positioning: Supine or lateral decubitus with the affected side up. Apply the ultrasound transducer in axial orientation perpendicular to the skin at approximately the midaxillary line between the costal margin and iliac crest (Figure 19.9a). After identifying the three layers of the abdominal wall (external oblique, internal oblique, and transversus abdominis muscles), direct the needle anterior-to-posterior[30] or posterior-to-anterior until the needle tip enters the plane between the internal oblique and transversus abdominis muscles (Figure 19.9b). Approximately 20 ml of local anesthetic solution injected via the placement needle will produce reliable anesthesia of the ipsilateral T10 to L1 dermatomes.[50,51] For postoperative local anesthetic infusion, a flexible epidural-type catheter can be placed into the tranversus abdominis plane (TAP) through the placement needle with midline incisions requiring bilateral TAP catheters.[30]

Pearls: The use of bilateral TAP catheters is not a replacement for epidural analgesia. However, for patients in whom epidural analgesia is not indicated, TAP blocks have demonstrated efficacy in reducing postoperative pain following various abdominal and pelvic procedures.[52–55] Insertion of the TAP catheter from the posterior approach offers the advantage of further displacement away from the surgical field, therefore permitting preoperative placement. To date, the optimal infusion regimen for TAP catheters is yet to be determined.

Conclusion

Ultrasound-guided CPNBs and subsequent perineural local anesthetic infusions offer superior pain relief for a variety of surgical indications. The application of ultrasound guidance has improved the success rate and efficiency of CPNB procedures,[19–21] but the effect, if any, on the optimal perineural infusion rates and drug dosage remains unknown. Further research exploring various catheter types (e.g., stimulating vs. nonstimulating), placement needles, ultrasound transducers and machines, infusion regimens for specific ultrasound-guided perineural catheter locations, and application of new technology is required.

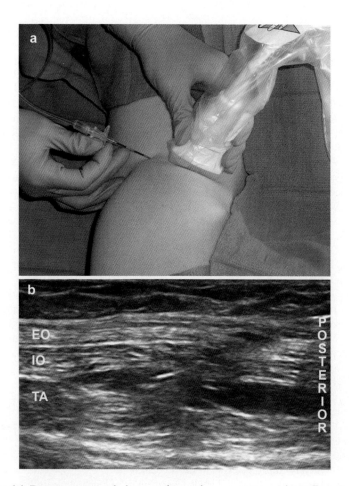

Figure 19.9. (a) Demonstration of ultrasound transducer position and needle insertion site for right transversus abdominis plane perineural catheter insertion. The patient is positioned left lateral decubitus. (b) Sample image from ultrasound-guided transversus abdominis plane perineural catheter insertion. *EO* external oblique muscle, *IO* internal oblique muscle, *TA* transversus abdominis muscle.

References

1. Ilfeld BM, Morey TE, Enneking FK. Continuous infraclavicular brachial plexus block for postoperative pain control at home: a randomized, double-blinded, placebo-controlled study. *Anesthesiology.* 2002;96:1297–1304.
2. Ilfeld BM, Morey TE, Wang RD, Enneking FK. Continuous popliteal sciatic nerve block for postoperative pain control at home: a randomized, double-blinded, placebo-controlled study. *Anesthesiology.* 2002;97:959–965.
3. Ilfeld BM, Morey TE, Wright TW, Chidgey LK, Enneking FK. Continuous interscalene brachial plexus block for postoperative pain control at home: a randomized, double-blinded, placebo-controlled study. *Anesth Analg.* 2003;96:1089–1095.
4. Singelyn FJ, Deyaert M, Joris D, Pendeville E, Gouverneur JM. Effects of intravenous patient-controlled analgesia with morphine, continuous epidural analgesia, and continuous three-in-one block on postoperative pain and knee rehabilitation after unilateral total knee arthroplasty. *Anesth Analg.* 1998;87:88–92.
5. Ganapathy S, Wasserman RA, Watson JT, et al. Modified continuous femoral three-in-one block for postoperative pain after total knee arthroplasty. *Anesth Analg.* 1999;89:1197–1202.

6. Ilfeld BM, Ball ST, Gearen PF, et al. Ambulatory continuous posterior lumbar plexus nerve blocks after hip arthroplasty: a dual-center, randomized, triple-masked, placebo-controlled trial. *Anesthesiology.* 2008;109:491–501.

7. Ilfeld BM, Le LT, Meyer RS, et al. Ambulatory continuous femoral nerve blocks decrease time to discharge readiness after tricompartment total knee arthroplasty: a randomized, triple-masked, placebo-controlled study. *Anesthesiology.* 2008;108:703–713.

8. Ilfeld BM, Wright TW, Enneking FK, Morey TE. Joint range of motion after total shoulder arthroplasty with and without a continuous interscalene nerve block: a retrospective, case-control study. *Reg Anesth Pain Med.* 2005;30:429–433.

9. Ilfeld BM, Vandenborne K, Duncan PW, et al. Ambulatory continuous interscalene nerve blocks decrease the time to discharge readiness after total shoulder arthroplasty: a randomized, triple-masked, placebo-controlled study. *Anesthesiology.* 2006;105:999–1007.

10. Ilfeld BM, Wright TW, Enneking FK, Vandenborne K. Total elbow arthroplasty as an outpatient procedure using a continuous infraclavicular nerve block at home: a prospective case report. *Reg Anesth Pain Med.* 2006;31:172–176.

11. Ilfeld BM, Gearen PF, Enneking FK, et al. Total hip arthroplasty as an overnight-stay procedure using an ambulatory continuous psoas compartment nerve block: a prospective feasibility study. *Reg Anesth Pain Med.* 2006;31:113–118.

12. Ilfeld BM, Gearen PF, Enneking FK, et al. Total knee arthroplasty as an overnight-stay procedure using continuous femoral nerve blocks at home: a prospective feasibility study. *Anesth Analg.* 2006;102:87–90.

13. Ilfeld BM, Mariano ER, Williams BA, Woodard JN, Macario A. Hospitalization costs of total knee arthroplasty with a continuous femoral nerve block provided only in the hospital versus on an ambulatory basis: a retrospective, case-control, cost-minimization analysis. *Reg Anesth Pain Med.* 2007;32:46–54.

14. Grant SA, Nielsen KC, Greengrass RA, Steele SM, Klein SM. Continuous peripheral nerve block for ambulatory surgery. *Reg Anesth Pain Med.* 2001;26:209–214.

15. Boezaart AP, De Beer JF, Nell ML. Early experience with continuous cervical paravertebral block using a stimulating catheter. *Reg Anesth Pain Med.* 2003;28:406–413.

16. Pham-Dang C, Kick O, Collet T, Gouin F, Pinaud M. Continuous peripheral nerve blocks with stimulating catheters. *Reg Anesth Pain Med.* 2003;28:83–88.

17. Sandhu NS, Capan LM. Ultrasound-guided infraclavicular brachial plexus block. *Br J Anaesth.* 2002;89:254–259.

18. Mariano ER, Afra R, Loland VJ, et al. Continuous interscalene brachial plexus block via an ultrasound-guided posterior approach: a randomized, triple-masked, placebo-controlled study. *Anesth Analg.* 2009;108:1688–1694.

19. Mariano ER, Cheng GS, Choy LP, et al. Electrical stimulation versus ultrasound guidance for popliteal-sciatic perineural catheter insertion: a randomized controlled trial. *Reg Anesth Pain Med.* 2009;34:480–485.

20. Mariano ER, Loland VJ, Bellars RH, et al. Ultrasound guidance versus electrical stimulation for infraclavicular brachial plexus perineural catheter insertion. *J Ultrasound Med.* 2009;28:1211–1218.

21. Mariano ER, Loland VJ, Sandhu NS, et al. Ultrasound guidance versus electrical stimulation for femoral perineural catheter insertion. *J Ultrasound Med.* 2009;28:1453–1460.

22. Swenson JD, Bay N, Loose E, et al. Outpatient management of continuous peripheral nerve catheters placed using ultrasound guidance: an experience in 620 patients. *Anesth Analg.* 2006;103:1436–1443.

23. Dhir S, Ganapathy S. Use of ultrasound guidance and contrast enhancement: a study of continuous infraclavicular brachial plexus approach. *Acta Anaesthesiol Scand.* 2008;52:338–342.

24. Antonakakis JG, Sites BD, Shiffrin J. Ultrasound-guided posterior approach for the placement of a continuous interscalene catheter. *Reg Anesth Pain Med.* 2009;34:64–68.

25. Mariano ER, Loland VJ, Ilfeld BM. Interscalene perineural catheter placement using an ultrasound-guided posterior approach. *Reg Anesth Pain Med.* 2009;34:60–63.

26. Fredrickson MJ, Danesh-Clough TK. Ambulatory continuous femoral analgesia for major knee surgery: a randomised study of ultrasound-guided femoral catheter placement. *Anaesth Intensive Care.* 2009;37:758–766.

27. Koscielniak-Nielsen ZJ, Rasmussen H, Hesselbjerg L. Long-axis ultrasound imaging of the nerves and advancement of perineural catheters under direct vision: a preliminary report of four cases. *Reg Anesth Pain Med.* 2008;33:477–482.

28. van Geffen GJ, Gielen M. Ultrasound-guided subgluteal sciatic nerve blocks with stimulating catheters in children: a descriptive study. *Anesth Analg.* 2006;103:328–333.

29. Luyet C, Eichenberger U, Greif R, Vogt A, Szucs Farkas Z, Moriggl B. Ultrasound-guided paravertebral puncture and placement of catheters in human cadavers: an imaging study. *Br J Anaesth.* 2009;102:534–539.

30. Gucev G, Yasui GM, Chang TY, Lee J. Bilateral ultrasound-guided continuous ilioinguinal-iliohypogastric block for pain relief after cesarean delivery. *Anesth Analg.* 2008;106:1220–1222.

31. Sites BD, Brull R, Chan VW, et al. Artifacts and pitfall errors associated with ultrasound-guided regional anesthesia. Part I: understanding the basic principles of ultrasound physics and machine operations. *Reg Anesth Pain Med.* 2007;32:412–418.

32. Gray AT. Ultrasound-guided regional anesthesia: current state of the art. *Anesthesiology.* 2006; 104:368–373.

33. Dhir S, Ganapathy S. Comparative evaluation of ultrasound-guided continuous infraclavicular brachial plexus block with stimulating catheter and traditional technique: a prospective-randomized trial. *Acta Anaesthesiol Scand.* 2008;52:1158–1166.

34. Fredrickson MJ, Ball CM, Dalgleish AJ, Stewart AW, Short TG. A prospective randomized comparison of ultrasound and neurostimulation as needle end points for interscalene catheter placement. *Anesth Analg.* 2009;108:1695–1700.

35. Tsui BC, Ozelsel TJ. Ultrasound-guided anterior sciatic nerve block using a longitudinal approach: "expanding the view". *Reg Anesth Pain Med.* 2008;33:275–276.

36. Hebl JR, Neal JM. Infectious complications: a new practice advisory. *Reg Anesth Pain Med.* 2006;31:289–290.

37. Mariano ER, Ilfeld BM, Cheng GS, Nicodemus HF, Suresh S. Feasibility of ultrasound-guided peripheral nerve block catheters for pain control on pediatric medical missions in developing countries. *Paediatr Anaesth.* 2008;18:598–601.

38. Fredrickson MJ, Ball CM, Dalgleish AJ. A prospective randomized comparison of ultrasound guidance versus neurostimulation for interscalene catheter placement. *Reg Anesth Pain Med.* 2009;34:590–594.

39. Davis JJ, Swenson JD, Greis PE, Burks RT, Tashjian RZ. Interscalene block for postoperative analgesia using only ultrasound guidance: the outcome in 200 patients. *J Clin Anesth.* 2009;21: 272–277.

40. Swenson JD, Davis JJ, DeCou JA. A novel approach for assessing catheter position after ultrasound-guided placement of continuous interscalene block. *Anesth Analg.* 2008;106:1015–1016.

41. Sandhu NS, Maharlouei B, Patel B, Erkulwater E, Medabalmi P. Simultaneous bilateral infraclavicular brachial plexus blocks with low-dose lidocaine using ultrasound guidance. *Anesthesiology.* 2006;104:199–201.

42. Desgagnes MC, Levesque S, Dion N, et al. A comparison of a single or triple injection technique for ultrasound-guided infraclavicular block: a prospective randomized controlled study. *Anesth Analg.* 2009;109:668–672.

43. Ilfeld BM, Le LT, Ramjohn J, et al. The effects of local anesthetic concentration and dose on continuous infraclavicular nerve blocks: a multicenter, randomized, observer-masked, controlled study. *Anesth Analg.* 2009;108:345–350.

44. Nader A, Malik K, Kendall MC, Benzon H, McCarthy RJ. Relationship between ultrasound imaging and eliciting motor response during femoral nerve stimulation. *J Ultrasound Med.* 2009;28:345–350.

45. Chan VW, Nova H, Abbas S, McCartney CJ, Perlas A, Xu DQ. Ultrasound examination and localization of the sciatic nerve: a volunteer study. *Anesthesiology.* 2006;104:309–314.

46. Karmakar MK, Kwok WH, Ho AM, Tsang K, Chui PT, Gin T. Ultrasound-guided sciatic nerve block: description of a new approach at the subgluteal space. *Br J Anaesth.* 2007;98:390–395.

47. Taboada M, Rodriguez J, Valino C, et al. A prospective, randomized comparison between the popliteal and subgluteal approaches for continuous sciatic nerve block with stimulating catheters. *Anesth Analg.* 2006;103:244–247.

48. Hadzic A, Vloka JD, Singson R, Santos AC, Thys DM. A comparison of intertendinous and classical approaches to popliteal nerve block using magnetic resonance imaging simulation. *Anesth Analg.* 2002;94:1321–1324.

49. Ilfeld BM, Loland VJ, Gerancher JC, et al. The effects of varying local anesthetic concentration and volume on continuous popliteal sciatic nerve blocks: a dual-center, randomized, controlled study. *Anesth Analg.* 2008;107:701–707.

50. Shibata Y, Sato Y, Fujiwara Y, Komatsu T. Transversus abdominis plane block. *Anesth Analg.* 2007;105:883.

51. Tran TM, Ivanusic JJ, Hebbard P, Barrington MJ. Determination of spread of injectate after ultrasound-guided transversus abdominis plane block: a cadaveric study. *Br J Anaesth.* 2009;102: 123–127.

52. El-Dawlatly AA, Turkistani A, Kettner SC, et al. Ultrasound-guided transversus abdominis plane block: description of a new technique and comparison with conventional systemic analgesia during laparoscopic cholecystectomy. *Br J Anaesth.* 2009;102:763–767.

53. McDonnell JG, Curley G, Carney J, et al. The analgesic efficacy of transversus abdominis plane block after cesarean delivery: a randomized controlled trial. *Anesth Analg.* 2008;106:186–191.

54. McDonnell JG, O'Donnell B, Curley G, Heffernan A, Power C, Laffey JG. The analgesic efficacy of transversus abdominis plane block after abdominal surgery: a prospective randomized controlled trial. *Anesth Analg.* 2007;104:193–197.

55. O'Donnell BD, McDonnell JG, McShane AJ. The transversus abdominis plane (TAP) block in open retropubic prostatectomy. *Reg Anesth Pain Med.* 2006;31:91.

20

Ultrasound-Guided Cervical Sympathetic Block

Philip W.H. Peng

Introduction

Stellate ganglion block (SGB) is performed for the management of patients for a variety of pain conditions, including complex regional pain syndrome and peripheral vascular disease.[1,2] The most widely practiced approach to SGB is the paratracheal approach, in which the needle is inserted toward the anterior tubercle of cervical sixth vertebra (Chassaignac tubercle).[3] This approach is essentially a blockade of the cervical sympathetic chain in proximity to the middle cervical ganglion instead of the stellate ganglion, which is located opposite to the neck of the first rib (Figure 20.1).[4] Thus, the classical approach is better termed cervical sympathetic block.

P.W.H. Peng (✉)
Department of Anesthesia, University of Toronto, Toronto Western Hospital,
McL 2-405, 399 Bathurst Street, Toronto, ON, Canada M5T2S8
e-mail: philip.peng@uhn.on.ca

S.N. Narouze (ed.), *Atlas of Ultrasound-Guided Procedures in Interventional Pain Management*,
DOI 10.1007/978-1-4419-1681-5_20, © Springer Science+Business Media, LLC 2011

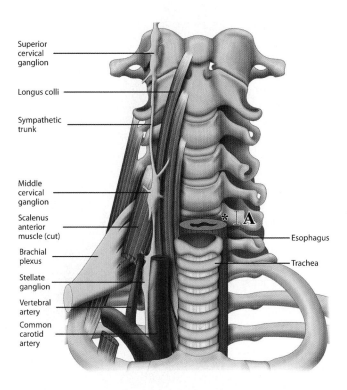

Figure 20.1. Prevertebral region of the neck. The target site for needle insertion in classical approach is marked as *asterisk*. The breadth of the transverse process is marked as **A**. Reproduced with permission from USRA (www.usra.ca).

Anatomy

The sympathetic outflow arises from the preganglionic neurons located at the lateral gray horn of the spinal cord at the thoracic and upper two lumbar spinal segments. The sympathetic fibers for the head, neck, upper limbs, and the heart arise from the first few thoracic segments, ascend through the sympathetic chains, and synapse in the superior, middle, and inferior cervical ganglion.[4,5] The stellate ganglion, formed by fusion of the inferior cervical and first thoracic ganglion, extends from the level of the head of the first rib to the inferior border of the transverse process of C7 and lies medial or sometimes posterior to the vertebral artery immediately adjacent to the dome of pleura (Figure 20.1). The postganglionic fibers from the stellate ganglion to the cervical nerves (seventh and eighth) and the first thoracic nerve provide sympathetic innervation to the upper limbs.[4-7] The preganglionic fibers of the head and neck region continue to travel cephalad to the superior and middle cervical ganglion through the cervical sympathetic trunk (CST). Injection of local anesthetic around the stellate ganglion interrupts the sympathetic outflow to the head, neck, and upper limbs through inactivation of both preganglionic and postganglionic fibers, while injection of local anesthetic around the CST results only in sympathetic blockade of head and neck regions.[5,6] The CST is located dorsal to the posterior fascia of the carotid sheath anteriorly and is embedded in the prevertebral fascia (personal communication Dr. E Civelek).[8-10]

Existing Techniques

As stated above, the popular approach is anterior paratracheal approach at sixth cervical vertebral level with or without fluoroscopic guidance because of the close relation of the stellate ganglion to the pleura and vertebral artery. These indirect approaches to CST assume that the medication will spread caudally to the stellate ganglion. A few concerns about these approaches are examined below.

The breadth (cephalocaudal distance) of the Chassaignac tubercle can be as narrow as 6 mm (Figure 20.1).[3] Thus, it can be easily missed with needle advancement with conventional technique. A consequence of this is potential puncture of the vertebral artery or nerve root, which is usually protected by the anterior tubercle of the C6. However, once the needle is in contact with the bone, the vertebral artery can still be at risk. The vertebral artery usually ascends and enters the foramen in the transverse process of C6 vertebra. Unfortunately, a cadaver study demonstrated that this arrangement applied in 90–93% of the cadavers examined and the vertebral artery may enter at the transverse process of C4 or C5.[11,12] Although contrast injection in fluoroscopy-guided technique helps to avoid inadvertent injection of local anesthetic into this artery, the intravascular injection can be recognized only *after* the artery has been punctured. A modified fluoroscopy-guided oblique approach may minimize the risk of vertebral artery puncture as the needle is directed to the junction of the uncinate process and the vertebra body.[13] However, this technique directs the needle much closer to the esophagus (see below).

Both landmark-based technique and fluoroscopy-guided technique do not reveal the soft tissues transverse by the needle path.[14] In most of the anatomy atlas, the esophagus is often seen as a structure located behind the cricoid and trachea. However, literature contradicts those assumptions. Esophagus is found deviated from the midline in 53% of the subjects.[15] In 5% of the subjects, approximately 40–60% of the esophagus is unopposed by the cricoid and lies ventral to the medial part of the transverse process, which is part of the needle path (Figure 20.2).[15] Mediastinitis can result especially if the patient has an unrecognized diverticulum.[16] Moreover, this probably is the cause of the "foreign body" sensation that is often attributed in the past to the blockade of external laryngeal branch of superior laryngeal nerve or recurrent laryngeal nerve.[17]

Certain artery, especially inferior thyroidal artery, can be seen passing in the needle path (Figure 20.3).[18] Another artery that can be found anterior to transverse process of C6 of C7 is the ascending cervical artery, which has been described to form an anastomosis with either vertebral artery or anterior spinal artery.[19] The major consequence of not recognizing this variation will be the formation of hematoma.[20,21] As a matter of fact, hematoma was fairly commonly encountered (25%) in the first case series comparing ultrasound-guided with "blind" injection technique.[22] The consequence of larger hematoma can be life threatening, as demonstrated by a review of those patients with retropharyngeal hematoma following SGB.[23]

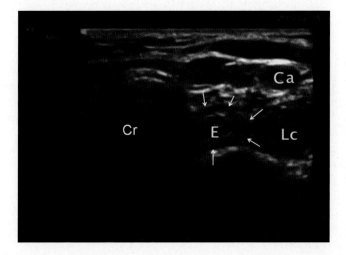

Figure 20.2. Ultrasonographic image of neck at C6 showing the deviation of esophagus (outlined by *line arrows*). *Cr* cricoid, *Lc* longus colli muscle, *E* esophagus, *Ca* carotid artery. Reproduced with permission from USRA (www.usra.ca).

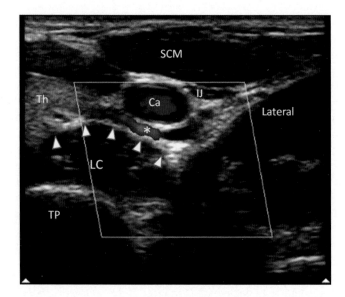

Figure 20.3. Ultrasonographic image with color Doppler. The inferior thyroidal artery was indicated with *asterisk*; the prevertebral fascia is marked by *solid arrowheads*. *TP* transverse process of C6, *Th* thyroid, *LC* longus colli muscle, *IJ* internal jugular vein. Reproduced with permission from USRA (www.usra.ca).

The key to the success of the blockade of CST is to deposit the local anesthetic around the CST with caudal spread of the local anesthetic to the stellate ganglion. The location of CST is in the prevertebral fascia which is a loose connective tissue. Without reference to this key anatomy landmark, both the landmark-based and fluoroscopy-guided techniques rely on the surrogate landmark, C6 or C7 transverse process, as the target. The technique involves directing the needle to the bone and withdrawing the needle. The spread of solution following "bone contact and needle withdrawal" has been studied and the injectate spread anterior to the prevertebral fascia and in the paratracheal space in most of the patients, without much caudal spread.[24] It has been suggested that subfascial injection results in more caudal spread, higher rate of sympathetic block of upper limb, and lower risk of hoarseness.[25,26] Too deep an injection into the longus colli muscle also renders the sympathetic block ineffective.[27] Given the anatomical position of the CST, the ideal location is into prevertebral fascia.

Technique for Ultrasound-Guided Injection

The patient is placed in the supine position with the neck in slight extension. A high-frequency linear transducer (6–13 MHz) is placed at the level of C6 to allow cross-sectional visualization of anatomic structures, including the transverse process and anterior tubercle of C6, longus colli muscle and prevertebral fascia, and carotid artery and thyroid gland (Figures 20.4 and 20.5).[14,17] A prescan is important in planning the path of needle insertion as the presence of the esophagus and the inferior thyroidal artery may obviate the needle insertion path between the carotid artery and trachea.[28] In that situation, the needle may be inserted lateral to the carotid artery, which is the author's preferred route.

For the lateral approach, the tip of the needle is directed to the prevertebral fascia between the carotid artery and the tip of C6 anterior tubercle (Figure 20.6). This needle path will avoid hitting the cervical nerve root. The internal jugular vein can be visualized by decreasing the probe pressure and avoided by "pushing" way with the needle. A total of 5 ml of local anesthetic is injected. Visualization of the spread of injectate under real-time scanning is important, as the absence of this may suggest unsuspected intravascular injection.

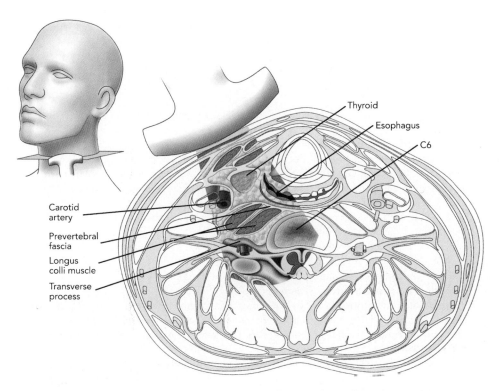

Figure 20.4. Cross section of the neck at the sixth cervical vertebral level correlating with the ultrasonographic image. Reproduced with permission from USRA (www.usra.ca).

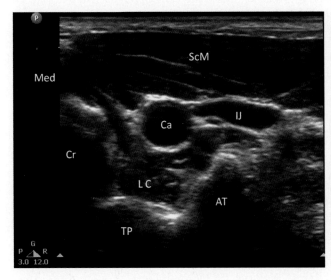

Figure 20.5. Ultrasonographic image of neck at C6. *ScM* sternocleidomastoid muscle, *Ca* carotid artery, *TP* transverse process of C6, *AT* anterior tubercle, *LC* longus colli muscle, *IJ* internal jugular vein, *Cr* cricoids, *Med* medial. Reproduced with permission from USRA (www.usra.ca).

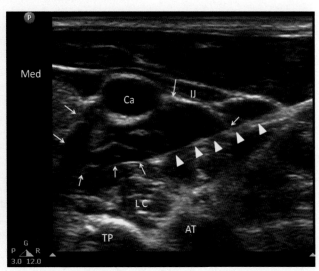

Figure 20.6. Ultrasonographic image of neck at C6 as in Figure 20.5 following injection of local anesthetic. The needle was indicated by *solid arrows* and the local anesthetic was outlined by the *line arrows*. *Ca* carotid artery, *IJ* internal jugular vein, *LC* longus colli muscle, *TP* transverse process, *AT* anterior tubercle. Reproduced with permission from USRA (www.usra.ca).

REFERENCES

1. Stanton-Hicks MD, Burton AW, Bruehl SP, et al. An updated interdisciplinary clinical pathway for CRPS: report of an expert panel. *Pain Pract.* 2002;2:1–16.
2. Elias M. Cervical sympathetic and stellate ganglion blocks. *Pain Physician.* 2000;3:294–304.
3. Janik JE, Hoeft MA, Ajar AH, Alsofrom GF, Borrello MT, Rathmell JP. Variable osteology of the sixth cervical vertebra in relation to stellate ganglion block. *Reg Anesth Pain Med.* 2008;33:102–108.
4. Williams PL. *Gray's Anatomy.* 38th ed. New York: Churchill Livingstone; 1995.
5. Fitzgerald MJT. *Neuroanatomy: Basic and Clinical.* 3rd ed. London: WB Saunders; 1996.
6. Tubbs RS, Loukas M, Remy AC, Shoja MM, Salter EG. The vertebral nerve revisited. *Clin Anat.* 2007;20:644–647.
7. Hogan QH, Erickson SJ. MR imaging of the stellate ganglion: normal appearance. *AJR Am J Roentgenol.* 1992;158:655–659.
8. Civelek E, Kiris T, Hepgul K, Canbolat A, Ersoy G, Cansever T. Anterolateral approach to the cervical spine: major anatomical structures and landmarks. *J Neurosurg Spine.* 2007;7:669–678.
9. Honma M, Murakami G, Sato TJ, Namiki A. Spread of injectate during C6 stellate ganglion block and fascial arrangement in the prevertebral region: an experimental study using donated cadavers. *Reg Anesth Pain Med.* 2000;25:573–583.
10. Kiray A, Arman C, Naderi S, Güvencer M, Korman E. Surgical anatomy of the cervical sympathetic trunk. *Clin Anat.* 2005;18:179–185.
11. Matula C, Trattnig S, Tschabitscher M, Day JD, Koos WT. The course of the prevertebral segment of the vertebral artery: anatomy and clinical significance. *Surg Neurol.* 1997;48:125–131.
12. Bruneau M, Cornelius JF, Marneffe V, Triffaux M, George B. Anatomical variations of the V2 segment of the vertebral artery. *Neurosurgery.* 2006;59:20–24.
13. Abdi S. A new and easy technique to block the stellate ganglion. *Pain Physician.* 2004;7:327–331.
14. Peng P, Narouze S. Ultrasound-guided interventional procedures in pain medicine: a review of anatomy, sonoanatomy and procedures. Part I: non-axial structures. *Reg Anesth Pain Med.* 2009;34:458–474.
15. Smith KJ, Dobranowski J, Yip G, Dauphin A, Choi PT. Cricoid pressure displaces the esophagus: an observational study using magnetic resonance imaging. *Anesthesiology.* 2003;99:60–64.
16. Narouze S, Vydyanathan A, Patel N. Ultrasound-guided stellate ganglion block successfully prevented esophageal puncture. *Pain Physician.* 2007;10:747–752.
17. Peng P. How I do it? Stellate ganglion block. ASRA Newsletter 2010 May: 16–18
18. Narouze S. Beware of the "serpentine" inferior thyroid artery while performing stellate ganglion block. *Anesth Analg.* 2009;109:289–290.
19. Huntoon MA. The vertebral artery is unlikely to be the sole source of vascular complications occurring during stellate ganglion block. *Pain Pract.* 2010;10:25–30.
20. Mishio M, Matsumoto T, Okuda Y, Kitajima T. Delayed severe airway obstruction due to hematoma following stellate ganglion block. *Reg Anesth Pain Med.* 1998;23:516–519.
21. Takanami I, Abiko T, Koizumi S. Life-threatening airway obstruction due to retropharyngeal and cervicomediastinal hematomas following stellate ganglion block. *Thorac cardiovasc Surg.* 2009;57:311–312.
22. Kapral S, Krafft P, Gosch M, Fleischmann D, Weinstabl C. Ultrasound imaging for stellate ganglion block: direct visualization of puncture site and local anesthetic spread. *Reg Anesth.* 1995;20:323–328.
23. Higa K, Hirata K, Hirota K, Nitahara K, Shono S. Retropharyngeal hematoma after stellate ganglion block. *Anesthesiology.* 2006;105:1238–1245.
24. Hogan QH, Erickson SJ, Haddox JD, Abram SE. The spread of solutions during stellate ganglion block. *Reg Anesth.* 1992;17:78–83.
25. Shibata Y, Fujiwara Y, Komatsu T. A new approach of ultrasound-guided stellate ganglion block. *Anesth Analg.* 2007;105:550–551.
26. Christie JM, Martinez CR. Computerized axial tomography to define the distribution of solution after stellate ganglion nerve block. *J Clin Anesth.* 1995;7:306–311.
27. Atez Y, Asik I, Özgencil E, Açar HI, Yağmurlu B, Tekdemir I. Evaluation of the longus colli muscle in relation to stellate ganglion block. *Reg Anesth Pain Med.* 2009;34:219–223.
28. Gofeld M, Bhatia A, Abbas S, Ganapathy S, Johnson M. Development and validation of a new technique for ultrasound-guided stellate ganglion block. *Reg Anesth Pain Med.* 2009;34:475–479.

21

Ultrasound-Guided Peripheral Nerve Blockade in Chronic Pain Management

Anuj Bhatia and Philip W.H. Peng

P.W.H. Peng (✉)
Department of Anesthesia and Pain Management, University of Toronto, Toronto Western Hospital,
McL 2-405, 399 Bathurst Street, Toronto, ON, Canada M5T2S8
e-mail: Philip.Peng@uhn.on.ca

S.N. Narouze (ed.), *Atlas of Ultrasound-Guided Procedures in Interventional Pain Management*,
DOI 10.1007/978-1-4419-1681-5_21, © Springer Science+Business Media, LLC 2011

Introduction

Application of ultrasound in pain medicine (USPM) is a rapidly growing medical field in interventional pain management.[1] In general, the application of USPM can be divided into three areas: peripheral, axial, and musculoskeletal structures. In this chapter, we will review the relevant anatomy, sonoanatomy, and the injection techniques of three peripheral structures: lateral femoral cutaneous nerve (LFCN), intercostal nerve (ICN), and suprascapular nerve (SSN).

Lateral Femoral Cutaneous Nerve Block

The LFCN provides sensory innervation to the skin of the anterior and lateral parts of the thigh as far as the knee (Figure 21.1). Regional block of the LFCN is performed for acute pain relief following surgical procedures and for the diagnosis and treatment of meralgia paresthetica.[2,3] Meralgia paresthetica refers to a symptom complex of pain, numbness, tingling, and paresthesia in the anterolateral thigh. The incidence in a primary care setting was estimated at 4.3 per 10,000 person-years.[4]

Anatomy

The LFCN is a purely sensory nerve that arises from branches of dorsal divisions of the second and third lumbar nerves. It emerges from the lateral border of the psoas major and crosses the iliacus muscle obliquely, toward the anterior superior iliac spine (ASIS).[5] The nerve then passes under the inguinal ligament at a distance 36 ± 20 mm medial to the ASIS, and after entering the thigh, the LFCN turns laterally and downward, where it typically divides into the anterior and posterior branches (Figure 21.1).[6] The course and location of the LFCN as it crosses the inguinal ligament has been found to be quite variable. While the nerve courses medial to the ASIS most of the time, it can pass over or even

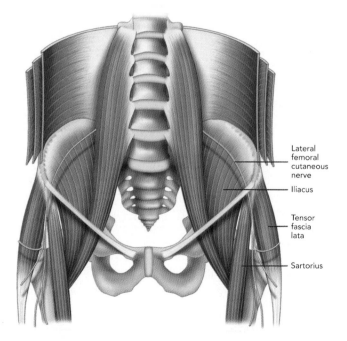

Lateral
femoral
cutaneous
nerve

Iliacus

Tensor
fascia
lata

Sartorius

Figure 21.1. The pathway of a typical course of lateral femoral cutaneous nerve is shown. Note that the nerve course beneath the inguinal ligament and runs superficially to the sartorius muscle and then in between this muscle and tensor fascia lata muscle. Reproduced with permission from USRA (www.usra.ca).

posterior to the ASIS in up to 25% of patients.[5-7] Though in the vast majority of cases, the LFCN enters the thigh superficial to the sartorius muscle beneath the fascia lata, in 22% of cases the LFCN passes through the muscle itself.[8] The LFCN has been shown to cross under the inguinal ligament as far as 4.6–7.3 cm medial to the ASIS.[6,9,10] The LFCN divides into an anterior and a posterior branch in the thigh. The anterior branch becomes superficial at a variable distance below the inguinal ligament, and divides into branches that are distributed to the skin of the anterior and lateral parts of the thigh, as far as the knee. The posterior branch pierces the fascia lata, and subdivides into filaments that pass backward across the lateral and posterior surfaces of the thigh, supplying the skin from the level of the greater trochanter to the middle of the thigh.[11]

Literature Review of Injection Techniques

The traditional approach to blocking the LFCN is a blind, landmark-assisted technique. The success of this method is variable, quoted success rates being as low as 38%.[12] The low success rate of the block can be attributed to the wide anatomic variability in the course of the LFCN, as well as to the lack of any predictable relationship of the LFCN to palpable vascular structures or bony landmarks.[3]

There are a few published reports of the use of ultrasound to identify and block the LFCN.[3,13-16] One of these was a study that demonstrated greater accuracy in identifying the LFCN with ultrasound in both cadavers and volunteers.[13] In the cadavers, 16 out of 19 needles (84.2%) inserted with ultrasound guidance were in contact with the LFCNs compared with 1 out of 19 (5.3%) where needles were inserted according to landmarks. In the same study, 16 out of 20 (80%) marked positions identified using ultrasound imaging corresponded to the LFCN position in human volunteers identified by percutaneous nerve stimulator compared to 0 out of 20 positions marked by anatomic landmarks.

In a case series of 10 patients with a mean BMI of 31, the author reported that the LFCN could be visualized by ultrasound in all patients and that sensory block was successful in all cases.[3] The technique was not complicated by coincidental blockade of any nearby nerves, nor did any patients complain of paresthesia from the needle coming into direct contact with the LFCN.

Ultrasound-Guided Block Technique

Locating this nerve with ultrasound can be a challenge as the LFCN is a small nerve and its course is highly variable. However, a few important principals may assist the beginners to locate the nerve:

1. A sound knowledge of anatomy of the course and direction of the LFCN as well as the structures around LFCN.[16]
2. The nerve is better appreciated with dynamic scanning or sweeping view because of the size of the nerve and its proximity with fascia layer.[3,16]
3. The LFCN may appear as hyperechoic, hypoechoic, or mixed structure, depending on the course of the nerve itself (under or through the inguinal ligament, or over the iliac crest), the special tissue architecture in the corresponding area, and the frequency of the transducer used (the higher frequency probe is likely to produce artifacts).[3,13,14,16]
4. In patients with severe or advanced symptoms of meralgia paresthetica, the LFCN is likely to be swollen or enlarged (pseudoneuroma) and likely to be picked up ultrasonography.[8]
5. The LFCN can be usually found in the infra-inguinal region, either superficial to the sartorius muscle or between sartorius and tensor of fascia lata muscles.

With the patient in the supine position, the ASIS and the inguinal ligament are marked on the skin. Using a high-frequency linear array transducer (6–13 MHz), the ultrasound probe is placed over the ASIS initially with the long axis view of the inguinal ligament,

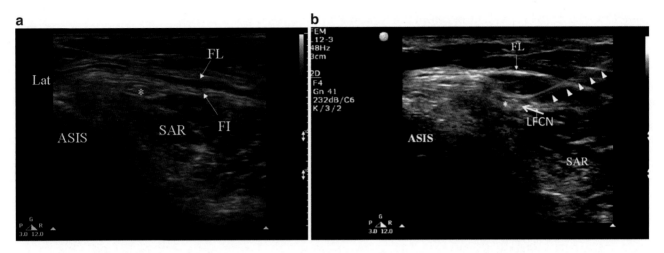

Figure 21.2. Ultrasonographic image of lateral femoral cutaneous nerve (LFCN) (**a**) before and (**b**) after injection. *FL* fascia lata, *FI* fascia iliaca, *SAR* sartorius muscle, *ASIS* anterior superior iliac spine. *Solid arrow head* indicates path of the needle; LFCN is indicated by *asterisk*. Reproduced with permission from Lippincott Williams & Wilkins.

and is then moved distally. The ASIS is visualized a hyperechoic structure with posterior acoustic shadowing (Figure 21.2). The sartorius muscle will be seen as an inverted triangular shape structure. Attention is paid to the orientation of the probe to the course of the nerve. The LFCN will appear as one or more hypoechoic structures in the short axis view superficial to the sartorius muscle. In some situation, it will be in a more medial position sandwiched between the fascia lata and fascia iliaca (Figure 21.2). When the nerve cannot be found in this area, one can look for the LFCN in the angle between the tensor of the fascia lata and the sartorius muscle. Once the LFCN has been identified, a 22 G 2.5 in. needle is advanced in plane with the ultrasound probe. Alternatively, the needle can be advanced out of plane using a nerve-stimulating needle to confirm placement.

If it is difficult to identify the LFCN, two other methods can be employed. One is to inject dextrose 5% solution to hydro-dissect the plane between the fascia lata and the fascia over the sartorius and iliacus muscles.[15] The other is to locate the nerve with a transdermal nerve stimulator or to use a stimulating needle.[13] Once the nerve is identified, injection is commenced. The injectate should be visualized by ultrasound as it spreads around the nerve circumferentially and in a cephalad manner, and a total volume of 5–10 ml is usually adequate to ensure complete blockade.

Suprascapular Nerve Block

First described in 1941,[17] SSN block has been performed over the years by anesthesiologists, rheumatologist, and pain specialists for the management of acute and chronic shoulder pain.[1,18,19] Indications for performing this block in interventional pain practice include adhesive capsulitis, frozen shoulder, rotator cuff tear, and glenohumeral arthritis secondary to degeneration or inflammation.[20] There has been renewed interest in the technique of performing SSN block under ultrasound guidance and descriptions of this method have appeared in recent published medical literature.[21–23]

Anatomy

The SSN originates from the superior trunk of the brachial plexus (formed by the union of the fifth and sixth cervical nerves), runs parallel to the omohyoid muscle, and courses under the trapezius (Figure 21.3) before it passes under the transverse scapular ligament in the suprascapular notch. It then passes beneath the supraspinatus, and curves around the lateral border of the spine of the scapula (spinoglenoid notch) to the infraspinatous fossa

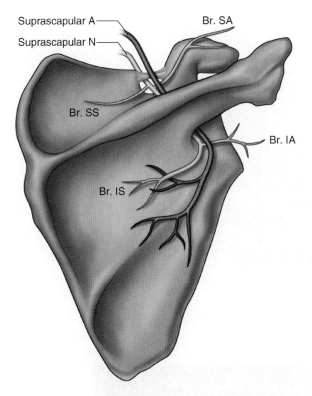

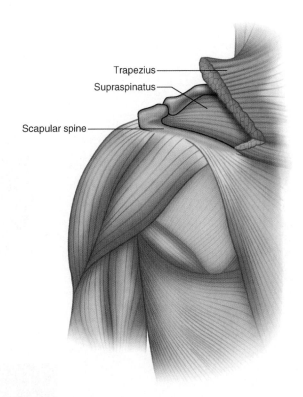

Figure 21.3. Suprascapular nerve and its branches. Superior articular branch (Br. SA) supplies the coracohumeral ligament, subacromial bursa and posterior aspect of the acromioclavicular joint capsule; Inferior articular branch (Br. IA) supplies the posterior joint capsule; *Br. SS* branch to the supraspinatus muscle, *Br. IS* branch to the infraspinatous muscle.

Figure 21.4. Left shoulder showing the muscle layers in the suprascapular fossa.

(Figure 21.4). In the supraspinatous fossa it gives off two branches to the supraspinatus muscle, and an articular branch to the shoulder joint; and in the infraspinatous fossa it gives off two branches to the infraspinatous muscle, besides some branches to the shoulder joint and scapula. The sensory component of the SSN provides fibers to about 70% of the shoulder joint.

The "U" or "V" shaped suprascapular notch is located on the superior margin of the scapula, medial to the coracoid process (Figure 21.5). However, the notch is absent in up to 8% of cadavers.[24] Above the notch run the suprascapular artery and vein, although rarely the artery travels along with the SSN through the notch.[25] The supraspinous fossa is bordered by the spine of the scapula dorsally, by the plate of the scapula ventrally and by the supraspinous fascia superiorly, forming a classic compartment, the only exit through which is the suprascapular fossa.[26,27]

Literature Review of Injection Techniques

The targets for most of the techniques are either at the suprascapular notch or on the floor of the scapular spine. Without image guidance, techniques relying on identification of the suprascapular notch have the potential for SSN block failure and/or adverse effects. The risk of pneumothorax is approximately 1%, and this complication usually arises from the needle being inserted too deep.[28,29] If the needle is placed blindly into the notch, the needle tip is unlikely to approximate the notch as demonstrated by a study using CT to confirm the position of the needle.[30] With the use of fluoroscopy, the position of the needle in the notch can be assured. However, there is a potential of spilling of local anesthetic to the brachial plexus.[26] A superior approach has been described in which the needle is inserted vertically into the suprascapular fossa. Large volumes of solution (10 ml or more)

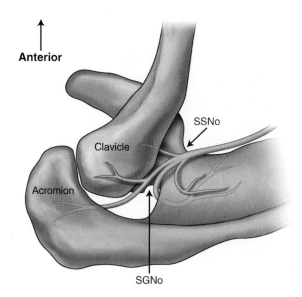

Figure 21.5. Superior view of the left shoulder. The course of the suprascapular nerve enters the suprascapular fossa through the suprascapular notch (SSNo) and then enters the infrascapular fossa through the spinoglenoid notch (SGNo).

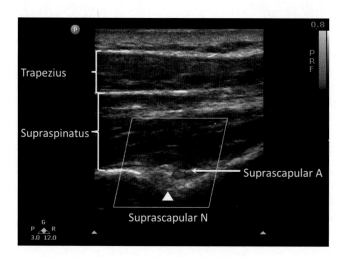

Figure 21.6. Ultrasonographic image of the suprascapular nerve on the floor of the scapular spine between suprascapular notch and spinoglenoid notch. Both suprascapular nerve and artery run underneath the fascia of supraspinatus muscle. Reproduced with permission from USRA (www.usra.ca).

will accomplish this, but according to a recent study in cadavers, there will be spread to the axillary fossa in a minority of these cases.[27]

Thus, the ideal site to perform the SSN injection is at the floor of the scapular spine between the suprascapular notch and spinoglenoid notch (Figures 21.5 and 21.6). First, this technique is independent of the notch as a target. Thus, it avoids the risk of pneumothorax if one considers the direction of the needle. This technique is also feasible in individuals without a suprascapular notch (8% of the population). Second, the suprascapular fossa forms a compartment and retains the local anesthetic around the nerve. One of the easiest ways to visualize this soft tissue plane is by the use of ultrasound.[31]

To date there is one case report detailing ultrasound-guided block of the suprascapular nerve[22] and one case series evaluating the ultrasonographic morphology of the suprascapular notch.[23] The latter reported results of measurement of the notch width, depth and distance between skin and notch base in 50 volunteers. The authors were able to visualize the transverse scapular ligament in 96% and the artery–vein complex in 86% of the vol-

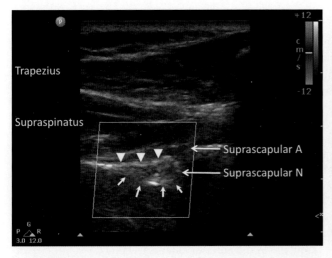

Figure 21.7. Ultrasonographic image of suprascapular nerve in the suprascapular notch (indicated by *line arrows*). Note that at this level, the suprascapular artery is above the transverse scapular ligament (*solid arrow heads*). A artery; N nerve. Reproduced with permission from USRA (www.usra.ca).

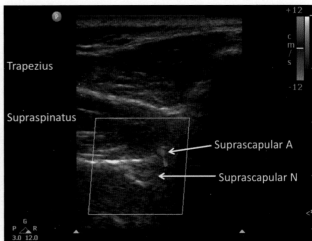

Figure 21.8. Ultrasonographic image of the suprascapular nerve slightly posterior to the plane obtained in Figure 21.7. The suprascapular artery can be seen running toward the floor of the scapular spine. Reproduced with permission from USRA (www.usra.ca).

unteers. Although visualization of the transverse scapular ligament is feasible, the probe has to be steady in a very narrow angle, making the needle advancement a very challenging technique (Figures 21.7 and 21.8). The authors in the other case report[22] claimed the visualization of the transcapular ligament and suprascapular notch. As a matter of fact, the area they were showing was the floor of the scapular spine in between the scapular notch and spinoglenoid notch (Figure 21.6).

Ultrasound-Guided Block Technique

The patient can be in sitting or in prone position. The scapula spine, coracoid process, and acromion are used as landmarks. Ultrasound scanning is performed with a linear ultrasound probe (7–13 MHz) placed in a coronal plane over the suprascapular fossa with a slight anterior tilt. The probe is placed in an orientation such that it is in the short axis to the line joining coracoid process and acromion (reflecting the position of the spinoglenoid notch).[1] The supraspinatus and trapezius muscles and the bony fossa underneath them should come into view (Figure 21.6). By adjusting the angle of the ultrasound probe in a cephalo-caudad direction, the SSN and artery should be brought into view in the trough of the floor. The nerve can sometimes be difficult to visualize as it has an approximate diameter of 25 mm. A 22-G, 80-mm needle is inserted along the longitudinal axis of the ultrasound beam. The needle is inserted either in-plane or out of plane from the medial aspect of the probe as the presence of the acromion process on the lateral side makes it difficult to angulate the needle. Because of the proximity of the nerve, an injectate volume of 5–8 ml is usually sufficient.

Intercostal Nerve Block

The ICNs supply skin and musculature of chest and abdominal wall. ICN block is performed for the treatment of acute and chronic pain conditions affecting the thorax and upper abdomen.[33] ICN blockade provides excellent analgesia for pain from rib fractures[34] and from chest and upper abdominal surgery.[35] Neurolytic ICNB may be used to manage chronic pain conditions such as postmastectomy and postthoracotomy pain.[36,37]

Anatomy

The ICNs originate from the first 12 thoracic nerves. Emerging from their respective intervertebral foramen, the thoracic nerves divide into posterior cutaneous rami that supply skin and muscle in the paravertebral region, and ventral rami that become the ICNs (Figure 21.9). ICNs are mixed sensory-motor nerves. After exiting from the spine it is located between the pleura and the posterior intercostal membrane and subsequently traverses the membrane to lie deep to or in the internal intercostal muscle (Figure 21.10). The intercostal vein and artery run in close proximity in this groove, just superior to the nerve (Figure 21.11).[38] The neurovascular bundle lies in the intercostal space but runs deep to the subcostal grove at the angle of rib. At a distance of about 5– 8 cm anterior to the angle of the rib, the groove ends and blends into the surface of the lower edge of the rib.[39] The lateral cutaneous branch of the ICN, which supplies the skin of the chest, branches off and pierces the external intercostal muscle in the region between the posterior and mid-axillary line. As the ICNs approaches the midline anteriorly, it pierces the overlying muscles and skin to terminate as the anterior cutaneous branch.

However, there are some exceptions – the first ICN has no anterior cutaneous branch, usually has no lateral cutaneous branch, and most of its fibers leave the intercostal space by crossing the neck of the first rib to join those from C8, while a smaller bundle continues on as a genuine ICN to supply the muscles of the intercostal space. Some fibers of the second and third ICNs give rise to the intercostobrachial nerve, which innervates the axilla and the skin of the medial aspect of the upper arm as far distal as the elbow. The ventral rami of the 12th ICN is similar to the other ICNs but is called a subcostal nerve because it is not in between two ribs.

Literature Review of Injection Techniques

The classic landmark-based technique is performed with the patient in the sitting or prone position. ICN block is usually performed at the angle of the rib to ensure that the tissues

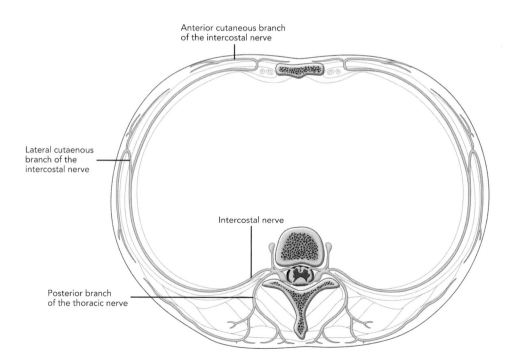

Figure 21.9. Branches of the typical intercostal nerves. Reproduced with permission from USRA (www.usra.ca).

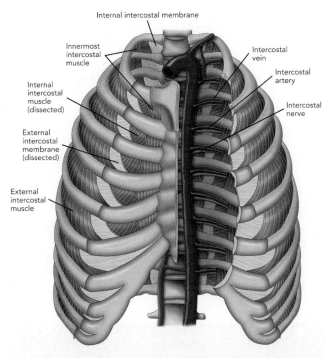

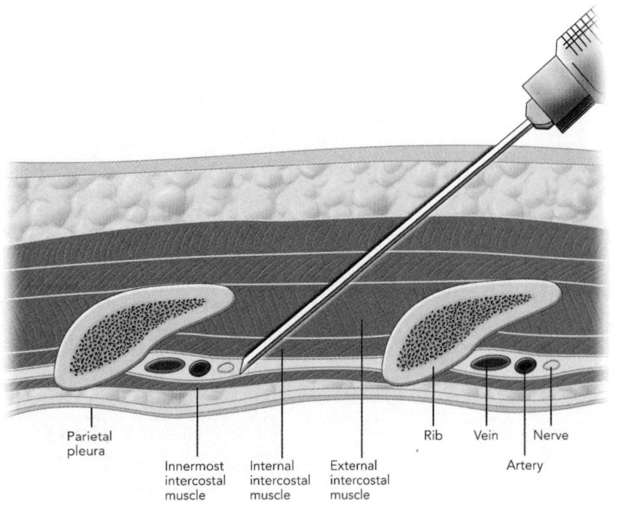

Figure 21.11. Cross section of chest wall showing intercostal muscles and neurovascular bundles. Reproduced with permission from USRA (www.usra.ca).

Figure 21.10. Intercostal muscles in the chest wall. Reproduced with permission from USRA (www.usra.ca).

innervated by the lateral cutaneous nerve are blocked. The needle is angled slight cephalad and walked off the inferior margin of the rib into the subcostal grove, where the needle is advanced 2–3 mm further. The small distance (as little as 0.5 cm) between the rib's inferior margin and the pleura cannot be over-emphasized.[37] The injection is performed after negative aspiration for air and blood but this maneuver cannot reliably prevent pneumothorax and/or hemothorax. The incidence of pneumothorax ranges anywhere from 0.09% to 8.7%.[33,40,41]

The fluoroscopic technique is performed with the patient in prone position. The appropriate rib is identified under fluoroscopic AP view and the needle is introduced in the inferior margin of the rib. Following negative aspiration, a contrast injection is performed to ensure appropriate spread prior to injection.[42] This technique does not theoretically minimize the risk of pneumothorax because the pleura cannot be visualized with fluoroscopy.

The feasibility of US-guided ICN injection has been confirmed in a small cadaver study.[43] A small case series also confirmed the feasibility and technical advantages of US-guided cryoablation of the ICNs in four patients with postthoracotomy pain syndrome.[37]

Ultrasound-Guided Block Technique

With the patient in prone position, a 6–13 MHz linear transducer is placed in the short axis to the ribs so that two consecutive ribs are simultaneously observed. The best site for injection is the angle of the rib (6–7.5 cm from the vertebral spinous process) where the costal groove is at its broadest and deepest and the lateral branch of the ICN has not yet branched.[1] The ribs are easily identified with their typical dorsal shadowing. The key structures in the scan are internal and external intercostal muscles, and the pleura which appears as a prominent hyperechoic line with gliding action during respiration

(Figure 21.12). The intercostal space of interest is located by scanning upwards from the 12th rib. The needle target is the internal intercostal muscle as the innermost internal intercostal is an ill-defined layer of muscle under ultrasonography. A 22 G needle can be inserted either in-plane or out-of-plane to the plane just deep to the internal intercostal muscle or "into" the intercostal muscle. In-plane technique is the authors' preferred technique since it will allow visualization of the needle tip, which needs to be placed 2–3 mm proximal to the pleura.[44] The needle entry site is the upper margin of the rib one level caudal to the targeted ICN. Because of the precision required, and the adverse consequences of advancing the needle too deep (i.e., pneumothorax), it is prudent to inject a small amount of solution upon reaching the external intercostal muscle to confirm needle tip position.[1] The needle is then advanced a few millimeters further into the internal intercostal muscle and the spread of local anesthetic is visualized in real-time as it is injected. If the injectate is seen pushing the external intercostal muscle upward, the needle position is still superficial. Usually, 2 ml of local anesthetic is sufficient to fill the intercostal space, which allows blockade of several ICNs with minimal risk of toxic effects.

Once the ICN block is complete, the probe is used to check for absence of pneumothorax. The ultrasound probe should be placed in the nondependent area. Normally, the pleura appears to glide with respiratory movement. Artifacts presenting as horizontal

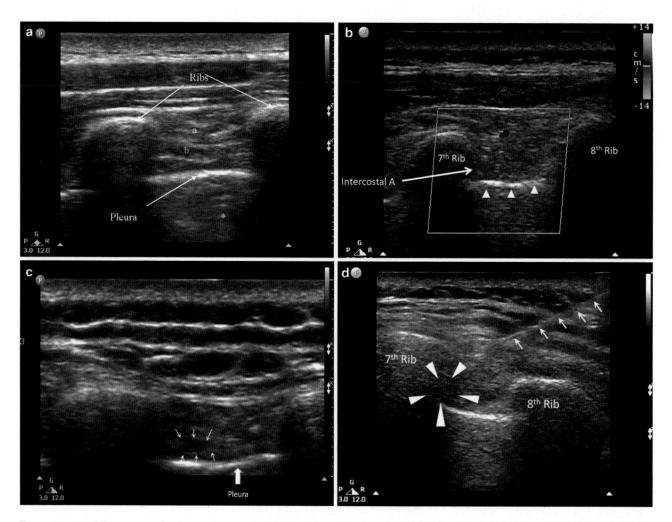

Figure 21.12. Ultrasonographic image showing the intercostal muscles and pleura at the angle of rib. (a) External intercostal muscle; (b) internal intercostal muscle; * reverberation artifact. (b) A similar image taken 2 cm medial to the angle of rib. The intercostal artery is seen in the intercostal space. The pleura, appears as a hyperechoic line, is indicated by the *solid arrow heads*. (c) Ultrasonographic image following injection. The *small arrows* outline the collection of local anesthetic. (d) Intercostal space following injection. The needle is indicated by the *line arrows* and the local anesthetic by the *arrow heads*. Reproduced with permission from USRA (www.usra.ca).

lines parallel to the pleural interface and vertical "comet tails" are also seen. Comet tail artifacts (CTAs) indicate the presence of an intact lung surface. When a pneumothorax is present, the pleura no longer glides with respiration (loss of "gliding sign") and there is a loss of CTAs. Using these signs, the sensitivity and specificity of ultrasound for detecting pneumothorax approaches 100%.[45]

Conclusion

Application of ultrasound in the field of interventional pain management allows the visualization of soft tissues and vessels, which in turn improves the accuracy of the needle placement. Ultrasound in pain management faces many of the same challenges it faced, and continues to face, in the perioperative setting, namely visualization of thin needles, poor image quality in obese patients, and the need to invest time and money in training so that the procedures are effective and safe. However, the benefits to be derived are likely to make ultrasound a very attractive option, and with further research and training, ultrasound may well become a standard of care.

REFERENCES

1. Peng P, Narouze S. Ultrasound-guided interventional procedures in pain medicine: a review of anatomy, sonoanaotmy and procedures. Part I: non-axial structures. *Reg Anesth Pain Med.* 2009;34:458–474.
2. Grossman MG, Ducey SA, Nadler SS, et al. Meralgia paresthetica: diagnosis and treatment. *J Am Acad Orthop Surg.* 2001;9:336–344.
3. Hurdle MF, Weingarten TN, Crisostomo RA, et al. Ultrasound-guided blockade of the lateral femoral cutaneous nerve: technical description and review of 10 cases. *Arch Phys Med Rehabil.* 2007;88:1362–1364.
4. van Slobbe AM, Bohnen AM, Bernsen RM, Koes BW, Bierma-Zeinstra SM. Incidence rates and determinants in meralgia paresthetica in general practice. *J Neurol.* 2004;251:294–297.
5. de Ridder VA, de Lange S, Popta J. Anatomical variations of the lateral femoral cutaneous nerve and the consequences for surgery. *J Orthop Trauma.* 1999;13:207–211.
6. Grothaus MC, Holt M, Mekhail AO, et al. Lateral femoral cutaneous nerve: an anatomic study. *Clin Orthop Relat Res.* 2005;437:164–168.
7. Murata Y, Takahashi K, Yamagata M, et al. The anatomy of the lateral femoral cutaneous nerve, with special reference to the harvesting of iliac bone graft. *J Bone Joint Surg Am.* 2000;82: 746–747.
8. Dias Filho LC, Valença MM, Guimarães Filho FAV, et al. Lateral femoral cutaneous neuralgia: an anatomical insight. *Clin Anat.* 2003;16:309–316.
9. Hospodar PP, Ashman ES, Traub JA. Anatomic study of the lateral femoral cutaneous nerve with respect to the ilioinguinal surgical dissection. *J Orthop Trauma.* 1999;13:17–19.
10. Ropars M, Morandi X, Huten D, et al. Anatomical study of the lateral femoral cutaneous nerve with special reference to minimally invasive anterior approach for total hip replacement. *Surg Radiol Anat.* 2009;31:199–204.
11. Gray H. *Anatomy of the Human Body.* Philadelphia: Lea & Febiger; 1918. Bartleby.com, 2000. <www.bartleby.com/107/212.html>. Accessed 16.12.09.
12. Shannon J, Lang SA, Yip RW. Lateral femoral cutaneous nerve block revisited: a nerve stimulator technique. *Reg Anesth.* 1995;20:100–104.
13. Ng I, Vaghadia H, Choi P, et al. Ultrasound imaging accurately identifies the lateral femoral cutaneous nerve. *Anesth Analg.* 2008;107:1070–1074.
14. Damarey B, Demondion X, Boutry N, et al. Sonographic assessment of the lateral femoral cutaneous nerve. *J Clin Ultrasound.* 2009;37:89–95.
15. Tumber PS, Bhatia A, Chan V. Ultrasound-guided lateral femoral cutaneous nerve block for meralgia paresthetica. *Anesth Analg.* 2008;106:1021–1022.
16. Bodner G, Bernathova M, Galiano K, et al. Ultrasound of the lateral femoral cutaneous nerve. Normal findings in a cadaver and in volunteers. *Reg Anesth Pain Med.* 2009;34:265–268.

17. Wertheim HM, Rovenstine EA. Suprascapular nerve block. *Anesthesiology*. 1941;2:541–545.

18. Ritchie ED, Tong D, Chung F, et al. Suprascapular nerve block for postoperative pain relief in arthroscopic shoulder surgery: a new modality? *Anesth Analg*. 1997;84:1306–1312.

19. Wassef MR. Suprascapular nerve block. A new approach for the management of frozen shoulder. *Anaesthesia*. 1992;47:120–124.

20. Karatas GK, Meray J. Suprascapular nerve block for pain relief in adhesive capsulitis: comparison of 2 different techniques. *Arch Phys Med Rehabil*. 2002;83:593–597.

21. Gofeld M. Ultrasonography in pain medicine: a critical review. *Pain Pract*. 2008;8:226–240.

22. Harmon D, Hearty C. Ultrasound-guided suprascapular nerve block technique. *Pain Physician*. 2007;10:743–746.

23. Yucesoy C, Akkaya T, Ozel O, et al. Ultrasonographic evaluation and morphometric measurements of the suprascapular notch. *Surg Radiol Anat*. 2009;31:409–414.

24. Natsis K, Totlis T, Tsikaras P, et al. Proposal for classification of the suprascapular notch: a study on 423 dried scapulas. *Clin Anat*. 2007;20:135–139.

25. Tubbs RS, Smyth MD, Salter G, et al. Anomalous traversement of the suprascapular artery through the suprascapular notch: a possible mechanism for undiagnosed should pain? *Med Sci Monit*. 2003;9:116–119.

26. Brown DE, James DC, Roy S. Pain relief by suprascapular nerve block in gleno-humeral arthritis. *Scand J Rheumatol*. 1988;17:411–415.

27. Feigl GC, Anderhuber F, Dorn C, et al. Modified lateral block of the suprascapular nerve: a safe approach and how much to inject? A morphological study. *Reg Anesth Pain Med*. 2007;32:488–494.

28. Moore DC. Block of the suprascapular nerve. In: Thomas CC, ed. *Regional Nerve Block*. Springfield, MA: Charles C. Thomas; 1979:300–303.

29. Dangoisse MJ, Wilson DJ, Glynn CJ. MRI and clinical study of an easy and safe technique of suprascapular nerve blockade. *Acta Anaesthesiol Belg*. 1994;45:49–54.

30. Schneider-Kolsky ME, Pike J, Connell DA. CT-guided suprascapular nerve blocks: a pilot study. *Skeletal Radiol*. 2004;33:277–282.

31. Peng P, Wiley MJ, Liang J, et al. Ultrasound-guided suprascapular nerve block: a correlation with fluoroscopic and cadaveric findings. *Can J Anaesth*. 2010;57:143–148.

32. Moore DC, Bridenbaugh LD. Intercostal nerve block in 4333 patients: indications, technique and complications. *Anesth Analg*. 1962;41:1–10.

33. Karmakar MK, Ho AMH. Acute pain management of patients with multiple fractured ribs. *J Trauma*. 2003;54:612–615.

34. Kopacz DJ, Thompson GE. Intercostal blocks for thoracic and abdominal surgery. *Tech Reg Anesth Pain Manag*. 1998;2:25–29.

35. Green CR, de Rosayro M, Tait AR. The role of cryoanalgesia for chronic thoracic pain: results of a long-term follow up. *J Natl Med Assoc*. 2002;94:716–720.

36. Byas-Smith MG, Gulati A. Ultrasound-guided intercostal nerve cryoablation. *Anesth Analg*. 2006;103:1033–1035.

37. Gray H. *Anatomy of the Human Body*. Philadelphia: Lea & Febiger; 1918. Bartleby.com, 2000. <www.bartleby.com/107/211.html>. Accessed 16.12.2009.

37. Moore DC. Anatomy of the intercostal nerve: its importance during thoracic surgery. *Am J Surg*. 1982;144:371–373.

39. Knowles P, Hancox D, Letheren M, et al. An evaluation of intercostal nerve blockade for analgesia following renal transplantation. *Eur J Anaesthesiol*. 1998;15:457–461.

40. Shanti CM, Carlin AM, Tyburski JG. Incidence of pneumothorax from intercostal nerve block for analgesia in rib fractures. *J Trauma*. 2001;51:536–539.

41. Cohen SP, Sireci A, Wu CL, Larkin TM, Williams KA, Hurley RW. Pulsed radiofrequency of the dorsal root ganglia is superior to pharmacotherapy or pulsed radiofrequency of the intercostal nerves in the treatment of chronic postsurgical thoracic pain. *Pain Physician*. 2006;9:227–235.

42. Bhatia A, Gofeld M, Ganapathy S, et al. A comparison of surface landmark technique and ultrasound-guided injection of intercostal nerves in cadavers. *Presented as an abstract at Shield's Day, University of Toronto, May 2009*.

43. Curatolo M, Eichenberger U. Ultrasound-guided blocks for the treatment of chronic pain. *Tech Reg Anesth Pain Manag*. 2007;11:95–102.

44. Reissig A, Kroegel C. Accuracy of transthoracic sonography in excluding post-interventional pneumothorax and hydropneumothorax: comparison to chest radiography. *Eur J Radiol*. 2005;53:463–470.

V

Musculoskeletal (MSK) Ultrasound

22

Ultrasound-Guided Shoulder Joint and Bursa Injections

Michael P. Schaefer and Kermit Fox

M.P. Schaefer (✉)
Case Western Reserve University, Metro Health Rehabilitation Institute of Ohio,
2500 Metro Health Dr, Cleveland, OH 44109, USA
e-mail: mschaefer@metrohealth.org

S.N. Narouze (ed.), *Atlas of Ultrasound-Guided Procedures in Interventional Pain Management*,
DOI 10.1007/978-1-4419-1681-5_22, © Springer Science+Business Media, LLC 2011

Introduction

Shoulder pain is commonly encountered in pain management practices. Although the rotator cuff and the subacromial structures are thought to contribute to the majority of shoulder pain presentations, there are a number of other structures that generate pain. Fortunately, all these structures are easily accessible with office-based procedures, and injections are useful to confirm the diagnosis and provide analgesia.

Ultrasound (US) is particularly suited for addressing shoulder problems. The majority of pain-generating shoulder structures can be visualized with basic US equipment. In particular, the superficial tendons such as long-head biceps, supraspinatus, and infraspinatus show excellent echogenicity and structural resolution.[1] Ultrasound permits visualization of soft tissue adjacent to orthopedic hardware, such as total shoulder arthroplasty components.[1,2] It also gives the clinician the ability to do dynamic assessment of the joint under real-time sonographic imaging.[3] Occult clefts or tendon subluxation may become evident with sonographic assessment during joint motion.[2]

Injections of the shoulder must be directed by clinical history, examination, and other imaging modalities. Although US is excellent for imaging the soft tissues, it provides little information about interosseous structures and those shielded by bone. Therefore, plain-film imaging is essential for any suspicion of intra-articular pathology (i.e., degenerative joint disease) or osseous pathology such as fractures or bony metastasis. Likewise, sonographic assessment of ligamentous or cartilaginous structures such as the glenoid labrum is very challenging, particularly in large-shouldered patients. Therefore, MRI scanning should be utilized in any case with suspected sinister pathology. In cases with a suspicion for labral tear (posttraumatic or dislocation/subluxation), MRI with intra-articular gadolinium is recommended.[4,5]

Patient safety concerns are minimal for US-guided shoulder injections. Direct complications of shoulder joint injections are extremely rare, although caution should be taken to avoid neurovascular structures, particularly with injections in the anterior shoulder region. The pleura may be at risk for deep injections in the superior shoulder. Finally, injection directly into tendon tissue should be avoided, due to suspected risk of rupture.[6–10] Fortunately, ultrasound allows continuous visualization of the needle tip, which minimizes risk of inadvertent tendon injection, and assists the clinician in avoiding neurovascular structures.[1,2,11,12] With any injection into a joint or bursa, particular care should be taken to avoid infection. In our current practice, we use a sterile transducer cover on every patient, with iodine gel as the conduction medium between the transducer cover and the skin. We also use sterile gel inside the cover because of two occasions (during resident training), where the needle was accidentally placed through the transducer cover and then into the skin. Most manufacturers will caution against the use of alcohol or iodine/betadine containing products against the transducer due to risk of damage or discoloration. In cases of iodine allergy, we use sterile gel as the conduction medium after skin preparation with chlorhexidine. We also use sterile technique with an operative drape on every patient. Although it is possible to direct a sterile needle under an uncovered probe, we do not recommend this technique, as inadvertent patient movement can easily contaminate the needle and field. In addition, keeping a sterile field allows the clinician to freely adjust transducer position, perform multiple needle passes, and to change the approach if unexpected findings are encountered.

Chapter 23 describes the most common shoulder joint injections with sonographic guidance. As in other regions, appropriate sonographic assessment is essential for the guidance of the needle. Major sonographic landmarks and associated pathology will be demonstrated. Transducer placement and needle approaches will be described according to the preferences of the authors, keeping in mind that there are multiple effective approaches for most joints. Finally, and most importantly, the patient's symptoms and a physical examination must be followed to direct these interventions. Although a complete review of shoulder assessment is outside the scope of this chapter, we have included a brief description of clinical presentation and physical examination findings for each of the syndromes described.

Subacromial/Subdeltoid Bursa

The subacromial bursa is the most commonly injected structure in the shoulder. Indications include rotator cuff pathology, impingement syndrome, and subacromial bursitis. Subacromial injection of lidocaine is often used to diagnose impingement and offers rationale for subacromial decompression surgery.

Anatomy

The subacromial and subdeltoid bursa typically communicate and effectively function as one bursa.[13] The distal aspect of bursa sits on the upper surface of the supraspinatus muscle, immediately under the deep surface of the deltoid. The bursa functions to protect the supraspinatus as it passes beneath the overlying structures, most notably the acromion process.

Clinical Presentation

Shoulder abduction and internal rotation can potentially impinge the bursa between the humeral head (greater tubercle) and the arch of the acromion and coracoacromial ligament. This action is reproduced clinically with the Neer and Hawkins–Kennedy impingement tests.[14] In a positive test, pain is reproduced when the humerus is passively elevated (Neer: full flexion in scapular plane with arm internally rotated. Hawkins: flexion to 90 in. in forward plane with arm neutral and elbow bent 90 in. followed by passive internal rotation of the humerus). Impingement can be present with either subacromial bursitis or rotator cuff tendinopathy. However, rotator cuff tendinopathy will typically be more painful with active abduction even within a short arc, while bursitis will be more painful in "impingement" positions, and may not be provoked with active abduction below 90°.

Limitations of the Blind Approach

Despite being the largest bursa in the body,[13] the accuracy of blind injections has been reported to be as low as 29%,[15] suggesting a high occurrence of false-negative injections. Erroneous placement of the needle in the deltoid muscle, glenohumeral joint, or directly into the cuff tendons has been described.[16] Other studies report accuracy as high as 70%[17,18] and 83%.[16] Studies have compared the various approaches to the subacromial bursa,[18,19] and currently, there is no universal consensus on which approach is superior.

Ultrasound-Guided Technique

Ultrasound imaging of the subacromial bursa typically starts with the transducer oriented in the coronal/scapular plane and positioned just over the tip of the acromion (Figure 22.1a). The supraspinatus tendon should be visualized emerging from beneath the acromion and

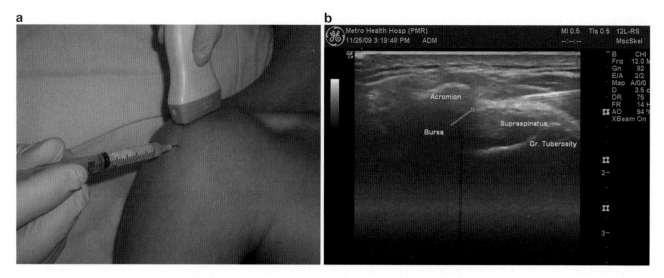

Figure 22.1. Subacromial/subdeltoid bursa. (**a**) Transducer positioned over the lateral tip of the acromion and supraspinatus tendon, with needle insertion toward the lateral subacromial space. (**b**) Needle approaching subacromial bursa. *Asterisk* indicates ideal end position of needle tip within the subacromial bursa.

running over the humerus to attach to the greater tuberosity (Figure 22.1b). The tendon is hyperechoic when appropriately aligned with the transducer. If the transducer is rocked in a heel–toe motion, the tendon fibrils become less visible (the phenomenon known as "anisotropy"), which may falsely give the appearance of tendon disruption.[20] The bursa is seen as a thin anechoic fluid layer immediately above the tendon (as shown in Figure 22.1b), or it may be very thin with intermediate echogenicity. In active bursitis, it may appear thickened relative to the contralateral side. Dynamic assessment may be helpful to visualize the tendon sliding smoothly under the acromion. With gentle active or passive abduction, a "catch" or snap may be appreciated in the presence of mechanical impingement. Dynamic assessment may also reveal clefts in the tendon, which indicate partial or full thickness tears. In the event of a large full thickness tear, the tendon may be absent, atrophic, or retracted. In this instance, an injection in the bursa will communicate directly with the glenohumeral space.[20]

The sonographer should also make note of calcific densities or clefts within the tendon, which may indicate tendinopathy or tear. Aspiration and lavage of these calcifications under ultrasound guidance has been reported.[21] Ultrasound has been found to be as effective as fluoroscopic guidance for localization of calcifications, and ultrasound can provide a measure of insight into deposit density, which may carry prognostic value.[21]

Injection of the subacromial bursa is performed with the patient in the seated position with the arm hanging at their side (Figure 22.1a). This allows the joint to be pulled open by the weight of the shoulder. Gentle downward traction on the arm may assist in opening the joint space, and the patient should be reminded to relax the shoulder. Alternatively, the patient's arm may be placed in the Crass position, with the elbow flexed to 90°, arm supinated and the palm of the hand placed over the ipsilateral hip (as if hand was being placed in the back pocket of pants). The transducer remains in the coronal plane and the needle is advanced in long axis starting approximately 1 cm lateral to the end of the transducer, maintaining an anterior path between the lateral border of the acromion and the greater tuberosity of the humerus. The needle angle should be adjusted to allow bursal entry just lateral to the acromion (Figure 22.1a), but bursa entry more distally will typically communicate with the proximal bursa. In very large shoulders, a spinal needle may be necessary, although a 1.5 in. needle is usually sufficient. We typically use a mixture of 1 ml triamcinolone (40 mg/ml) and 2 ml of local anesthetic. Ideally, the injectate is visualized distending the entire bursa with real-time sonography. Fluid may be seen running under the acromion or distally under the deltoid. The diagnosis of impingement or so-called "impingement test" is confirmed when the patient is reassessed after approximately 15 min and examination shows reduction in pain with the impingement maneuvers.

Biceps Tendon Sheath (Biceps – Long Head)

Anatomy

The long head of the biceps tendon originates at the supraglenoid tubercle of the glenoid labrum and crosses the humerus anteriorly. The head of the humerus has two anterior prominences or tubercles, the lesser tubercle being medial to the greater tubercle. The intertubercular groove runs between the tubercles and houses the bicipital tendon (long head), and is covered by the intertubercular ligament (including extensions of the fibers of the subscapularis muscle). The short head of the biceps originates on the coracoid process in conjunction with the tendon of the coracobrachialis (conjoint tendon). The tendon sheath of the long-head tendon communicates proximally with the glenohumeral joint. Therefore injection of the sheath may fill upward into the joint, especially if large volumes of injectate are used. Likewise, glenohumeral joint fluid may flow distally along the tendon in the setting of shoulder joint effusion.

Clinical Presentation

The long head is the most commonly injured portion of the muscle, and tears of the long head usually occur at the proximal end. Biceps tendon tears can be transverse or longitudinal (split), and may also include tearing or fraying of the anterior/superior labrum or "SLAP lesion". Complete rupture of the long head gives the "Popeye" arm appearance with a balled up muscle in the distal arm. Bicipital tendinopathy typically presents with pain in the anterior shoulder that is increased with active flexion or passive extension of the limb. The "Speed" test (active forward flexion of the arm with the palm up) typically reproduces the patient's pain. However, rotator cuff pathology will usually be painful with this maneuver also, and the patient should be asked to localize symptoms as precisely as possible. Tenderness to palpation directly over the bicipital groove is often present, although in large shoulders localization may be difficult. Sonographically-assisted palpation is often helpful to localize the area of greatest tenderness.

Ultrasound-Guided Technique

The long head is first visualized sonographically in cross section with a linear transducer held in the transverse plane directly over the anterior shoulder (Figure 22.2a). The tendon and sheath can then be imaged longitudinally by rotating the probe into the sagittal plane. In this view, the lesser and greater tuberosities are seen "popping up" on either side of the bicipital groove as the transducer is slowly passed from medial to lateral, respectively. With tendon pathology or glenohumeral joint effusion, the tendon sheath will be filled with synovial fluid. If it is nondistended, the sheath may offer less than 2 mm clearance to place a needle.[3]

Injection of the bicipital groove can be performed in the short-axis (transverse or out of plane) approach or the longitudinal approach. The short-axis approach is more common and technically easier but does not allow for visualization of the entire length of the needle. After appropriate setup, the medial side of the bicipital groove is placed in the center of the field of view, and the needle is inserted in the midline of the transducer (Figure 22.2a). The target is the small space between the tendon and the lesser tuberosity of the humerus, just medial to the tendon (Figure 22.2b). The needle should be directed deep enough (at minimum) to be through the intertubercular ligament, and typically is advanced all the way down to contact bone on the floor or medial wall of the groove. Injecting directly over or against the tendon should be avoided with the short-axis approach, as the position of the needle tip may sometimes be in question, and injection of steroid directly into the tendon may lead to rupture.[6–10] Injection on the lateral aspect of the groove is equally effective as the medial side, but caution should be taken to avoid the ascending branch of the circumflex humeral artery which typically runs up the lateral side

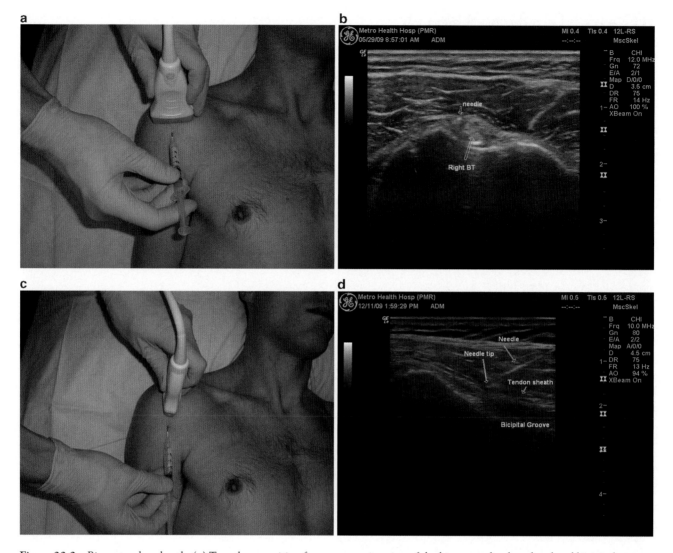

Figure 22.2. Biceps tendon sheath. (**a**) Transducer position for transverse imaging of the biceps tendon long head and bicipital groove, and needle insertion just medial to the tendon. (**b**) Transverse image showing the needle tip just medial to the tendon, deep to the intertubercular ligament. (**c**) Transducer position for longitudinal approach. (**d**) Longitudinal view showing the needle approaching the distal aspect of the bicipital groove, directed from distal to proximal (just medial to tendon).

of the groove, and may be difficult to see due to its small size. If available, power Doppler imaging should be utilized to visualize this structure.

Alternatively, the needle may be advanced in the longitudinal or "in plane" approach, with the tendon visualized along the entire field of view (Figure 22.2c, d). This approach may be more appropriate for aspiration of the fluid in the sheath, but in our experience this is rarely clinically necessary. With either approach, the injection is typically completed with a volume of 0.5 ml triamcinolone (40 mg/ml) and 1 ml of local anesthetic. The injectate should be visualized flowing along and around the tendon.

Acromio-Clavicular Joint

Anatomy

The acromio-clavicular or "AC" joint is formed by the articulation of the distal end of the clavicle and the acromion process of the scapula. It is easily palpable by following the clavicle distally until small osteophytes are encountered at the joint margin or a bony step-off is palpated at the joint. In cases of shoulder separation, the step-off may be pronounced, and the clavicle may be high-riding due to tearing of the coracoclavicular ligaments. While this joint may seem easy to localize because of its superficial position, it is often narrowed or shielded by osteophytes. Thus, ultrasound guidance is very helpful. The subacromial bursa and supraspinatus tendon lie directly beneath the joint, often predisposing them to damage from inferiorly-directed osteophytes (or needles placed inadvertently through this very small joint).

Clinical Presentation

AC joint pain typically presents with superior shoulder pain and tenderness directly over the joint. Pain is reproduced with active elevation of the arm (e.g., changing a light bulb), or with the "scarf" test, where the humerus is passively positioned in crossed-arm adduction (as if throwing a scarf over the contralateral shoulder). Patients who have suffered a shoulder separation, or those that do repetitive upper limb movements, particularly overhead, are prone to AC joint pain. Athletes who do excessive overhead weight-lifting are prone to osteolysis of the distal clavicle, which may present very similarly, but will not show on ultrasound imaging, and should not be treated with steroid injection.

Ultrasound-Guided Technique

The AC joint is visualized by placing a linear transducer in line with the clavicle and following the clavicle distally until the joint is seen (Figure 22.3a). The appearance is typically a "V" shape (Figure 22.3b), with the clavicle often projecting superficially compared to the acromion (Figure 22.3c). The joint is covered by a thin capsule (acromio-clavicular ligament), and may be distended if effusion is present. A small hyperechoic fibrocartilaginous disk can sometimes be visualized within the joint space. There are no significant vascular or neural structures to consider in this injection, but the skin is often thin and friable over the AC joint, so care should be taken not to deposit steroids superficially above the joint.

The patient is best positioned for injection in the seated position with the arm hanging at their side. This allows the joint to be pulled open by the weight of the shoulder. Gentle downward traction on the arm may be helpful to open the joint space, but is usually not needed with appropriate sonographic guidance. For accurate needle placement, the "V" of the joint should be positioned precisely in the middle of the image, and then the needle is inserted in short-axis orientation, just adjacent to the midline of the transducer from either the anterior or posterior side of the transducer. The needle is directed underneath the transducer so that the tip of the needle is visualized as a bright "dot" as it enters the field of view. Depth is then adjusted by the "walk-down" technique to position the needle tip deep to the capsule, typically, directly between the articulating bony surfaces. Care should be taken to avoid passing the needle completely through the joint, so it is acceptable to position the needle against either wall of the joint. The joint is often completely distended by a very small volume of injectate, so the smallest possible mixture should be used, particularly if the injection is meant for diagnostic purposes. We typically use a mixture of 0.25 ml triamcinolone (40 mg/ml) and 0.75 ml of local anesthetic.

Glenohumeral Joint

Anatomy

The glenohumeral joint or "true shoulder joint" is formed by an articulation between the proximal humeral head and the glenoid cavity. While the true articulation surface is small and shallow, the joint surface area is greatly increased by the presence of the cartilaginous glenoid labrum. The joint is surrounded by a thin fibrous articular capsule, and while

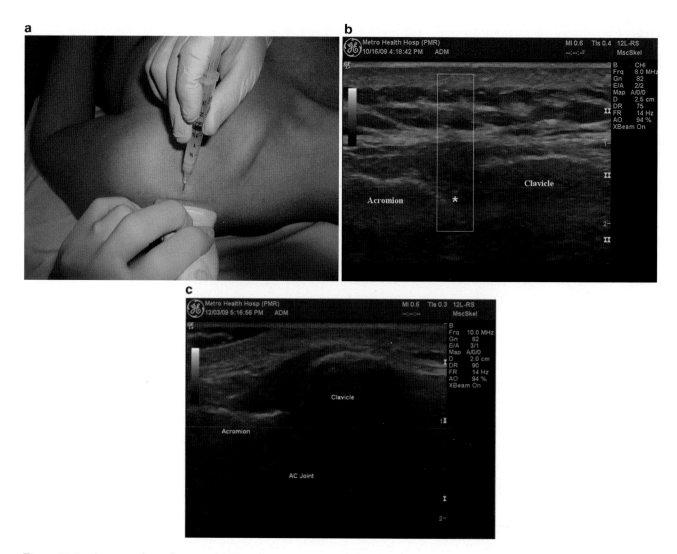

Figure 22.3. Acromio-clavicular joint. (**a**) Transducer position parallel to the clavicle spanning across the joint with needle insertion at midline of the transducer. (**b**) Transverse image of AC joint showing the needle shadow and tissue displacement (*open rectangle*) with needle tip just above *asterisk*. (**c**) High-riding clavicle.

strengthened by three glenohumeral ligaments, it remains relatively weak. This allows for a large range of motion at the cost of joint stability. As described under biceps injection above, it should be noted that the joint synovium also extends down the bicipital sheath into the intertubercular groove. Occasionally, the joint capsule also communicates with a subscapular bursa lying on the anterior surface of the scapula.

Glenohumeral joint entry is most commonly performed for injection of degenerative joint disease and adhesive capsulitis.[22] Injections may also be useful for articular-sided rotator cuff disease and labral pathology. When effusion is present, aspiration is also very helpful to exclude septic, autoimmune, or crystalline disease of the joint. In many cases, effusion is small and ultrasound guidance is essential for appropriate localization. Also, periarticular ganglia can often be diagnosed and aspirated with ultrasound guidance.[2]

Clinical Presentation

Glenohumeral pathology typically presents with painful and restricted range of motion of the joint. The most reliable finding is reduced external rotation with the arm held at the patient's side, whereas in other shoulder pathologies, the external rotation range of motion is preserved. As with other shoulder pathology, external rotation is nonpainful or minimally painful. It is also very common for glenohumeral disorders to mimic cervical radiculopathy, with referred pain and paresthesias down the entire upper limb, even into the digits. In these cases, the Spurling maneuver (neck extension and ipsilateral head rotation toward the affected side) will not change the patient's pain, while glenohumeral motion will worsen the pain.[14] Glenohumeral pathology often coexists with rotator cuff and biceps pathology, but the pain from the glenohumeral joint typically makes isolation of other coexisting entities clinically difficult.

Limitations of the Blind Approach

As with subacromial bursa injections, studies have shown poor accuracy for blind injections of the glenohumeral joint. Sethi et al reported 26.8% accuracy using an anterior approach.[22] Eustace et al reported success in 10 of 24 shoulder injections (42%), and Jones et al reported success in 2 of 20 (10%) attempted injections, though the approach was not disclosed in either study.[15,23] In contrast, Rutten reported a first attempt success of 94% using ultrasound to guide glenohumeral joint injections.[24] In the same study, Rutten also noted having similar success with the anterior (24 of 25) and posterior (23 of 25) approaches.

Ultrasound-Guided Technique

The glenohumeral joint is visualized by a posterior view with the transducer just caudal and parallel to the spine of the scapula (Figure 22.4a). The circular humeral head is seen abutting the glenoid fossa with the less-echogenic triangular-shaped labrum between them (Figure 22.4b). Gentle rotation of the joint will demonstrate the humeral head rolling on the glenoid and labrum. For very large shoulders, a curvilinear probe with a lower frequency (5–6 MHz) may be necessary. A deeper beam focus and lower frequency is always used relative to other shoulder structures.

Injection of the joint is performed via a posterior approach with the humerus adducted across the thorax, thus opening the posterior joint space (Figure 22.4a). It is also very helpful to ask the patient to retract the scapula (i.e., sit or lie with shoulder pulled back in good posture). The transducer is placed as described above, and the needle is inserted in long-axis approach, approximately 2 cm lateral to the lateral heel of the transducer. This lateral entry permits a more shallow-angle approach and facilitates visualization of the entire shaft of the needle (Figure 22.4b). The target is the space between the glenoid labrum and the humeral head. If the labrum is not well visualized, the needle should be directed toward the humeral head to avoid piercing the labrum or deflecting off the glenoid and away from the joint. Depending upon shoulder size, a 3- or 4-in. (7.5–10 cm) needle is often needed to reach the necessary depth. For larger shoulders, a steeper approach angle may also be required. We have found it helpful to bend the tip of the needle approximately 30°. This facilitates walking of the needle off the posterior aspect of the humeral head. The bent needle is then rotated so that the tip points anteriorly (toward the glenoid) and the needle follows the contour of the humeral head until it lodges deep into the joint. Typically, 1 ml of triamcinolone (40 mg/ml) and 2–5 ml of local anesthetic are injected. Injectate is seen distending the joint capsule, but *not* flowing extra-articularly or dorsally. Resistance to injection suggests that the needle is embedded into cartilage, and very slight retraction of the needle (with steady pressure on the plunger) will allow free flow of injectate into the joint.

The Rotator Interval Approach

Anterior visualization of the glenohumeral joint is difficult with most portable equipment, due to increased depth and overlying dense structures. This approach, however, may be worthwhile in patients with joint effusions that present with anterior swelling, or in patients with altered anatomy, positioning limitations, or habitus that prohibits posterior joint visualization. For anterior joint entry, the authors recommend a "Rotator Interval approach". The rotator interval is a triangular space bordered by the corocoid process, the anterior-most

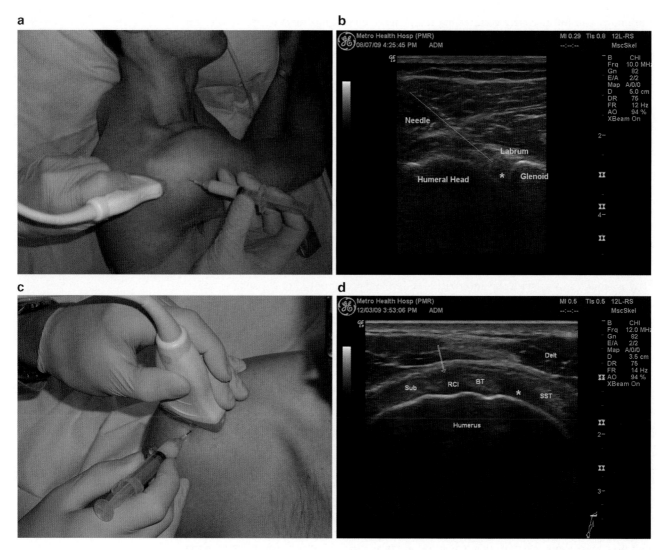

Figure 22.4. Glenohumeral Joint. (**a**) Transducer positioned on the posterior shoulder, just beneath the spine of the scapula with the arm adducted. (**b**) Longitudinal needle insertion behind the humeral head (*above line*), entering the posterior joint just under the glenoid labrum. *Asterisk* indicates ideal position of needle tip. (**c**) Transducer position for anterior joint entry through the "rotator interval". (**d**) Rotator interval (RCI) with desired needle position (*arrow*) between the biceps tendon and subscapularis (Sub) tendon. Alternative position indicated by *asterisk* between *SST* supraspinatus tendon and biceps tendon. *Delt* deltoid.

portion of the supraspinatus and the superior border of the subscapularis tendon. Contained within this triangular space are the biceps tendon, glenohumeral capsule, coracohumeral ligament, and glenohumeral ligament. Recently, Lim et al reported injecting the GHJ through the rotator interval using ultrasound guidance with good results.[25]

The rotator interval injection is performed with the arm resting at patient's side and the shoulder placed in slight external rotation. The transducer is positioned in the transverse plane on the superior/anterior shoulder just cranial to the greater and lesser tuberosities of the humerus (Figure 22.4c). This position can be found by following the biceps (long head) tendon proximally above the bicipital groove. The transducer is positioned to visualize the intra-articular course of the biceps tendon between the supraspinatus and subscapularis tendons (Figure 22.4d). The superior glenohumeral ligament may be visualized between the biceps and subscapularis tendons, whereas the coracohumeral ligament is between the biceps and supraspinatus tendons. The injection is performed after the needle is advanced into the rotator interval between the biceps tendon and the subscapularis tendon (indicated as arrow in Figure 22.4d). Alternatively, the needle may be placed between the biceps tendon and the supraspinatus tendon ("asterisk" in Figure 22.4d). Real-time visualization should show fluid dispersing freely along the humerus, and *not* down the bicipital sheath or anteriorly away from the space. Resistance to injection may indicate that the needle tip has entered a tendon or ligament. Injecting into the rotator interval may be advantageous in very large shoulders. This approach (relative to an injection in the middle of the anterior joint) also avoids many anterior structures such as the subcoracoid bursa, subscapularis muscle and tendon, and the inferior glenohumeral ligament. Furthermore, the needle avoids the anterosuperior labrum by staying lateral to the joint space.

Subscapularis Tendon/Subscapularis Bursa

Anatomy

The subscapularis muscle originates from the subscapular fossa of the scapula and inserts on the lesser tuberosity of the humerus in the anterior shoulder. Some of its fibers continue across the bicipital groove to attach to the greater tuberosity, thereby forming the roof of the bicipital groove. The subscapularis is the only rotator cuff muscle that acts to internally rotate the shoulder. The subscapularis bursa lies deep to the tendon against the neck of the scapula. The bursa usually communicates with the shoulder joint; therefore, it may be distended in the presence of shoulder joint effusion. However, the bursa may be swollen or inflamed in isolation. Occasionally, ganglion cysts or cartilaginous loose bodies are found in this region.

Clinical Presentation

Subscapularis tendinopathy usually presents with pain in the anterior shoulder and is provoked with active internal rotation or passive external rotation of the shoulder. However, this syndrome is relatively rare and usually does not occur in isolation. Therefore, it is more common for patients to present with diffuse shoulder pain and impingement signs along with localized pain in the region of the subscapularis tendon and bursa.

On physical examination, the patient may have increased tenderness deep in the anterior shoulder just inferior and lateral to the coracoid process. Keep in mind that even normal, asymptomatic patients are tender in this region; so contralateral comparison is essential. Shoulder range of motion is usually preserved. Passive external motion (with the arm at the patient's side) will stretch the tendon across the anterior shoulder to facilitate palpation, but the deep location of the tendon makes it difficult to palpate. Rarely, a snapping sound or mechanical clunk is detected in this region, which may signify impingement of the subscapularis bursa, a subluxing biceps tendon, a glenoid labral tear, or a loose body in the joint.

Strength of the subscapularis is assessed with the "Lift off test."[14] The examiner places the affected hand behind the patient's back (at the level of the waist) with the palm facing posteriorly. Then the patient is asked to lift the hand off the back by internally rotating. Lack of ability to lift the hand indicates subscapularis weakness, tendon rupture, or inadequate range of motion. Pain with this motion is common, so the patient should be asked to precisely localize the painful region.

Ultrasound-Guided Technique

Imaging of the subscapularis usually starts with localization of the bicipital groove (see above section on Biceps tendon sheath). A linear transducer is held in the transverse position relative to the humerus and bicipital groove (Figure 22.5a), and the subscapularis is seen traveling from its deep, medially located muscle belly to attach to the lesser tuberosity. External rotation will pull the tendon across the field of view, and the distal muscular tissue will be seen surrounding the tendon. When the probe is rotated 90° to show the musculotendinous junction, multiple tendon fascicles are seen within the muscle belly,

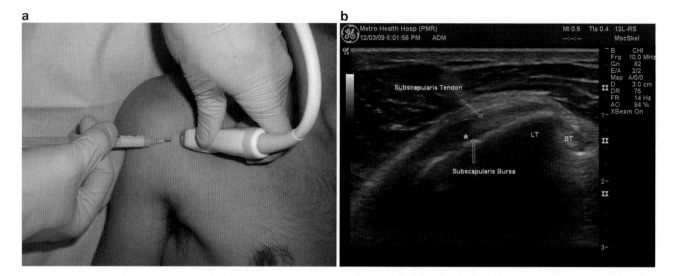

Figure 22.5. Subscapularis tendon/bursa. (**a**) Transducer positioned longitudinal to the tendon over the anterior shoulder. (**b**) Ultrasound image shows the humerus in external rotation with tendon, underlying bursa, and desired needle tip position indicated by *asterisk*.

coalescing laterally into the tendon just prior to insertion. The subscapularis bursa may be seen between the tendon and the scapular neck, and in distended shoulder joints the bursa is commonly seen communicating with the anterior glenohumeral joint.

The tendon and bursa injection can be performed in either the short-axis (transverse or "out of plane") approach or the longitudinal approach. In the longitudinal approach, a lateral starting position is preferred to avoid the pectoralis muscles and deep neurovascular structures of the axilla. To facilitate visualization and entry, the shoulder should be gently externally rotated (approximately 45°). For the tendon sheath injection, the needle should stop just short of the tendon, with the injectate deposited just anterior to it (indicated as "*asterisk*" in Figure 22.5b). The bursa is reached by advancing the needle through the tendon, at which time a subtle "pop" or give-way is detected. (We typically use a mixture of 0.5 ml triamcinolone (40 mg/ml) and 1 ml of local anesthetic.) When a larger volume is injected in this region, the bursa may be seen distending, or the injectate may flow directly into the glenohumeral joint.

Sternoclavicular Joint

Anatomy

The sternoclavicular or "SC" joint is formed by the articulation of the proximal end of the clavicle with the clavicular fossa in the superior lateral aspect of the sternum. It is easily palpable by following the clavicle proximally where its medial end is usually positioned just anterior to the sternum. With scapular retraction (asking the patient to pull their shoulders back and chest out), the end of the clavicle becomes more prominent, while with protraction (or hunching forward), the clavicle protrudes less. In cases of SC dislocation, the entire end of the clavicle may project anterior and medial to the border of the sternum. The great vessels of the chest and the pleura lie deep to the joint, so care is needed to avoid excessive penetration of the needle.

Clinical Presentation

SC joint pain typically presents with chest wall pain, swelling, and tenderness directly over the joint. Crepitation or subluxation in this region is very common and is not considered pathological unless accompanied by pain or swelling. Pain is reproduced with scapular protraction/retraction, arm elevation, or with the "scarf" test as described for AC joint pain. Patients who have suffered a clavicle fracture, shoulder separation, or those that do excessive weight-lifting (especially bench presses) are prone to SC joint disease.

Ultrasound-Guided Technique

The SC joint is visualized by placing a linear transducer in line with the clavicle and following the clavicle proximally until the joint is seen. The appearance is typically a small notch with the clavicle projecting superficially compared to the sternum. The joint is covered by a very thin capsule and may be distended if effusion is present. The patient is best positioned in the seated position with the arm hanging at their side. Gentle retraction of the scapula may be helpful to open the joint space. A small hyperechoic fibrocartilaginous disk can sometimes be visualized within the joint space, and seen subluxing with excessive joint movement.

For SC joint injection, the needle is inserted in short-axis orientation, just adjacent to the transducer. For accuracy, the notch of the joint should both be positioned precisely in the middle of the image, and the needle lined up with the corresponding position along the transducer (Figure 22.6a). The needle tip is visualized as a bright "dot" as it enters the field of view, hopefully just superficial to the joint (a very shallow angle of approach is required, as the joint is usually very superficially located). Depth is then adjusted by the "walk-down" technique to position the needle tip deep to the capsule, typically, directly between the articulating bony surfaces (indicated as "asterisk" in Figure 22.6b). Care should be taken to avoid passing the needle completely through the joint, so that it is acceptable and usually prudent to direct the needle from medial to lateral and stopping if bony contact is made with the end of the clavicle, or adequate depth is visualized. The joint is often completely distended by a very small volume of injectate, so that the smallest possible mixture should be used. We typically use a mixture of 0.25 ml triamcinolone (40 mg/ml) and 0.75 cm^3 of local anesthetic.

Conclusion

Currently, musculoskeletal ultrasound is still a new and emerging tool. As techniques are further developed, better and varying approaches are expected to develop. Already, there is compelling evidence supporting the merits of ultrasound-guided shoulder injections over "blind" injections[15–18] and even fluoroscopic guidance.[21,24] These merits include (but are not limited to) real-time assessment of soft-tissue anatomy, no radiation exposure,

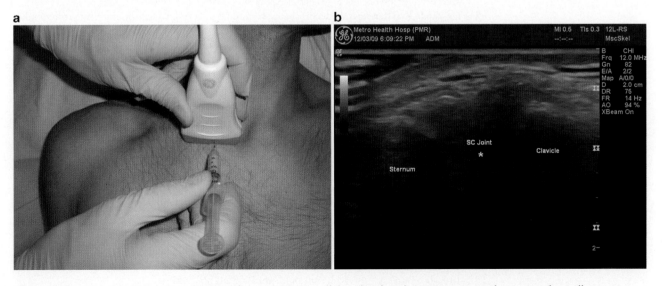

Figure 22.6. Sternoclavicular joint. (**a**) Transducer position parallel to the clavicle spanning across the joint with needle insertion at midline of the transducer. (**b**) Transverse image of AC joint injection showing desired needle tip position indicated by *asterisk*.

direct visualization of needle placement, and flow of injectate.[3,26] The procedures that have been described are powerful tools in the diagnosis and treatment of shoulder disorders. To provide the best outcome, however, they should be combined with a rehabilitation program to address underlying biomechanical deficits and restore optimal function.

References

1. Smith J, Finnoff J. Diagnostic and interventional musculoskeletal ultrasound: part 2. Clinical applications. *PMR.* 2009;1:162–177.
2. Jacobson J. *Fundamentals of Musculoskeletal Ultrasound (p.75–79 for rotator cuff), and (p.87–91 for paralabral cyst).* Philadelphia: Saunders; 2007.
3. Adler RS, Allan A. Percutaneous ultrasound guided injections in the shoulder. *Tech Shoulder Elbow Surg.* 2004;5(2):122–133.
4. Huber DJ, Sauter R, Mueller E, Requardt H, Weber H. MR imaging of the normal shoulder. *Radiology.* 1986;158:405–408.
5. Chandnani VP, Yeager TD, DeBerardino T, et al. Glenoid labral tears: prospective evaluation with MRI imaging, MR arthrography, and CT arthrography. *AJR Am J Roentgenol.* 1993;161: 1229–1235.
6. Balasubramaniam P, Prathap K. The effect of injection of hydrocortisone into rabbit calcaneal tendons. *J Bone Joint Surg Br.* 1972;54–B:729–734.
7. Ford LT, DeBender J. Tendon rupture after local steroid injection. *South Med J.* 1979;72:827–830.
8. Gottlieb NL, Riskin WG. Complications of local corticosteroid injections. *JAMA.* 1980;243: 1547–1548.
9. Shrier I, Matheson GO, Kohl HW. Achilles tendonitis: are corticosteroid injections useful or harmful? *Clin J Sport Med.* 1996;6:245–250.
10. Unverferth LJ, Olix ML. The effect of local steroid injections on tendon. *J Sports Med.* 1973;1:31–37.
11. Grassi W, Farina A, Filippucci E, et al. Sonographically guided procedures in rheumatology. *Semin Arthritis Rheum.* 2001;30:347–353.
12. Sofka CM, Collins AJ, Adler RS. Use of ultrasonographic guidance in interventional musculo-skeletal procedures: a review from a single institution. *J Ultrasound Med.* 2001;20:21–26.
13. Van Holsbeeck M, Strouse PJ. Sonography of the shoulder: evaluation of the subacromial-subdeltoid bursa. *AJR Am J Roentgenol.* 1993;160:561–564.
14. McGee D. *Orthopedic Physical Assessment.* 5th ed. Philadelphia: Saunders; 2008:293–294, 312.
15. Eustace JA, Brophy DP, Gibney RP, Bresnihan B, FitzGerald O. Comparison of the accuracy of steroid placement with clinical outcome in patients with shoulder symptoms. *Ann Rheum Dis.* 1997;56:59–63.
16. Partington PF, Broome GH. Diagnostic injection around the shoulder: hit and miss? A cadaveric study of injection accuracy. *J Shoulder Elbow Surg.* 1998;7:147–150.
17. Yamakado K. The targeting accuracy of subacromial injection to the shoulder: an arthrographic evaluation. *Arthroscopy.* 2002;18:887–891.
18. Kang MN, Rizio L, Prybicien M, et al. The accuracy of subacromial corticosteroid injections: a comparison of multiple methods. *J Shoulder Elbow Surg.* 2008;17(suppl):61S–66S.
19. Henkus HE, Cobben LP, Coerkamp EG, et al. The accuracy of subacromial injections: a prospective randomized magnetic resonance imaging study. *Arthroscopy.* 2006;22:277–282.
20. Farin PU, Rasanen H, Heikki J, Arvi H. Rotator cuff calcifications: treatment with ultrasound-guided percutaneous needle aspiration and lavage. *Skeletal Radiol.* 1996;25:551–554.
21. Weiss J, Ting M. Arthrography-assisted intra-articular injection of steroids in treatment of adhesive capsulitis. *Arch Phys Med Rehabil.* 1978;59:285–287.
22. Sethi PM, Kingston S, Elattrache N. Accuracy of anterior intra-articular injection of the glenohumeral joint. *Arthroscopy.* 2005;21:77–80.
23. Jones A, Regan M, Ledingham J, et al. Importance of placement of intraarticular steroid injections. *BMJ.* 1993;307:1329–1330.
24. Rutten MJ, Collins JM, Maresch BJ, et al. Glenohumeral joint injection: a comparative study of ultrasound and fluoroscopically guided techniques before MR arthrography. *Eur Radiol.* 2009;19: 722–730.
25. Lim JB, Kim YK, Kim SW, Sung KW, Jung I, Lee C. Ultrasound guided shoulder joint injection through rotator cuff interval. *Korean J Pain.* 2008;21(1):57–61.
26. Christensen RA, Van Sonnenberg E, Casola G, et al. Interventional ultrasound in the musculo-skeletal system. *Radiol Clin North Am.* 1988;26:145–156.

23

Ultrasound-Guided Hand, Wrist, and Elbow Injections

Marko Bodor, John M. Lesher, and Sean Colio

M. Bodor (✉)
Department of Neurological Surgery, University of California San Francisco, and
Physical Medicine and Rehabilitation, Sports Medicine, Electrodiagnostic Medicine,
3421 Villa Lane 2B, Napa, CA, USA
e-mail: mbodormd@sbcglobal.net

S.N. Narouze (ed.), *Atlas of Ultrasound-Guided Procedures in Interventional Pain Management*,
DOI 10.1007/978-1-4419-1681-5_23, © Springer Science+Business Media, LLC 2011

Introduction

Patients with pain, numbness, and weakness in the upper extremity are frequently referred to pain specialists. Carpal tunnel syndrome (CTS) combined with shoulder impingement can easily mimic cervical radiculopathy and disk herniation.[1,2] Chronic pain at the thenar eminence following carpal tunnel surgery may stem from occult trigger thumb or carpo-metacarpal (CMC) joint arthritis. Median neuropathy at the wrist combined with impingement of the flexor pollicis longus (FPL) tendon on a fixation plate screw following fracture of the radius can mimic the pain, burning, and weakness of complex regional pain syndrome (CRPS). These and other conditions of the hand, wrist, and elbow can be effectively diagnosed and treated with diagnostic ultrasonography and ultrasound-guided injections.

A few general principles apply with regard to ultrasound-guided injections in the hand, wrist, and elbow. The structures are small and superficial, so a small high-frequency transducer (>12 MHz) is best because of its maneuverability and high resolution. Adequate gel is necessary to maintain good skin contact while scanning over bony structures. The tip of a curved hemostat or other small instrument or the examiner's little finger can be used to help determine which specific structures are tender, such as the CMC joint of the thumb or the adjacent scaphoid–trapezium–trapezoid (STT) joint. A model of the hand, wrist, and elbow placed next to the patient and ultrasound machine can be useful for teaching purposes and visualization of complex anatomy, such as the bony contours of the carpal bones.[3]

Ultrasound-Guided Carpal Tunnel Injections

Anatomy

The carpal tunnel contains the median nerve and nine tendons, including the flexor digitorum superficialis (FDS), profundus (FDP), and pollicis longus (FPL) (Figure 23.1). The tendons are retained by the flexor retinaculum, which extends from the tubercle of the trapezium and scaphoid to the hook of the hamate and pisiform. The FDS and FDP tendons are surrounded by a common synovial sheath, while the FPL has a separate sheath. The location of the median nerve is just beneath the flexor retinaculum, medial to the flexor carpiradialis (FCR), superficial to the FPL, and lateral to the FDS, however it may

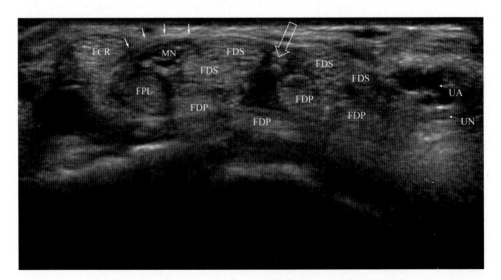

Figure 23.1. Normal carpal tunnel. Short-axis view at the distal wrist crease and opening of the carpal tunnel showing typical anatomy in an unaffected individual. The FCR is separated from the median nerve (MN) and FPL by the transverse retinaculum (*solid arrows*). A cleft or opening (*open arrow*) is seen between FDS tendons halfway between the median and ulnar nerve (UN) and artery (UA).

be located up to a centimeter or more medially, thus even the best performed blind carpal tunnel injections may injure the nerve. The normal median nerve moves in response to finger movements, which can be seen with dynamic ultrasound imaging.

CTS is the most common peripheral nerve entrapment syndrome. The symptoms include numbness in the hand at night, pain, weakness, and a feeling that the hand is swollen. Sensation is decreased in the volar aspect of the thumb, index, middle, and radial half of the ring finger. The gold standard for diagnosis remains nerve conduction studies and electromyography, but ultrasound criteria for CTS have been developed and include median nerve cross-sectional area (CSA) at the distal wrist crease[4] >15 mm[2,] median nerve CSA ratio between distal wrist crease and 12 cm proximally >1.5 (we use >2.0 for greater specificity),[5] and bowing of the flexor retinaculum.[6]

Literature Review on Ultrasound-Guided Carpal Tunnel Injections

Grassi et al described a short-axis technique for carpal tunnel injection in a case of CTS caused by rheumatoid synovitis in which the needle was directed into the interval between the median nerve and the FCR tendon.[7] In our experience, this interval is too narrow to allow easy access to the carpal tunnel in most people but is an option when the median nerve is located more medially (Figure 23.2).

Smith et al described a long-axis ultrasound-guided carpal tunnel injection technique which is performed at the level of the pisiform.[8] The needle is inserted just superficial and lateral to the ulnar nerve and artery and directed toward the median nerve at a shallow angle. Hydrodissection is used to peel the median nerve away from any adhesions. Smith et al performed over 50 injections using this technique with no complications. The long-axis technique ensures that the needle tip and shaft are seen at all times. We have found this technique to be especially useful in cases of failed carpal tunnel surgery, when injecting directly into the transverse carpal ligament or into the middle of the carpal tunnel where the nerve and tendons are closely packed.

At this time, there are no outcome studies comparing ultrasound-guided vs. blind carpal tunnel injections. A recent review of blind carpal tunnel corticosteroid injections found that 75% of patients treated with carpal tunnel release surgery had excellent outcomes, while 8% got worse. With injections 70% of patients had excellent short-term outcomes, but 50% relapsed at 1 year.[9]

Armstrong et al discovered improvement of nerve function; specifically return of absent median sensory nerve action potentials 2 weeks following blind carpal tunnel corticosteroid injections, findings which are of potential significance to all pain specialists, particularly those treating the spine.[10]

The advantage of a short-axis technique is that it deploys the thinnest possible needle the shortest distance. When performed correctly it is nearly painless, however if the needle is jabbed into a tendon the patient will experience pain. We have used the following

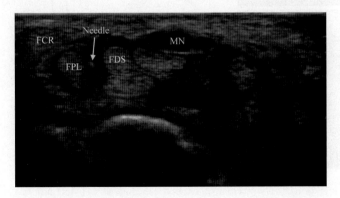

Figure 23.2. Carpal tunnel syndrome (short-axis injection) – medially displaced median nerve. The median nerve (MN) is medially displaced and an opening is present between FPL and FDS tendons allowing passage of the needle (*arrow*).

technique in over 1,800 ultrasound-guided carpal tunnel injections with only one complication (infection in a patient with a previous history of infection).

Ultrasound-Guided Technique for Carpal Tunnel Injection

The patient is seated across from the pain interventionist with the wrist and hand in supination resting on a pillow. The patient is seated next to the ultrasound machine so that the interventionist does not have to turn his head or significantly alter his gaze, factors which could affect the accuracy of needle placement.

The fingers are flexed and the hand is relaxed to maximize space between tendons, then a short-axis view at the distal wrist crease is obtained. An opening between the flexor tendons, usually a vertical or slightly diagonal cleft located halfway between the median and ulnar nerves and most often between the middle and ring finger FDS tendons, is identified (Figures 23.1 and 23.3a–c). When performing an ultrasound-guided injection in either the short or long axis, it is important to remember that the site of needle insertion always lies outside of view of the ultrasound screen. Thus, it is necessary to briefly scan over the intended needle insertion site to make sure any sensitive structures, such as the median or ulnar nerve or artery, are not in the way.[3] The median nerve can be differentiated from the tendons on the basis of their anisotropy or change in appearance from light to dark as the transducer is tipped back and forth in the sagittal plane. It should also be noted that the median nerve can sublux medially or laterally depending on transducer orientation and position.

After the target is centered on the ultrasound screen, the distance between needle insertion site and target is calculated using the ultrasound machine caliper tool or estimated on the basis of the scale on the screen. We typically insert a 30-gauge, 25-mm needle in the short axis and slightly obliquely to pass through the cleft with minimal to no contact with tendons. We hold the syringe lightly in the hand in order to sense the needle slipping between tendons instead of jabbing into them. When the tip of the needle is within the superficial row of tendons, approximately 1.5 ml of 20-40 mg triamcinolone acetonide and normal saline are injected (Figure 23.3b, c). If the medication is not well mixed or the needle jabs into a tendon, clogging may occur and require insertion of another possibly larger gauge needle.

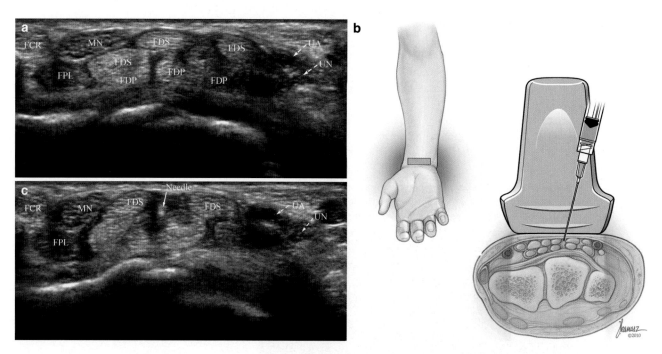

Figure 23.3. Carpal tunnel syndrome (short-axis injection). (**a**) Note enlargement of the median nerve (MN) and the opening between FDS tendons. (**b**) Illustration showing needle and transducer position prior to injection. Medical Illustrations by Joseph Kanasz, BFA (**c**) Ultrasound image obtained during injection shows needle tip (*arrow*) surrounded by anechoic injectate.

After the needle is withdrawn, the patient is asked to fully extend the fingers, thus drawing medication into the carpal tunnel. Combined with use of a wrist splint at night and avoidance of exacerbating activities, the injection can provide complete relief of symptoms in mild to moderate cases of CTS for up to 6 months or longer in our experience.

Ultrasound-Guided Trigger Finger Injections

Anatomy

Triggering occurs at the first annular (A1) pulley, where there is an increase in friction or a mismatch in size between the flexor tendons and pulley. The A1 pulley consists of annular bands of connective tissue located at and proximal to the metacarpophalangeal (MCP) joint and contiguous with the tendon sheath.[11] The mean length of the A1 pulley is 12 mm for the adult index, middle, and ring fingers and 10 mm for the little finger.[12] Ultrasound imaging findings of trigger finger include swelling of the tendons, hypoechoic thickening of the A1 pulley, hypervascularization, synovial sheath effusion, and dynamic changes in the shape of the sheath during flexion and extension.[11,13,14]

On axial ultrasound views, the A1 pulley is hypoechoic and shaped like an inverted parabola overlying the FDS and FDP tendons and volar plate. In thumbs, the A1 pulley has a more circular shape because of only one tendon present, the FPL.[11]

Trigger finger is a common hand problem, with a lifetime prevalence of 2.6% in the general population and 10% among those with diabetes. Symptoms may range from a vague sense of tightness in the fingers or pain in the palm of the hand to overt triggering and locking. Tenderness is almost always present at the A1 pulley and in mild cases may be the only clue as to the presence of the disorder.[11] Trigger finger can be graded according to the Quinnell scale as follows: 0, normal movement; 1, uneven movement; 2, actively correctable locking; 3, passively correctible locking; and 4, fixed deformity of the digit.[15]

Literature Review on Ultrasound-Guided Trigger Finger Injections

Godey et al published a long-axis technique and demonstrated deposition of steroid below and above the pulley in a single patient.[16] Bodor and Flossman described a short-axis technique in their prospective study of 50 of 52 consecutive trigger fingers, noting complete resolution of symptoms in 94% of fingers at 6 months, 90% at 1 year, 65% at 18 months, and 71% at 3 years. The results were statistically significant and compared favorably to the 56% success rates reported at 1 year for blind injections.[11,17,18]

Ultrasound-Guided Trigger Finger Injection Technique

Using the short-axis technique, the target for injection is a triangle under the A1 pulley whose borders consist of the FDS and FDP tendons and volar plate, the distal metacarpal bone, and the pulley (Figure 23.4). The flexor tendons are identified in an axial view at the level of the proximal phalanx. At this location, the underlying surface of the bone appears concave. As the transducer is passed more proximally, the concave surface of the proximal phalanx gives way to the convex surface of the metacarpal bone as the MCP joint is crossed.

At this level, the A1 pulley and target triangle are identified and centered on the screen or slightly to the left of center for someone injecting with the right hand. It does not matter whether the triangle on the radial or ulnar side of the tendons is selected. This as well as other short-axis injections requiring such a high degree of accuracy can be facilitated by placing a mark on the side of the transducer indicating its exact center.

We use a distal-to-proximal approach and plan a trajectory to the hypotenuse of the triangle using an approximately 70° angle to horizontal in the axial plane and a 45° angle

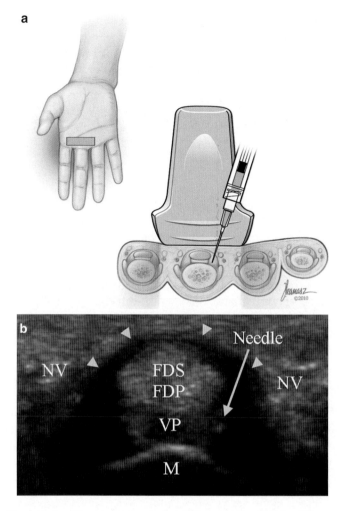

Figure 23.4. Trigger finger (short-axis injection). (**a**) Illustration and Medical Illustrations by Joseph Kanasz, BFA (**b**) short-axis view of the A1 pulley (*arrowheads*) with the tip of the needle inside the target triangle, consisting of the A1 pulley (*arrowheads*), FDS and FDP tendons, volar plate (VP), and distal metacarpal bone (M). The neurovascular bundles (NV) lie on both sides of the pulley.

in the sagittal plane. As soon as the 30-gauge needle punctures the skin, we inject with 0.25 ml of 4% lidocaine for immediate anesthesia then carefully advance the needle into the target triangle using real-time ultrasound guidance.

When the tip of the needle is inside the triangle, the syringes are switched and approximately 0.5–1.0 ml of 10–15 mg triamcinolone acetonide and lidocaine 2–4% are injected, making sure to visualize flow under the A1 pulley. If flow occurs outside the pulley or there is no flow, the needle is adjusted until flow is obtained. Sometimes initially high resistance to outflow is noted followed by a steep drop in resistance accompanied by visual distention of the pulley. The pulley can be tough to penetrate and the needle may clog, requiring insertion of another possibly larger gauge needle. Afterward, the patient is encouraged to resume usual activities.

Ultrasound-Guided Wrist Injections

Anatomy

The wrist consists of the distal radius and ulna, the proximal carpal row, including the scaphoid, lunate, triquetrum, and pisiform, the distal carpal row, including the trapezium, trapezoid, capitate, and hamate, and the bases of the metacarpal bones. The wrist joints are grouped as follows: distal radio-ulnar, radiocarpal, midcarpal, and carpo-metacarpal. The distal radio-ulnar joint allows the radius to pivot around the ulna during pronation and supination. The biconcave radiocarpal joint permits both wrist flexion and extension and radial and ulnar deviation. The proximal carpal row serves as a rigid intercalated segment within the wrist kinetic chain and forms a semirigid ring with the distal carpal row.[19] The distal carpal row serves as a solid base of support for the metacarpal bones, and a complex array of ligaments, description of which is beyond the scope of this chapter, connect and stabilize the carpal bones.[20]

The wrist is vulnerable to both acute and chronic injury, including dorsal and volar dislocations, chronic instabilities, rheumatoid and inflammatory arthritides and osteoarthritis. Osteoarthritis can be classified as primary or secondary. The most common site of primary osteoarthritis in the hand and wrist involves the CMC joint of the thumb. Secondary osteoarthritis typically occurs after fractures or following disruption of the two most important wrist ligaments, the scapholunate and lunotriquetral.[21] Approximately 95% of cases of secondary arthritis involve the scaphoid bone.[22]

Literature Review on Ultrasound-Guided Wrist Injections

Koski et al performed US-guided wrist injections in 50 patients with active rheumatoid arthritis (RA).[23] In the first group, patients were injected with triamcinolone hexacetonide 20 mg entirely into the radiocarpal joint, while in the second group half the dose was provided to the radiocarpal joint and half to the midcarpal joint. At 3 months, visual analog scores (VAS) improved in both groups, with 19 of 25 wrists in the first group being clinically assessed as better or normal and 22 of 25 in the second group.

Boesen et al injected the radiocarpal joint of each of 17 RA patients with 1 ml methylprednisolone 40 mg, 0.15 ml gadolinium, and 0.5 ml lidocaine 0.5% with the goal of assessing distribution of contrast among the four wrist compartments.[24] A short-axis approach was used with the transducer sagittally oriented between the distal radius and lunate. A value of 1 was assigned for complete spread within one compartment, 0.5 for partial spread, and 0 for no spread. The mean distribution score was 2.4, with greater distribution noted in patients with higher MRI synovitis scores and distribution in all four compartments noted in only two patients.

In their retrospective study of US-guided contrast injections for MR arthrography, Lohman et al noted that 101 of 108 (93.5%) injections were intra-articular.[25] Their injection technique involved placing the wrist in slight volar flexion and palpating for Lister's tubercle. Ultrasound scanning in the short axis was used to identify and mark the space between the third and fourth tendon compartments at the radiocarpal joint, the transducer was rotated 90° and the needle inserted in the long axis.

Umphrey et al performed US-guided short-axis injections of the trapeziometacarpal (TMC) or thumb CMC joint in cadavers.[26] Fluoroscopic images confirmed intra-articular contrast in 16 of 17 (94%) joints following a single attempt. Mandl et al reported similar success rates (91%) with blind injections, using ultrasound for confirmation.[27]

In a recent study of 18 patients, Salini et al provided a single ultrasound-guided injection of sodium hyaluronate 1% to the CMC joint of the thumb, noting at 1 month follow-up a reduction of pain from 1.8 to 0.5 at rest and 8 to 4 with activities, with the elimination of NSAID use in 9 patients and reduction of NSAID use (2.5–1 tablet per week) in 7 patients.[28]

In a well-controlled nonultrasound-guided study of 56 patients with thumb CMC joint arthritis, Fuchs et al compared one triamcinolone acetonide (TA) 10 mg injection to three 1 ml injections of sodium hyaluronate (SH) 1% given 1 week apart. The VAS score went from 61 to 20 to 48 in the TA group and from 64 to 30 to 28 in the SH group 3 weeks following the last injection and at 26 weeks final follow-up.[29]

Ultrasound-Guided Technique for Wrist Injections

A precise sonographic examination is advised before planning any injections. Thus, for example, if treating pain at the radial aspect of the wrist, the radial-scaphoid joint is visualized and centered on the screen and careful palpation performed over the joint to confirm that it is the pain generator. To facilitate precise sonopalpation, we recommend use of a small probe or the tip of one's little finger. If a specific joint is the pain generator we expect it to be tender relative to adjacent structures. We find this technique to be especially useful in identifying pain arising from small and difficult to access structures such as the piso-triquetral (PT) and STT joints.

Two techniques of wrist injections will be described, the first using a long-axis and the second using a short-axis approach.

For the long-axis approach to the radio-carpal joint, the patient is seated next to the ultrasound machine facing the physician. The wrist is in pronation, slight volar flexion, and resting on a pillow. Lister's tubercle is identified in the short axis. Next to it on the ulnar side is the extensor pollicis longus (EPL) followed by the extensor digitorum communis (EDC). The interval between EPL and EDC tendons is centered on the screen and the transducer moved distally until the bony cortex of the radius disappears. Here the transducer is rotated 90° so that the underlying radial-scaphoid joint is seen in the long axis (Figure 23.5). A 27-gauge, 32-mm needle is then advanced in the long axis from distally to proximally until the tip of the needle enters the joint.

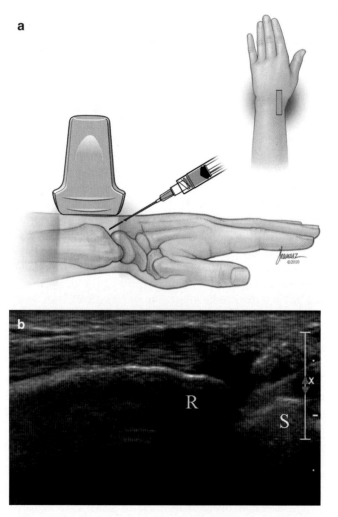

Figure 23.5. Wrist (radial-scaphoid) joint long-axis injection. (**a**) Illustration and Medical Illustrations by Joseph Kanasz, BFA (**b**) long-axis view of the joint and radius (R), scaphoid (S), and needle seen entering from the right. Injected fluid surrounds the tip of the needle.

For small and superficial joint injections such as the CMC joint of the thumb, a short-axis injection is easiest to perform. The wrist is placed in neutral, between pronation and supination and in slight ulnar deviation for a dorsal approach, and in supination, thumb adduction and slight ulnar deviation for a volar approach. The joint is centered on the screen and the distance between the skin and a point within the superficial part of joint is estimated. A 30-gauge, 12.5 or 25-mm needle is inserted in the short axis and directed toward the joint (Figure 23.6). When the needle is within the joint, 0.5–1.0 ml of corticosteroid, lidocaine or viscosupplement is injected. The advantage of the dorsal approach is that it avoids the sensitive skin of the volar aspect of the hand, whereas the volar approach, as described by Umphrey et al,[26] avoids the overlying thumb tendons.

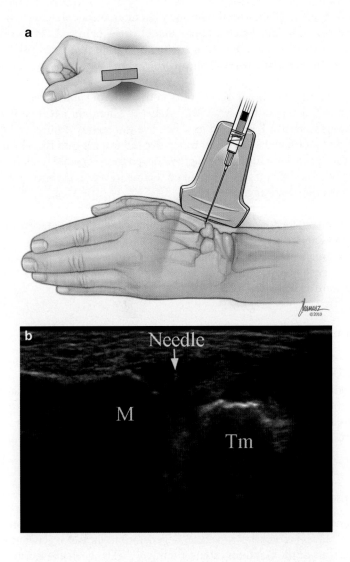

Figure 23.6. CMC joint of thumb injection (short-axis dorsal approach). (a) Illustration and Medical Illustrations by Joseph Kanasz, BFA (b) short-axis view of the needle (*arrow*), the proximal metacarpal bone (M) and trapezium (Tm) during injection. The medication is being injected via a 30-gauge needle resulting in high velocity and air bubbles being injected deep into the joint producing a somewhat brighter appearance of the fluid between M and Tm.

Ultrasound-Guided Injections for Tendon Dysfunction

Anatomy

The extensor tendons are divided into six compartments at the dorsal wrist and forearm: E1, abductor pollicis longus (APL) and extensor pollicis brevis (EPB); E2, extensor carpi radialis longus and brevis (ECRL and ECRB); E3, EPL; E4, EDC; E5, extensor digiti minimi (EDM); and E6, extensor carpi ulnaris (ECU). The tendons are prone to friction, overuse, effusions, and degenerative changes. The common extensor tendon of the ECRB, EDC, EDM, and ECU originates from the lateral epicondyle of the humerus. The anatomy of the flexor tendons is discussed in the carpal tunnel section.

de Quervain's Tenosynovitis

Fritz de Quervain described stenosing tenosynovitis of the first compartment tendons, the APL and EPB, in 1895.[30] Pain with thumb and wrist motion and tenderness over the radial styloid are present. The incidence is approximately 0.94–6.3 per 1,000 person-years,[31,32] and women, older individuals, and African-Americans are at greater risk.[32] Ultrasound findings include tendon and synovial sheath thickening with peritendinous edematous changes.[33]

Zingas et al performed blind injections of cortiocosteroid and radiographic dye in 19 patients with de Quervain's tenosynovitis.[34] Relief of symptoms occurred in 11 of 16 in which dye was present in E1, in 4 of 5 in which dye was seen within E1 and around both APL and EPB tendons, and in 0 of 3 in which dye did not get into E1. The authors concluded that the optimal resolution of symptoms depends on accurate tendon sheath injections and hypothesized that if an unrecognized septum separates the smaller EPB from the larger APL, injections and surgery may fail.

Avci et al performed a randomized controlled trial in pregnant and lactating women demonstrating complete relief of pain in nine of nine patients treated with blind corticosteroid injections, and in zero of nine using thumb spica splints.[35]

Jeyapalan and Choudhary performed US-guided injections in 17 patients with de Quervain's tenosynovitis, noting significant resolution of symptoms in the 15 of 16 (94%) patients that were available for follow-up.[36]

Intersection Syndrome

Intersection or oarsman's syndrome occurs at the intersection of the E1 (APL and EPB) and E2 (ECRL and ECRB) tendon sheaths in the distal forearm. Focal tenderness to palpation confirms the diagnosis. Ultrasound findings may include thickening of the tendon sheaths or the presence of an effusion.[37] Ultrasound-guided corticosteroid injection and avoidance of direct pressure and exacerbating activities can help resolve this problem. A rarer friction syndrome can occur more distally at the intersection of E2 and E3.

Lateral Epicondylitis

Lateral epicondylitis (LE) or tennis elbow has an incidence of 0.4–0.7% among the general population.[38,39] LE is secondary to overuse, degeneration, lack of regeneration (tendinosis), or micro-tears of the common extensor tendon.[3,40] The deep fibers of the ECRB portion of the tendon are most often involved. Ultrasound findings include diffuse tendon enlargement, hypoechoic areas, linear and complex tears, intratendinous calcification, and adjacent bone irregularity.[3]

Recent systematic reviews[41,42] found that corticosteroid injections provide good short-term relief of symptoms, but no long-term benefit, whereas physical therapy slightly improves intermediate and long-term outcomes compared to no intervention. Risks of corticosteroids include common extensor tendon and lateral collateral ligament rupture.

Mishra et al performed the first randomized controlled trial of platelet-rich plasma (PRP) injections for chronic lateral epicondylitis in 20 patients who had failed corticosteroid injections and physical therapy.[43] After 8 weeks there was a 60% improvement in VAS score among the 15 patients in the PRP group, compared to 16% for the 5 patients in the bupivacaine group. At final follow-up an average of 25.6 months later there was a 93% improvement in the PRP group.

Recent systematic reviews[44,45] also concluded that prolotherapy, polidocanol, autologous whole blood, and PRP are all effective for LE with more studies underway. McShane et al reported good to excellent results in 92% of patients at an average of 22 months following sonographically guided percutaneous needle tenotomy for LE.[46]

Tendon Impingement

Arora et al reported on a series of 141 patients treated with a fixed-angle open reduction internal fixation (ORIF) palmar plate, noting two ruptures of the FPL tendon, nine cases of flexor tendon tenosynovitis, two EPL ruptures, four cases of extensor tendon synovitis, three CTS, and five with CRPS.[47] Casaletto et al described seven cases of FPL rupture associated with palmar plate fixation.[48] Adham et al described four cases of flexor tendon problems after volar plate fixation of distal radius fractures, all of which were associated with close contact of flexor tendons with screws or the distal edge of the plate.[49]

Ultrasound-Guided Technique for Tendon Dysfunction

US-guided injections for de Quervain's tenosynovitis are performed as follows: the APL and EPB tendons are identified in the short axis at the base of the thumb and followed proximally to the point of maximum tenderness, usually where they cross the radial styloid. The E1 tendon sheath is the target for injection, but each tendon can be targeted separately if a septum is present or flow does not spread throughout the sheath. After the cleft between tendons is centered on the screen, a short-axis injection is performed using a 27-gauge, 32-mm needle and 1–2 ml of lidocaine/corticosteroid (Figure 23.7).

US-guided injections for intersection syndrome are performed in a similar fashion. The E1 tendons are followed proximally up to the point where they cross the E2 tendons. A short-axis injection can be provided into the E1 tendon sheath between the APL and EPB tendons, followed by advancement of the needle into the space between E1 and E2 where more medication can be injected.

Ultrasonography for lateral epicondylitis is most useful to determine whether the common extensor tendon is swollen, degenerated, partially or completely torn, factors which are as likely to impact outcome as exact needle placement. Ultrasound guidance can be used in the short or long axis for an injection of PRP into a tear or for the assessment of spread of injectate (Figure 23.8).

US-guided injections for tendon impingement can be performed following the use of dynamic imaging to determine which tendon is being impinged and where. An injection of local anesthetic only is provided because corticosteroids increase the risk of tendon rupture. When the source of pain is identified, a decision can be made whether to remove the hardware. The injection technique for impingement of a tendon such as the FPL is similar to that for CTS. A short- or long-axis approach is used, but the needle is advanced beyond the superficial row of tendons so that the tip is positioned between the FPL and fixation plate or screw. At that point, 0.5–1.0 ml of lidocaine 4% or bupivacaine 0.75% is injected followed by the assessment of pain and function (Figure 23.9).

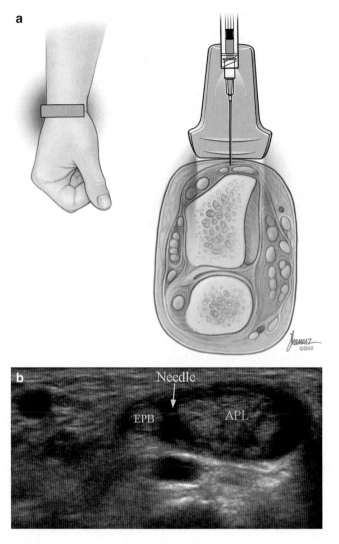

Figure 23.7. de Quervain's tenosynovitis (short-axis injection). (**a**) Illustration and Medical Illustrations by Joseph Kanasz, BFA (**b**) short-axis view of the tip of the needle (*arrow*) seen between the APL and EPB tendons.

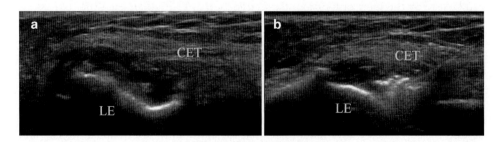

Figure 23.8. Lateral epicondylitis. (**a**) Long-axis view showing anechoic fluid between the origin of the common extensor tendon (CET) and the lateral epicondyle (LE) indicating a tear. (**b**) Long-axis view with needle showing PRP being injected into the tear.

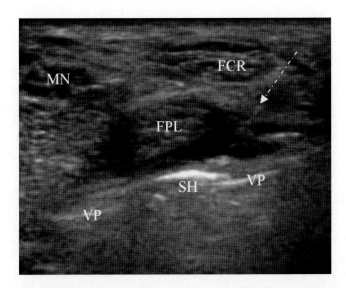

Figure 23.9. FPL tendon impingement. Short-axis view of the distal radius with a volar fixation plate (VP) and protruding screw head (SH) adjacent to the FPL. The image was taken during a diagnostic injection. The FPL tendon is being displaced away from the SH by local anesthetic injected via a long-axis approach. The needle is seen as a series of dots below the arrow and is difficult to see because of its high angle.

Ultrasound-Guided Elbow Injections

Anatomy

The elbow is a compound joint formed by the articulations of three bones including the humerus, radius, and ulna. The ulno-humeral articulation approximates a hinge joint, whereas the radio-ulnar and radio-humeral articulations allow for axial rotation. The joint capsule envelopes the entire elbow joint and is taut in elbow extension and lax in elbow flexion. It contains three fat pads, two of which are located in the capitellar and trochlear fossa, and the third in the olecranon fossa. When an elbow joint effusion is present, the fat pads are elevated, resulting in the radiographic signs of visible posterior and elevated anterior fat pads.

Numerous bursae are found around the elbow including the cubital and olecranon bursae. The cubital bursae include the bicipito-radial bursa and the interosseous bursa.[50] The cubital bursa is located between the distal biceps tendon and the radial tuberosity and decreases friction during forearm pronation. Cubital bursitis is rare and causes pain and swelling in the antecubital fossa.[51] Three bursae are found posteriorly including the superficial olecranon bursa that is located in the subcutaneous tissue posterior to the olecranon. This bursa is commonly inflamed following direct injury or repetitive trauma or with inflammatory disorders.

Knowledge of peripheral nerve anatomy around the elbow is important when performing interventional procedures in this area. The ulnar nerve is located medially between the olecranon process and medial epicondyle, and the radial nerve is located laterally under the brachioradialis muscle, where it bifurcates into deep and superficial branches. The deep branch of the radial nerve runs between the two heads of the supinator, and the superficial branch runs under the brachioradialis muscle on its way to the dorsal radial aspect of the hand.[52] The median nerve lies anteriorly, superficial to the brachialis muscle and medial to the brachial artery.[53]

Literature Review on Ultrasound-Guided Elbow Injections

Ultrasound-guided elbow joint injections are commonly performed for diagnosis and treatment of pain resulting from osteoarthritis, rheumatoid arthritis, crystal arthropathies, and infection. Ultrasound can be a valuable tool to the physician treating elbow pain since physical examination and blind aspiration often fail to reveal the presence of an effusion.

Louis et al and Bruyn et al described similar approaches with the elbow either flexed across the chest, or protruding behind the back with the hand resting on a flat surface.[54,55] The transducer is aligned with the long axis of the upper arm and moved laterally until just out of view of the triceps tendon. The needle is inserted using a long-axis approach. The median, radial, and ulnar nerves are not at risk for injury with this approach, and the key anatomical landmarks include the concave olecranon fossa of the humerus, the posterior fat pad, and the olecranon.

Ultrasound-Guided Elbow Injection Technique

The patient is seated facing away from the physician with a pillow doubled-up in the lap, the hand resting on the pillow and the elbow bent. A long-axis view of the olecranon and triceps tendon is obtained (Figure 23.10a). While maintaining the lower end of the transducer on the olecranon, the upper end is rotated 30° clockwise for the right or 30° counter clockwise for the left elbow. As the transducer is rotated, the convex surface of the lateral trochlea of the distal humerus with its thin layer of hypoechoic cartilage emerges into view. The joint space is the small notch between the olecranon and trochlea (Figure 23.10c).

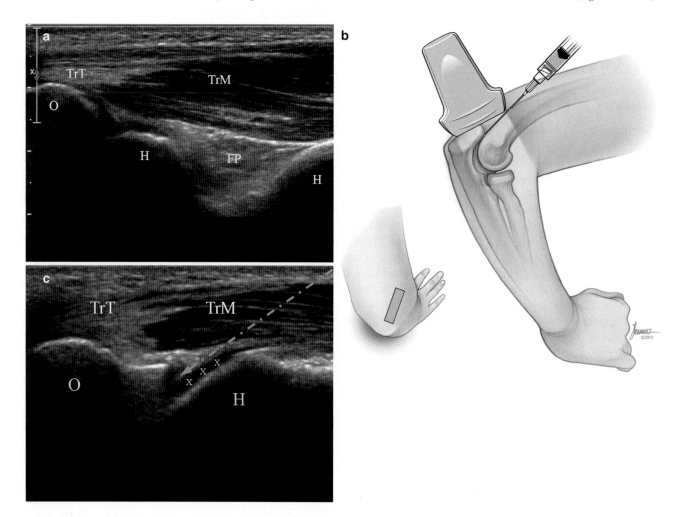

Figure 23.10. Elbow (long-axis injection). (**a**) Initial long-axis view of the triceps tendon (TrT), muscle (TrM), olecranon (O), humerus (H), hyaline cartilage (x), and posterior fat pad (FP). (**b**) Illustration of position after rotating the upper end of the transducer 30° laterally. Medical Illustrations by Joseph Kanasz, BFA (**c**) Ultrasound image (**b**) showing triceps tendon (TrT), muscle (TrM), and needle trajectory (*arrow*) which passes through the muscle and avoids the tendon.

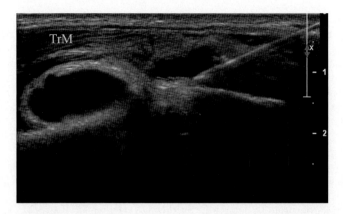

Figure 23.11. Elbow joint aspiration. Long-axis view of an 18-gauge needle taken during aspiration of 15 ml of synovial fluid from the elbow of a patient with gout. The effusion was located superiorly to the joint so all of the underlying bone seen in this image is the distal lateral humerus.

One must be careful not to rotate too far laterally – if the hypoechoic layer of cartilage is not seen, the bony surface seen superior to the olecranon may be the posterior lateral epicondyle. The transducer is then moved inferiorly to minimize the distance the needle needs to travel to the joint space. As usual, the thinnest possible needle is used and is inserted in the long axis from superiorly to inferiorly (Figure 23.10b). If an aspiration needs to be performed (Figure 23.11) the needle is withdrawn while anesthetizing its track and a larger gauge needle is inserted along its path.

REFERENCES

1. Bodor M. Shoulder pathokinesiology and rehabilitation. In: *Painful Shoulder, 2004 AAEM Course Symposia, American Association of Neuromuscular and Electrodiagnostic Medicine.*
2. Gorski JM, Schwartz LH. Shoulder impingement presenting as neck pain. *J Bone Joint Surg Am.* 2003;85-A(4):635–638.
3. Bodor M, Fullerton B. Ultrasonography of the hand, wrist and elbow. *Phys Med Clin N Am.* 2010 Aug;21(3):509–31.
4. Lee D, van Holsbeeck MT, Janevski PK, Ganos DL, Ditmars DM, Darian VB. Diagnosis of carpal tunnel syndrome. Ultrasound versus electromyography. *Radiol Clin North Am.* 1999;37(4): 859–872.
5. Hobson-Webb LD, Massey JM, Juel VC, Sanders DB. The ultrasonographic wrist-to-forearm median nerve area ratio in carpal tunnel syndrome. *Clin Neurophysiol.* 2008;119(6):1353–1357.
6. Beekman R, Visser LH. Sonography in the diagnosis of carpal tunnel syndrome: a critical review of the literature. *Muscle Nerve.* 2003;27(1):26–33. Review.
7. Grassi W, Farina A, Filippucci E, Cervini C. Intralesional therapy in carpal tunnel syndrome: a sonographic-guided approach. *Clin Exp Rheumatol.* 2002;20(1):73–76.
8. Smith J, Wisniewski SJ, Finnoff JT, Payne JM. Sonographically guided carpal tunnel injections: the ulnar approach. *J Ultrasound Med.* 2008;27(10):1485–1490.
9. Bland JD. Treatment of carpal tunnel syndrome. *Muscle Nerve.* 2007;36(2):167–171. Review.
10. Armstrong T, Devor W, Borschel L, Contreras R. Intracarpal steroid injection is safe and effective for short-term management of carpal tunnel syndrome. *Muscle Nerve.* 2004;29(1):82–88.
11. Bodor M, Flossman T. Ultrasound-guided first annular pulley injection for trigger finger. *J Ultrasound Med.* 2009;28(6):737–743.
12. Wilhelmi BJ, Snyder N IV, Verbesey JE, Ganchi PA, Lee WP. Trigger finger release with hand surface landmark ratios: an anatomic and clinical study. *Plast Reconstr Surg.* 2001;108:908–915.
13. Serafini G, Derchi LE, Quadri P, et al. High resolution sonography of the flexor tendons in trigger fingers. *J Ultrasound Med.* 1996;15:213–219.
14. Guerini H, Pessis E, Theumann N, et al. Sonographic appearance of trigger fingers. *J Ultrasound Med.* 2008;27(10):1407–1413.

15. Quinnell RC. Conservative management of trigger finger. *Practitioner*. 1980;24:187–190.
16. Godey SK, Bhatti WA, Watson JS, Bayat A. A technique for accurate and safe injection of steroid in trigger digits using ultrasound guidance. *Acta Orthop Belg*. 2006;72:633–634.
17. Fleisch SB, Spindler KP, Lee DH. Corticosteroid injections in the treatment of trigger finger: a level I and II systematic review. *J Am Acad Orthop Surg*. 2007;15:166–171.
18. Peters-Veluthamaningal C, Winters JC, Groenier KH, Jong BM. Corticosteroid injections effective for trigger finger in adults in general practice: a double-blinded randomised placebo controlled trial. *Ann Rheum Dis*. 2008;67(9):1262–1266.
19. Lichtman DM, Schneider JR, Swafford AR, Mack GR. Ulnar midcarpal instability-clinical and laboratory analysis. *J Hand Surg Am*. 1981;6(5):515–523.
20. Boutry N, Lapegue F, Masi L, Claret A, Demondion X, Cotten A. Ultrasonographic evaluation of normal extrinsic and intrinsic carpal ligaments: preliminary experience. *Skeletal Radiol*. 2005;34(9):513–521.
21. Taljanovic MS, Sheppard JE, Jones MD, Switlick DN, Hunter TB, Rogers LF. Sonography and sonoarthrography of the scapholunate and lunotriquetral ligaments and triangular fibrocartilage disk: initial experience and correlation with arthrography and magnetic resonance arthrography. *J Ultrasound Med*. 2008;27(2):179–191.
22. Watson HK, Ryu J. Evolution of arthritis of the wrist. *Clin Orthop Relat Res*. 1986;(202):57–67.
23. Koski JM, Hermunen H. Intra-articular glucocorticoid treatment of the rheumatoid wrist. An ultrasonographic study. *Scand J Rheumatol*. 2001;30(5):268–270.
24. Boesen M, Jensen KE, Torp-Pedersen S, Cimmino MA, Danneskiold-Samsøe B, Bliddal H. Intra-articular distribution pattern after ultrasound-guided injections in wrist joints of patients with rheumatoid arthritis. *Eur J Radiol*. 2009;69(2):331–338.
25. Lohman M, Vasenius J, Nieminen O. Ultrasound guidance for puncture and injection in the radiocarpal joint. *Acta Radiol*. 2007;48(7):744–747.
26. Umphrey GL, Brault JS, Hurdle MF, Smith J. Ultrasound-guided intra-articular injection of the trapeziometacarpal joint: description of technique. *Arch Phys Med Rehabil*. 2008;89(1):153–156.
27. Mandl LA, Hotchkiss RN, Adler RS, Ariola LA, Katz JN. Can the carpometacarpal joint be injected accurately in the office setting? Implications for therapy. *J Rheumatol*. 2006;33(6):1137–1139.
28. Salini V, De Amicis D, Abate M, Natale MA, Di Iorio A. Ultrasound-guided hyaluronic acid injection in carpometacarpal osteoarthritis: short-term results. *Int J Immunopathol Pharmacol*. 2009;22(2):455–460.
29. Fuchs S, Mönikes R, Wohlmeiner A, Heyse T. Intra-articular hyaluronic acid compared with corticoid injections for the treatment of rhizarthrosis. *Osteoarthritis Cartilage*. 2006;14(1):82–88.
30. de Quervain F. Uber eine form von chronischer tendovaginitis, Corresp.-Bl. f. Schweizer Arzte 1895;25:389–394.
31. Roquelaure Y, Ha C, Leclerc A, et al. Epidemiologic surveillance of upper-extremity musculoskeletal disorders in the working population. *Arthritis Rheum*. 2006;55:765–778.
32. Wolf JM, Sturdivant RX, Owens BD. Incidence of de Quervain's tenosynovitis in a young, active population. *J Hand Surg Am*. 2009;34:112–115.
33. Diop AN, Ba-Diop S, Sane JC, et al. Role of US in the management of de Quervain's tenosynovitis: review of 22 cases. *J Radiol*. 2008;89(9 pt 1):1081–1084. French.
34. Zingas C, Failla JM, Van Holsbeeck M. Injection accuracy and relief of De Quervain's tendinitis. *J Hand Surg Am*. 1998;23(1):89–96.
35. Avci S, Yilmaz C, Sayli U. Comparison of nonsurgical treatment measures for de Quervain's disease of pregnancy and lactation. *J Hand Surg Am*. 2002;27:322–324.
36. Jeyapalan K, Choudhary S. Ultrasound-guided injection of triamcinolone and bupivacaine in the management of De Quervain's disease. *Skeletal Radiol*. 2009;38(11):1099–1103.
37. De Maeseneer M, Marcelis S, Jager T, Girard C, Gest T, Jamadar D. Spectrum of normal and pathologic findings in the region of the first extensor compartment of the wrist: sonographic findings and correlations with dissections. *J Ultrasound Med*. 2009;28(6):779–786.
38. Plancher KD, Halbrecht J, Lourie GM. Medial and lateral epicondylitis in the athlete. *Clin Sports Med*. 1996;15:283–305.
39. Hamilton P. The prevalence of humeral epicondylitis: a survey in general practice. *J R Coll Gen Pract*. 1986;36:464–465.
40. Rineer CA, Ruch DS. Elbow tendinopathy and tendon ruptures: epicondylitis, biceps and triceps ruptures. *J Hand Surg Am*. 2009;34(3):566–576. Review.
41. Smidt N, Assendelft WJ, van der Windt DA, Hay EM, Buchbinder R, Bouter LM. Corticosteroid injections for lateral epicondylitis: a systematic review. *Pain*. 2002;96(1–2):23–40. Review.

42. Barr S, Cerisola FL, Blanchard V. Effectiveness of corticosteroid injections compared with physiotherapeutic interventions for lateral epicondylitis: a systematic review. *Physiotherapy.* 2009; 95(4):251–265.

43. Mishra A, Pavelko T. Treatment of chronic elbow tendinosis with buffered platelet-rich plasma. *Am J Sports Med.* 2006;34(11):1774–1778.

44. Rabago D, Best TM, Zgierska AE, Zeisig E, Ryan M, Crane D. A systematic review of four injection therapies for lateral epicondylosis: prolotherapy, polidocanol, whole blood and platelet-rich plasma. *Br J Sports Med.* 2009;43(7):471–481.

45. Fullerton BD, Reeves KD. Ultrasonography in regenerative injection (prolotherapy) using dextrose, platelet-rich plasma and other injectants. *Phys Med Clin N Am.* 2010 Aug;21(3):585–605.

46. McShane JM, Shah VN, Nazarian LN. Sonographically guided percutaneous needle tenotomy for treatment of common extensor tendinosis in the elbow: is a corticosteroid necessary? *J Ultrasound Med.* 2008;27:1137.

47. Arora R, Lutz M, Hennerbichler A, Krappinger D, Espen D, Gabl M. Complications following internal fixation of unstable distal radius fracture with a palmar locking-plate. *J Orthop Trauma.* 2007;21(5):316–322.

48. Casaletto JA, Machin D, Leung R, Brown DJ. Flexor pollicis longus tendon ruptures after palmar plate fixation of fractures of the distal radius. *J Hand Surg Eur Vol.* 2009;34(4):471–474.

49. Adham MN, Porembski M, Adham C. Flexor tendon problems after volar plate fixation of distal radius fractures. *Hand (N Y).* 2009;4(4):406–409.

50. Skaf AY, Boutin RD, Dantas RW, et al. Bicipitoradial bursitis: MR imaging findings in eight patients and anatomic data from contrast material opacification of bursae followed by routine radiography and MR imaging in cadavers. *Radiology.* 1999;212:111–116.

51. Sofka CM, Adler RS. Sonography of cubital bursitis. *AJR Am J Roentgenol.* 2004;183(1):51–55.

52. Nakamichi K, Tachibana S. Ultrasonographic findings in isolated neuritis of the posterior interosseous nerve: comparison with normal findings. *J Ultrasound Med.* 2007;26(5):683–687.

53. Finlay K, Ferri M, Friedman L. Ultrasound of the elbow. *Skeletal Radiol.* 2004;33(2):63–79.

54. Louis LJ. Musculoskeletal ultrasound intervention: principles and advances. *Radiol Clin North Am.* 2008;46(3):515–533, vi.

55. Bruyn GA, Schmidt WA. How to perform ultrasound-guided injections. *Best Pract Res Clin Rheumatol.* 2009;23(2):269–279.

24

Ultrasound-Guided Hip Injections

Hariharan Shankar and Swetha Simhan

Introduction

Hip pain is caused by many conditions, including osteoarthritis (OA), rheumatoid arthritis, and trauma. Incidence of hip OA is expected to increase over time with the aging population and with the increase in obesity in United States. Overall, 14.3% of the US adults aged 60 years and older reported significant hip pain on most days over the previous 6 weeks.[1] Management options for pain in the hip include analgesics, including nonsteroidal anti-inflammatory agents, intra-articular steroids, and visco-supplementation and hip replacement for advanced stages.[2] Intra-articular injections are performed based on landmarks, using fluoroscopy, computerized tomography, and with the use of ultrasound imaging.[2-8] This chapter discusses the various imaging methods, their advantages, and disadvantages and finally discuss the technique for ultrasound-guided intra-articular hip injections.

H. Shankar (✉)
Department of Anesthesiology, Clement Zablocki VA Medical Center & Medical College of Wisconsin,
5000 West National Avenue, Milwaukee, WI 53295, USA
e-mail: hshankar@mcw.edu

S.N. Narouze (ed.), *Atlas of Ultrasound-Guided Procedures in Interventional Pain Management*,
DOI 10.1007/978-1-4419-1681-5_24, © Springer Science+Business Media, LLC 2011

Anatomy of the Hip Joint

Hip joint is a synovial joint that permits movement in all directions because of the ball and socket configuration of the femoral head and the acetabulum. The depth of the acetabular cavity is enhanced by the fibro-cartilaginous labrum which lines the rim. The ligamentum teres femoris attaches the center of the femoral head to the acetabulum and hence is intra-articular. The capsule has various thickenings formed by ilio-femoral, ischio-femoral, and pubo-femoral ligaments.

The femoral neurovascular bundle is separated from the hip joint by the iliopsoas. It is located in the femoral triangle formed by the sartorius laterally, adductor longus medially, and the inguinal ligament superiorly. The femoral artery gives off the deep femoral artery which divides into the medial and lateral circumflex arteries supplying the femoral head and neck. The posterior division of the obturator artery also contributes a major branch traversing the ligamentum teres and supplying the head.

Articular branches to the hip joint are provided by branches from the femoral, obturator, and sciatic nerves.

Intra-Articular Hip Injections

Some of the commonly adopted methods of providing temporary pain relief in hip joint pain are the injection of local anesthetics, steroid, and visco-supplementation. Intra-articular injection of local anesthetics facilitates the identification of the source of pain.[9,10] Precision in the injection contributes significantly to its diagnostic value. Intra-articular steroid injections decrease pain and inflammation.[11] Robinson et al compared two different doses of steroids with fluoroscopic guidance in 120 patients and found that there is a dose response to the effectiveness of intra-articular steroid injections in increasing range of motion and pain relief.[12] Visco-supplementation is injecting hyaluronate into the joints to improve lubrication and pain relief and hence may delay joint replacement.[13] Although extensively studied for knee joint, few reports exist for the use of hip joint visco-supplementation. Two randomized controlled studies on the use of visco-supplementation did not find any benefit in hip OA.[14,15]

Limitations of the Blind Technique

Being a deeply located joint, blind landmark-based injections suffer from lack of accuracy in addition to the possibility for damage to neurovascular structures in proximity to the joint. With the anterior approach the needle is very close to the femoral nerve and may sometimes impale the nerve. The reported success rate with landmark-based injections varies from 50% to 80% depending on the technique and the practitioner. Leopold et al placed needles into the hip joints of cadavers based on landmarks and found that the needle passed within 4.5 mm of the femoral nerve with an anterior approach and 58.9 mm with the lateral approach.[3]

This begs for the use of image guidance for needle interventions to the hip. But, utilizing fluoroscopy or CT guidance for the performance of these injections entail cost considerations and the potential for radiation exposure both to the patient and the practitioner.[6,7] In addition, although extensively used for intra-articular injections fluoroscopy does not permit visualization of the neurovascular bundle.

Evidence for Ultrasound-Guided Hip Injections

Experimentation with the use of ultrasound led to its use in diagnostic musculoskeletal imaging and naturally transitioned to needle guidance. Ultrasound machines are portable, cheap, have no known major bioeffects in humans, and permit delineation of soft tissue structures besides bone. Sonography has been shown to be useful in diagnosing various pathologies, including arthritis, soft tissue masses, effusion, and labral tears besides facilitating joint aspiration of effusions.[16,17]

Sofka et al conducted a retrospective review of 358 adult hip ultrasound-guided aspirations/injections and found no cases of inadvertent vascular or femoral nerve puncture.[18] Similarly, Berman et al reported 800 successful sonographically guided hip injections and reported no major complications.[19] Few other smaller studies also exist to attest to the effectiveness of ultrasound guidance for intra-articular hip injections.[20] In a pilot study, Caglar-Yagci et al demonstrated the usefulness for approximately 90 days with ultrasound-guided hyaluronate injection using a lateral approach.[21] Other studies have demonstrated similar efficacy.[22,23] In addition, Pourbagher et al confirmed intra-articular hip hyaluronate injection under ultrasound guidance with postinjection computerized tomographic verification.[23]

Technique of Ultrasound-Guided Hip Injections

The author prefers the anterior longitudinal approach. The patient is positioned supine, hip maintained in the neutral position; a pillow beneath the knee may provide some comfort and relax the joint.

A linear array transducer is utilized to identify the superficial neurovascular structures to avoid accidental injury during the injection. In patients with a larger body habitus, a curvilinear transducer with lower frequencies may provide better penetration. The frequency is adjusted for the depth of penetration required to visualize the femoral head and neck. Commonly used frequencies are 3–5 and 7–12 MHz.

The target for injection is the anterior synovial recess. This is located at the junction of the neck and head. Effusions may sometimes be seen at this location as hypoechoic areas. The transducer is placed parallel to the neck overlying the femoral head. The femur is seen as a hyperechoic structure and is followed from the neck on to the head which appears as a slightly oval hyperechoic structure (Figure 24.1). Cephalad to the femoral head, the labrum may be seen as a triangular structure.

An initial scout scan is performed to identify the neurovascular bundle and the location of the femoral head and neck (Figure 24.2). Color Doppler sonography should be used to exclude any blood vessels in the needle path (Figure 24.3). The femoral neurovascular bundle is identified in a transverse view. Following this, the transducer is oriented sagittally. The transducer is moved from the lateral to medial side until the femoral head is identified as a hyperechoic globular structure (Figure 24.4). Subsequently, the orientation is adjusted to be in line with the femoral neck and head (Figure 24.5).

The skin is prepped with either chlorohexidine gluconate or betadine. Following this sterile drapes are placed. Following the identification of the location, orientation, and depth of the femoral head and neck, the transducer is placed in a sterile sheath with adequate amount of water-soluble gel. A sterile 3.5-in. spinal needle is introduced either in plane or out of plane depending on individual preference and comfort. Because of the depth of the joint, the needle may not be visualized in its entirety (Figure 24.6).

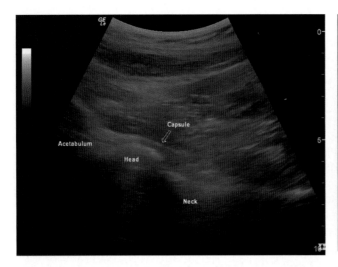

Figure 24.1. Anterior longitudinal ultrasound view of the hip joint showing the head of the femur, neck, acetabulum, and the capsule.

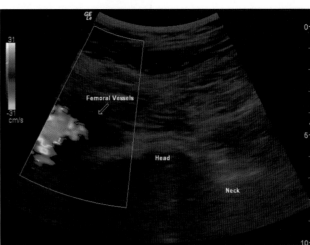

Figure 24.2. Ultrasound view of an internally rotated normal hip joint showing the femoral vessels with color flow Doppler. The transducer was placed more medially than normal to get the vessels and the joint in one view.

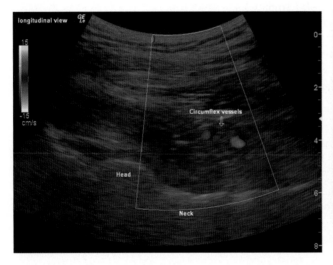

Figure 24.3. Anterior longitudinal sonographic view of the hip joint with color flow Doppler showing the circumflex vessels.

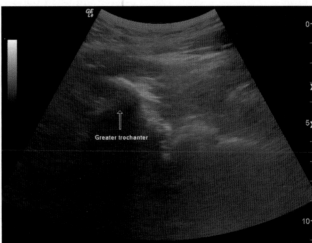

Figure 24.4. Sonographic view of the greater trochanter with the transducer in a lateral and sagittal position.

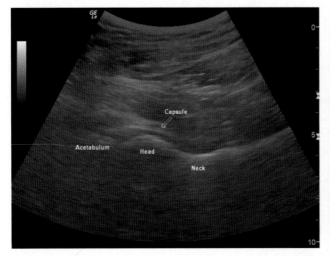

Figure 24.5. Ultrasound view of an arthritic hip showing narrowed joint space and slightly irregular head surface.

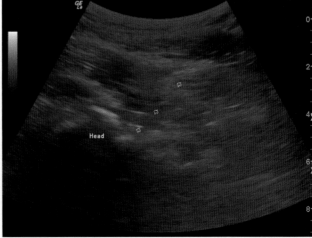

Figure 24.6. Ultrasound view of a severely arthritic hip showing the femoral head as an irregular hyperechoic shadow. The *arrow heads* indicate the 25-G spinal needle.

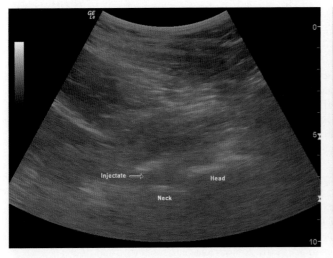

Figure 24.7. Ultrasound view of severely arthritic hip joint with significant destruction of the femoral head, which appears as an uneven discontinuous straight hyperechoic line. The injectate appears as a hypoechoic shadow over the neck.

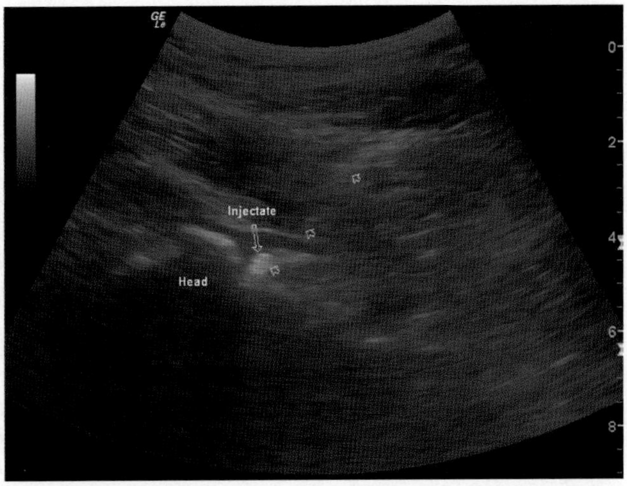

Figure 24.8. Ultrasound view of the hip joint after a steroid injection showing the injectate as a hyperechoic shadow. The *arrow heads* point to the 25-G spinal needle.

Hydrolocalization may permit identification of the location of the tip. Sometimes a distinct "pop" is felt when traversing through the ilio-femoral ligament. The ultrasound view of the femoral head may reveal arthritic changes (Figure 24.7). Injection should be with ease, otherwise suspect placement of needle in the periosteum or the ilio-femoral ligament. During real time injection the local anesthetic and steroid mixture may appear hyperechoic and spreads anteriorly in a nondependent fashion (Figure 24.8).

An alternative lateral approach has been described where the needle is advanced in plane from the lateral side with the patient lying with the affected side up and the transducer placed anteriorly.

Conclusion

Visualization of the target site and the surrounding structures ensures improved patient care and demonstrates evidence for the procedural competency of the operating clinician. Landmark-based and fluoroscopy-guided intra-articular injections although providing some visualization, have attendant risks associated with them. US imaging can safely and effectively provide real-time needle guidance for hip joint injections while avoiding neurovascular injury and radiation exposure.

References

1. Christmas C, Crespo CJ, Franckowiak SC, Bathon JM, Bartlett SJ, Andersen RE. How common is hip pain among older adults? Results from the Third National Health and Nutrition Examination Survey. *J Fam Pract.* 2002;51(4):345–348.
2. Zhang W, Moskowitz RW, Nuki G, et al. OARSI recommendations for the management of hip and knee osteoarthritis, Part II: OARSI evidence-based, expert consensus guidelines. *Osteoarthritis Cartilage.* 2008;16(2):137–162.
3. Leopold SS, Battista V, Oliverio JA. Safety and efficacy of intraarticular hip injection using anatomic landmarks. *Clin Orthop Relat Res.* 2001;391:192–197.
4. Kullenberg B, Runesson R, Tuvhag R, Olsson C, Resch S. Intraarticular corticosteroid injection: pain relief in osteoarthritis of the hip? *J Rheumatol.* 2004;31(11):2265–2268.

5. Brocq O, Tran G, Breuil V, Grisot C, Flory P, Euller-Ziegler L. Hip osteoarthritis: short-term efficacy and safety of viscosupplementation by hylan G-F 20. An open-label study in 22 patients. *Joint Bone Spine*. 2002;69(4):388–391.

6. Santos-Ocampo AS, Santos-Ocampo RS. Non-contrast computed tomography-guided intra-articular corticosteroid injections of severe bilateral hip arthritis in a patient with ankylosing spondylitis. *Clin Exp Rheumatol*. 2003;21(2):239–240.

7. Margules KR. Fluoroscopically directed steroid instillation in the treatment of hip osteoarthritis: safety and efficacy in 510 cases. *Arthritis Rheum*. 2001;44(10):2449–2450. author reply 2455–6.

8. Karim Z, Brown AK, Quinn M, et al. Ultrasound-guided steroid injections in the treatment of hip osteoarthritis: comment on the letter by Margules. *Arthritis Rheum*. 2004;50(1):338–339. author reply 339–40.

9. Crawford RW, Gie GA, Ling RS, Murray DW. Diagnostic value of intra-articular anaesthetic in primary osteoarthritis of the hip. *J Bone Joint Surg Br*. 1998;80(2):279–281.

10. Kleiner JB, Thorne RP, Curd JG. The value of bupivicaine hip injection in the differentiation of coxarthrosis from lower extremity neuropathy. *J Rheumatol*. 1991;18(3):422–427.

11. Neidel J, Boehnke M, Kuster RM. The efficacy and safety of intraarticular corticosteroid therapy for coxitis in juvenile rheumatoid arthritis. *Arthritis Rheum*. 2002;46(6):1620–1628.

12. Robinson P, Keenan AM, Conaghan PG. Clinical effectiveness and dose response of image-guided intra-articular corticosteroid injection for hip osteoarthritis. *Rheumatology (Oxford)*. 2007;46(2):285–291.

13. Fernandez Lopez JC, Ruano-Ravina A. Efficacy and safety of intraarticular hyaluronic acid in the treatment of hip osteoarthritis: a systematic review. *Osteoarthritis Cartilage*. 2001;14(12):1306–1311.

14. Qvistgaard E, Kristoffersen H, Terslev L, Danneskiold-Samsoe B, Torp-Pedersen S, Bliddal H. Guidance by ultrasound of intra-articular injections in the knee and hip joints. *Osteoarthritis Cartilage*. 2001;9(6):512–517.

15. Richette P, Ravaud P, Conrozier T, et al. Effect of hyaluronic acid in symptomatic hip osteoarthritis: a multicenter, randomized, placebo-controlled trial. *Arthritis Rheum*. 2009;60(3):824–830.

16. Sofka CM, Adler RS, Danon MA. Sonography of the acetabular labrum: visualization of labral injuries during intra-articular injections. *J Ultrasound Med*. 2006;25(10):1321–1326.

17. Cavalier R, Herman MJ, Pizzutillo PD, Geller E. Ultrasound-guided aspiration of the hip in children: a new technique. *Clin Orthop Relat Res*. 2003;415:244–247.

18. Sofka CM, Saboeiro G, Adler RS. Ultrasound-guided adult hip injections. *J Vasc Interv Radiol*. 2005;16(8):1121–1123.

19. Berman L, Fink AM, Wilson D, McNally E. Technical note: identifying and aspirating hip effusions. *Br J Radiol*. 1995;68(807):306–310.

20. Smith J, Hurdle MF, Weingarten TN. Accuracy of sonographically guided intra-articular injections in the native adult hip. *J Ultrasound Med*. 2009;28(3):329–335.

21. Caglar-Yagci H, Unsal S, Yagci I, Dulgeroglu D, Ozel S. Safety and efficacy of ultrasound-guided intra-articular hylan G-F 20 injection in osteoarthritis of the hip: a pilot study. *Rheumatol Int*. 2005;25(5):341–344.

22. Migliore A, Tormenta S, Massafra U, et al. 18-month observational study on efficacy of intraarticular hyaluronic acid (Hylan G-F 20) injections under ultrasound guidance in hip osteoarthritis. *Reumatismo*. 2006;58(1):39–49.

23. Pourbagher MA, Ozalay M, Pourbagher A. Accuracy and outcome of sonographically guided intra-articular sodium hyaluronate injections in patients with osteoarthritis of the hip. *J Ultrasound Med*. 2005;24(10):1391–1395.

25

Ultrasound-Guided Knee Injections

Mark-Friedrich B. Hurdle

Introduction

Intra-articular knee injections as well as other peripheral joint injections have been successfully utilized for several decades.[1] Knee injections may be completed for both diagnostic and therapeutic goals. More recently, in 1997 exogenous high molecular weight hyaluronan viscosupplementation was approved to treat knee osteoarthritis in the United States by the FDA.

Limitations of the Current Surface Landmarks Technique

Incorrect placement of hyaluronic acid may lead to increased pain and reduced therapeutic effect.[2] Unlike corticosteroids, hyaluronic acid has little effect if injected in periarticular tissue.[3] While injecting multiple joints and using contrast with follow-up radiographs to determine their accuracy, Jones et al demonstrated that 66% knee joint injections were intra-articular and almost a third of the injections were extra-articular.[4] In a study designed to measure the accuracy of intra-articular knee joint injections, Jackson et al demonstrated

M.-F.B. Hurdle (✉)
Department of Anesthesiology and Pain Medicine, Mayo Clinic,
200 First Street SW, Rochester, MN 55905, USA
e-mail: Hurdle.MarkFriedrich@mayo.edu

S.N. Narouze (ed.), *Atlas of Ultrasound-Guided Procedures in Interventional Pain Management*,
DOI 10.1007/978-1-4419-1681-5_25, © Springer Science+Business Media, LLC 2011

that blind injections through the lateral mid-patellar portal were most accurate 93% of the time while the anterior medial and anterior lateral approaches were only accurate 75% and 71%, respectively.[5] To date there is only one article evaluating the accuracy of ultrasound-guided intra-articular knee injections. Im et al reported 96% accuracy with US guidance vs. 77% accuracy with blind injections.[6]

Technique for Ultrasound-Guided Knee Joint Injection

The patient is placed in the supine position with a pillow or support under the knee so the joint is flexed roughly 30°. A high-frequency linear probe is utilized to scan the suprapatellar and lateral pouches for an effusion (Figures 25.1–25.7). If an effusion is localized, this hypoechioc fluid collection becomes the target for the aspiration and injection. Typically, a subclinical effusion can be visualized under the quadriceps tendon just proximal to the patella. These effusions can be visualized by placing a linear probe on the patella in the transverse position and gently sliding proximally until the quadriceps tendon is visualized (Figure 25.1). By avoiding excessive sono-palpation (compression), subtle effusions can be visualized without blotting out the capsular fluid. Deep to the quadriceps tendon between the quadriceps fat pad and prefemoral fat pad the collapsed joint recess or joint effusion can be visualized in the short axis by turning the probe 90° (Figure 25.2). The probe is kept in the transverse plane while the skin lateral to the probe is palpated (Figure 25.6). Based on this tissue movement with palpation lateral to the probe under US visualization, a needle pathway is predetermined to avoid having to stick a needle through the quadriceps tendon. This area is then marked and prepped in a sterile fashion. Drapes are then applied. To minimize pain, a 25–27-gauge needle is used to administer lidocaine subcutaneously. Next a 22- or 25-gauge needle is advanced into the joint recess or effusion.

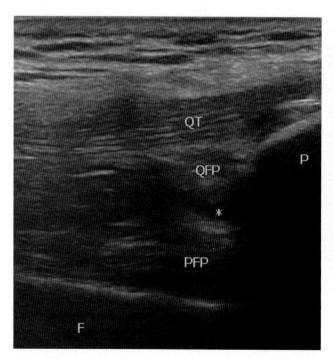

Figure 25.1. Long-axis view of the proximal anterior knee with a subclinical effusion (*asterisk*). QT quadriceps tendon, P patella, QFP quadriceps fat pad, PFP prefemoral fat pad, F femur.

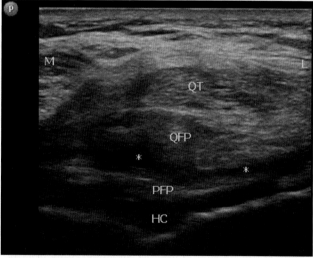

Figure 25.2. Short-axis view of the proximal anterior knee with a subclinical effusion (*asterisks*) in the suprapatellar pouch. QT quadriceps tendon, P patella, QFP quadriceps fat pad, PFP prefemoral fat pad, HC hypoechoic hyaline cartilage.

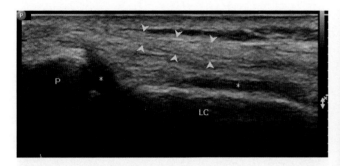

Figure 25.3. Transverse view on the lateral side of the patella. *Arrowheads* lateral patellar retinaculum, *P* patella, *LC* lateral femoral condyle, *asterisks* collapsed joint space.

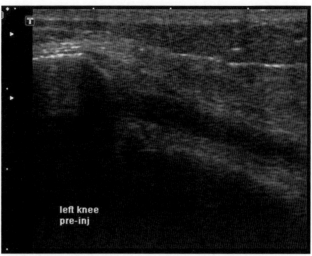

Figure 25.4. Transverse view of the lateral pouch with a well-defined effusion.

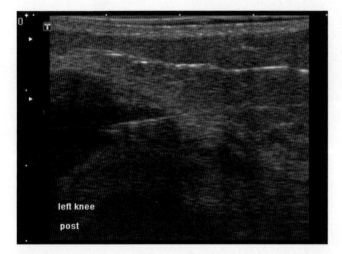

Figure 25.5. Transverse view of lateral patella and a needle placed in the medial portion of the lateral pouch.

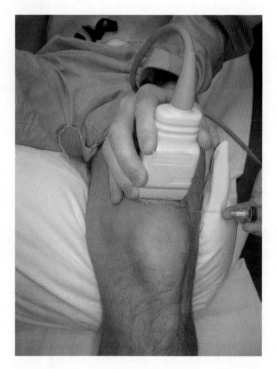

Figure 25.6. Short-axis approach to the suprapatellar pouch from lateral to medial.

A test dose containing 1–2 ml of local anesthetic can be utilized to confirm proper intra-synovial needle tip placement. Fluoroscopic confirmation can also be obtained with a lateral view of the knee joint (Figure 25.7). There should be minimal resistance while 2–6 ml of viscosupplementation or corticosteroid is injected. A medial patellar approach was also described with the knee fully extended[6] (Figures 25.8 and 25.9).

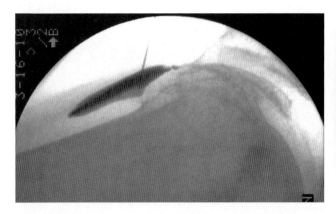

Figure 25.7. Fluoroscopic confirmation of suprapatellar pouch approach under US guidance.

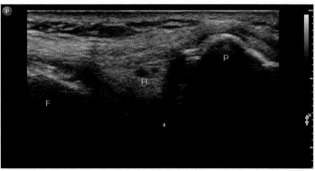

Figure 25.8. Transverse view of mid-medial patella. Site of the medial patellar portal approach described by Im. *F* femur, *H* Hoffa's fat pad, *P* patella, *asterisk* joint space.

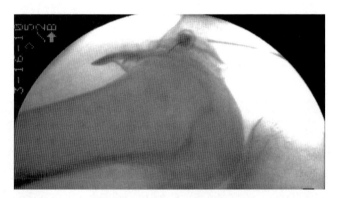

Figure 25.9. Fluoroscopically confirmed patellofemoral approach with contrast flowing freely between the patella and femur.

Conclusion

In conclusion, blind knee injections are relatively accurate in skilled hands. However, when a definitive diagnosis is needed, synovial fluid is required or viscosupplementation is utilized, guided injections should be seriously considered.

References

1. Hollander JL, Brown EM Jr, Jessar RA, Brown CY. Hydrocortisone and cortisone injected into arthritic joints: comparative effects of and use of hydrocortisone as a local antiarthritic agent. *J Am Med Assoc.* 1951;147(17):1629–1635.
2. Lussier A, Cividino AA, McFarlane CA, Olszynski WP, Potashner WJ, De Medicis R. Viscosupplementation with hylan for the treatment of osteoarthritis: findings from clinical practice in Canada. *J Rheumatol.* 1996;23(9):1579–1585.
3. Bliddal H. Placement of intra-articular injections verified by mini air-arthrography. *Ann Rheum Dis.* 1999;58(10):641–643.
4. Jones A, Regan M, Ledingham J, Pattrick M, Manhire A, Doherty M. Importance of placement of intra-articular steroid injections. *BMJ.* 1993;307(6915):1329–1330.
5. Jackson DW, Evans NA, Thomas BM. Accuracy of needle placement into the intra-articular space of the knee. *J Bone Joint Surg Am.* 2002;84-A(9):1522–1527.
6. Im SH, Lee SC, Park YB, Cho SR, Kim JC. Feasibility of sonography for intra-articular injections in the knee through a medial patellar portal. *J Ultrasound Med.* 2009;28(11):1465–1470.

VI

Advanced and New Applications of Ultrasound in Pain Management

26

Ultrasound-Guided Peripheral Nerve Stimulation

Marc A. Huntoon

Introduction

Peripheral nerve stimulation (PNS) is currently a topic of increased interest after decades of apparent decline. Some of this increased popularity can be attributed to the advent of new imaging techniques, including ultrasound. Two recent feasibility studies in fresh cadavers suggested that ultrasound (US) could be used to place electrodes without apparent nerve injury next to peripheral nerves, similar to nerve catheter placement.[1,2] These reports were followed by a small case series of patients receiving permanent implants, with generally good outcomes. US-guided placement allowed a percutaneous trial, preventing incision in

M.A. Huntoon (✉)
Department of Anesthesiology, Division of Pain Medicine, Mayo Clinic,
200 1st Street SW, Rochester, MN, USA
e-mail: Huntoon.Marc@mayo.edu

S.N. Narouze (ed.), *Atlas of Ultrasound-Guided Procedures in Interventional Pain Management*,
DOI 10.1007/978-1-4419-1681-5_26, © Springer Science+Business Media, LLC 2011

nonresponders, and in many cases produced durable analgesia beyond 1 year. Percutaneous leads designed for spinal cord stimulation placed via US allowed the intraoperative testing of multiple different stimulation parameters. US visualization also allowed electrode placement superior or inferior to the nerve, or even two parallel leads placed abreast of the nerve.[3]

Historical uses of PNS came about after publishing of the gate control theory.[4] Wall and Sweet's initial experiments with PNS essentially sought to put "gate control" to the test.[5] Early studies by multiple authors were promising, yet technical difficulties and patient selection problems were common.[6–9] Due to declining interest, lead design/technical improvement for peripheral nerve leads has lagged behind the comparative technical advances for spinal cord stimulation leads over the last two decades. Early versions of cuff electrodes and button electrodes have been largely replaced by the current commercial leads (flat lead with four circular contacts). Neurosurgical open procedures will likely continue to be the predominant method of placement of these devices. Whether the US-guided technique will serve as a method of trial only, will allow permanent placement in some anatomical areas, or will help develop the evidence basis for PNS remains to be answered.

Current Evidence

There are no major prospective studies to date, which has been chronicled recently by Bittar and Teddy.[10] Davis lamented this lack of evidence in an editorial on the subject of peripheral neuromodulation.[11] Questions regarding the role of neurolysis on the analgesia seen after PNS, placebo effects, physical therapy effects, analgesic drug changes, or merely increased attention to the patients' needs were all raised as possible confounding factors. The largest clinical series in print, are those from Eisenberg et al,[12] and the Cleveland Clinic.[9] In Eisenberg's series, 46 patients with isolated painful neuropathies received PNS. They reported good results in 78% of patients with 22% poor. Visual analog pain scores decreased from 69 ± 12 prior to surgery to 24 ± 28 postoperatively.[12] Four major etiologies were identified: nerve lesions following operation around the hip or knee; entrapment neuropathy; pain following nerve graft; or painful neuropathy after traumatic nerve injection.[12] In the Cleveland Clinic series, the most notable result was the high requirement for surgical revision; a mean of 1.6 operations per patient.[9] In some cases, a neuroma may be the cause of the neuropathic pain (Figure 26.1).

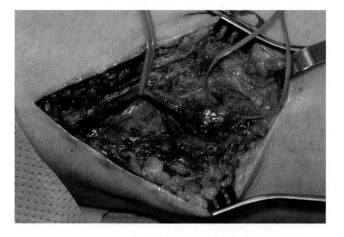

Figure 26.1. A peroneal nerve is depicted with large neuroma. Photo courtesy of Spinner, Robert J., M.D. Mayo Clinic

Patient Selection and Role of Neurolysis

Patient selection for peripheral nerve procedures is of paramount importance. It is important to properly diagnose the condition, as many disorders are categorized as complex regional pain or "neuropathic pain" due to imprecise terminology. Sympathetically maintained syndromes may respond well to PNS implants, particularly if the pain is predominately in one nerve distribution.[8,9] Pain that is resistant to previous surgical procedure such as transposition of the nerve, or a neuroma in continuity with good functional preservation are other possible candidates. Pain that persists despite previous external or internal neurolysis may also be good candidates. Patients should have previously failed good pharmacologic therapy with standard neuromodulatory drugs. External neurolysis refers to the removal of scar tissue around the nerve in circumferential fashion. If entrapment of the nerve is seen it is mobilized and freed. External neurolysis poses little risk of fascicular injury. Nerve action potentials can be utilized to better assess nerve function than clinical or standard EMG/nerve conduction studies. Internal neurolysis can be used for pain syndromes, especially if incomplete loss of nerve function distally is present. The risk of fascicular injury or disruption is higher with internal neurolysis.[13]

Anatomical Considerations

One issue that complicates any peripheral nerve electrode placement in the four extremities is that nerves must freely glide within fascial/muscle planes along with their vascular supply as the extremity moves. Nerves can be entrapped by scar tissue, and the rough edges of an external electrode could, over time, cause constriction and scarring. Mixed peripheral nerves are also characterized by a complex internal fascicular arrangement. Briefly, nerve trunks may have sensory, motor, and mixed axons at various locations within the peripheral nerve. This complex cross-sectional anatomical configuration means that optimal stimulation of the desired sensory fascicle might, for example, be at the medial aspect of the ulnar nerve in a supra-condylar placement, but change location within a matter of a few millimeters to a posterior location. If the amplitude of stimulation is too high above sensory threshold, motor fascicles deeper within the trunk may easily be activated causing muscle cramping and/or pain. A recent study looked at these issues more closely; specifically, the effects of the fascicle perineural thickness, diameter, and position within the nerve trunk on axonal excitation thresholds and neural recruitment. A model of human femoral nerve within a nerve circumferential cuff electrode was studied. The study showed that stimulation of target fascicles is strongly dependent upon the cross-sectional anatomy of the nerve being stimulated. The mean thickness of perineurium was $3.0 \pm 1.0\%$ of the fascicle diameter. Increased thickness of the human perineurium or larger fascicle diameter increases the threshold for electrical activation. If a large neighbor fascicle was present, it could also effect stimulation activation of the target fascicle by as much as $80 \pm 11\%$.[14]

Radial Nerve Stimulation

The radial nerve is very close to the lateral surface of the humerus at a point 10–14 cm proximal to the lateral epicondyle. The nerve is scaphoid shaped and superficial enough to be seen reasonably well under US. Ultrasound scanning usually begins at the elbow and, with the probe in a transverse orientation to the arm, continues proximally until the desired approach is identified. The needle can be advanced in-plane with the transducer to lie between the nerve and humerus. The lateral head of the triceps muscle is overlying the nerve here, and although one would desire to avoid transgression of large amounts of muscular tissue, there is no more optimal approach to the nerve in a superficial location above the humerus. Vascular structures including the profunda brachii artery and recurrent radial artery branch may be in anatomic proximity and should be scanned, as one would desire to avoid injuries to these structures.[14] The electrode(s) may be anchored in the superficial fascia of the triceps muscle. A tension loop at the site where the electrode exits the muscle is also desirable. Generator placement should be as close as possible to the leads to eliminate traction and lead migration. The fascicular arrangement of the radial nerve may not be favorable for the stimulation of more distal pain syndromes, e.g., the distal radial nerve sensory branch in locations above the elbow. In one patient in the first case series of US-guided stimulator placement, for example,[3] the patient's threshold between sensory and motor activation was too narrow to be therapeutic. A de Quervain's tenosynovectomy, for example, may have caused injury to the superficial distal radial branch nerve. Thus, a better approach to stimulate this distal radial branch was in the mid-forearm, immediately deep to the brachioradialis muscle. Ultimately, the patient above[3] required open placement of a flat electrode at the distal superficial radial branch to improve her analgesia. Open operative findings included perineural scarring and neuroma. This branch could have been visualized with ultrasound near the radial artery where imaging may be improved by using color flow Doppler.

Ulnar Nerve

The ulnar nerve is very near the surface of the skin, superficial to the medial head of the triceps muscle. In the recent anatomical feasibility studies,[1,2] the nerve was identified at a point 9–13 cm proximal to the medial epicondyle in the medial/posterior arm, a location in which it was usually easily identifiable and also in close proximity to the humerus. Ultrasound scanning can commence at the elbow and, with the probe in a transverse orientation to the arm, continue to scan more proximally until the nerve fascicular arrangements can be well identified. The needle may be advanced from posterior to anterior on the medial aspect of the arm to lie between nerve and humerus, staying superficial to the medial head of the triceps. Often, patients with ulnar nerve pain syndromes such as cubital tunnel syndrome status- post failed transposition surgery may be good candidates. In these cases, the nerve may have already been surgically transposed, making it more easily identifiable. US may allow large neuromas to be visualized. The nerve passes into the cubital tunnel after passing into the ulnar groove behind the medial epicondyle. The cubital tunnel is formed by the aponeurotic arch of the flexor carpi ulnaris as its ceiling where the aponeurosis attaches to the medial epicondyle and olecranon, with the floor formed by the medial ligaments of the elbow and the flexor digitorum profundus muscle.[14] This area is a potential area of compression of the nerve.

Median Nerve

The median nerve enters the antecubital fossa medial to the biceps muscle and its tendon, and next to the brachial artery. The artery serves as a good landmark to scan the neurovascular bundle, identify the median nerve, and continue to scan distally. In the upper forearm at a point approximately 4–6 cm distal to the antecubital crease, the nerve passes between the two heads of the pronator teres muscle, and then passes under the sublimis bridge of the two heads of the flexor digitorum superficialis (Figure 26.2). There are numerous potential neural fascicular communications between the median and ulnar nerves which are often in the forearm. The most important one is the Martin-Gruber anastomosis. Most of these Martin-Gruber anastomoses involve fibers from the median nerve passing to the

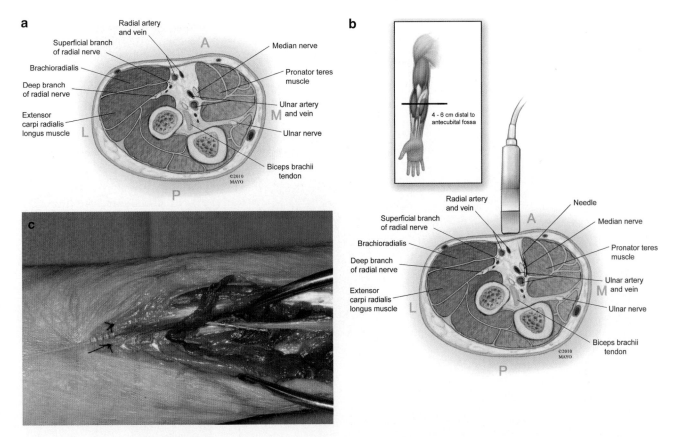

Figure 26.2. (a) Cross-sectional anatomy of median nerve approximately 4–6 cm distal to antecubital fossa in upper forearm. (b) A long axis in-plane US approach to the median nerve is depicted, keeping the needle and electrode closer to the muscle and avoiding the ulnar artery. (c) Fresh cadaver dissection after US-guided electrode placement. Anatomical entry site approximately 4–6 cm distal to the antecubital fossa (anchor sutured to superficial fascia) showing a lead placed longitudinally and lying anterior to the median nerve.

ulnar nerve, with the reverse much less common. Other anomalous connections may exist as well. Interestingly, the very first series of PNS[5] likely involved some type of abnormal connection, with both median and ulnar sensory distributions being stimulated by the application of stimulation to the ulnar nerve.

Median nerve stimulation may be accomplished either superior to the elbow, or inferior. Stimulation below the elbow might encounter one of these aberrant anastomoses, or stimulate the nerve between the pronator heads where compression may be more likely.

Sciatic Nerve at Popliteal Bifurcation

The common peroneal nerve may be identified at its branch point from the sciatic nerve, a point 6–12 cm proximal to the popliteal crease. Ultrasound scanning usually commences at the popliteal crease and, with the probe in a transverse orientation to the leg, continued proximally until the desired nerve is identified. Either transverse or longitudinal placement can be utilized, with transverse placement being more forgiving of movement, but a greater number of possible electrodes contacting the nerves with longitudinal placement. Location of the popliteal artery is noted to avoid vascular puncture during electrode placement. The needle may be advanced from posterolateral to anteromedial in a slightly oblique plane, attempting to avoid passing through the biceps femoris muscle (Figure 26.3). The area distal to the bifurcation of the sciatic nerve, a short distance beyond the tibial

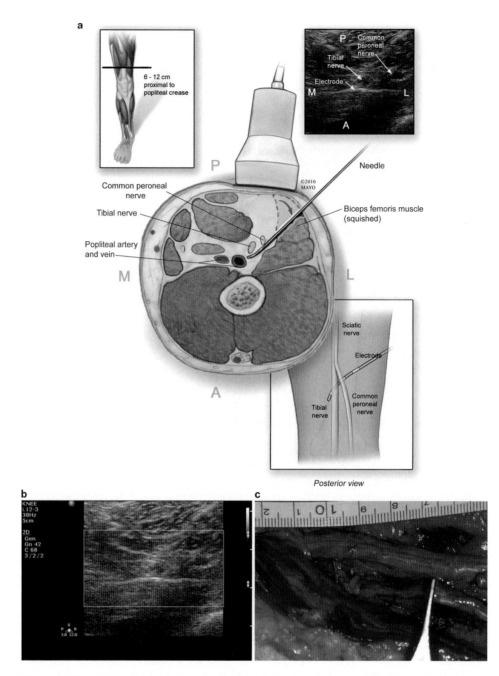

Figure 26.3. (a) Cross-sectional anatomy and technique of short-axis US visualization, with perpendicular electrode placement to cover both the tibial and common peroneal nerves. (b) An enlarged view of US view in (a). (c) Anatomical dissection of electrode placement just distal to sciatic bifurcation similar to (a) and (b) but passing between the tibial and common peroneal (CP) nerves. Note that two electrical contacts can be seen under the tibial and common peroneal nerve branches. The forceps are on the CP more distally.

branch is reasonably easily seen with ultrasound. The electrode can be anchored on the fascia of the biceps femoris muscle. During anatomical feasibility studies, the area near the fibular head was also evaluated for potential US-guided placements, but there is very little room to maneuver anatomically, and current leads are not well designed for this area. Supramalleolar areas may be attractive sites to target the superficial peroneal nerve, but have not yet been attempted.

Posterior Tibial Nerve

The posterior tibial nerve can also be approached more distally in the leg. Approximately 8–14 cm proximal to the medial malleolus, the nerve is in close proximity to the tibialis posterior muscle, the digitorum profundus, one or two large veins, and the flexor hallucis longus. Ultrasound scanning usually begins at the ankle near the medial malleolus, with the probe in a transverse orientation to the leg, then continued proximally until the desired approach is identified. Location of the posterior tibial artery is noted to avoid vascular puncture during electrode placement. The needle may be advanced from anterior to posterior along the medial aspect of the ankle to lie just superficial (or deep) to the nerve. Care should be taken to minimize trauma to surrounding tissues and avoid transgression of these muscular structures. The pulse generator may be placed superficial to the fascia of the medial gastrocnemius muscle.

Conclusion

PNS may be accomplished using minimally invasive guidance. In general, performing permanent implantations should continue to be done in open fashion until both significant clinical experience is accomplished, and long-term outcomes are clearer. Future prospective double blinded studies and development of new electrodes may be helpful in furthering this minimally invasive technique.

References

1. Huntoon MA, Hoelzer BC, Burgher AH, Hurdle MFB, Huntoon EA. Feasibility of ultrasound guided percutaneous placement of peripheral nerve stimulation electrodes and anchoring during simulated movement: part two, upper extremity. *Reg Anesth Pain Med.* 2008;33:558–565.
2. Huntoon MA, Huntoon EA, Obray JB, Lamer TJ. Feasibility of ultrasound guided percutaneous placement of peripheral nerve stimulation electrodes in a cadaver model: part one, lower extremity. *Reg Anesth Pain Med.* 2008;33:551–557.
3. Huntoon MA, Burgher AH. Ultrasound-guided permanent implantation of peripheral nerve stimulation (pns) system for neuropathic pain of the extremities: original cases and outcomes. *Pain Med.* 2009;10:1369–1377.
4. Melzack R, Wall PD. Pain mechanisms: a new theory. *Science.* 1965;150:971–979.
5. Wall PD, Sweet WH. Temporary abolition of pain in man. *Science.* 1967;155:108–109.
6. Nashold BS, Goldner JL, Mullen JB, Bright DS. Long-term pain control by direct peripheral nerve stimulation. *J Bone Joint Surg Am.* 1982;64:1–10.
7. Strege DW, Cooney WP, Wood MB, Johnson SJ, Metcalf BJ. Chronic peripheral nerve pain treated with direct electrical nerve stimulation. *J Hand Surg (Am).* 1994;19:931.
8. Hassenbusch SJ, Stanton-Hicks M, Schoppa D, Walsh JG, Covington EC. Long-term results of peripheral nerve stimulation for reflex sympathetic dystrophy. *J Neurosurg.* 1996;84:415–423.
9. Stanton-Hicks M, Rauck RL, Hendrickson M, Racz G. Miscellaneous and experimental therapies. In: Wilson PR, Stanton-Hicks M, Harden RN, eds. *CRPS: Current Diagnosis and Therapy, Progress in Pain Research and Management,* vol. 32. Seattle: IASP Press; 2005.
10. Bittar RG, Teddy PJ. Peripheral neuromodulation for pain. *J Clin Neurosci.* 2009;16(10): 1259–1261.
11. Davis GA. Commentary: peripheral neuromodulation for pain. *J Clin Neurosci.* 2009;16:1262.
12. Eisenberg E, Waisbrod H, Gerbershagen HU. Long-term peripheral nerve stimulation for painful nerve injuries. *Clin J Pain.* 2004;20:143–146.
13. Spinner RJ, Kline DG. Surgery for peripheral nerve and brachial plexus injuries or other nerve lesions. *Muscle Nerve.* 2000;23:680–695.
14. Grinberg Y, Schiefer MA, Tyler DJ, Gustafson KJ. Fascicular perineurium thickness, size, and position affect model predictions of neural excitation. *IEEE Trans Neural Syst Rehabil Eng.* 2008;16:572–581.

27

Ultrasound-Guided Occipital Stimulation

Samer N. Narouze

Introduction

Occipital neurostimulation (ONS) or greater occipital nerve (GON) stimulation offers the potential for a minimally invasive, low risk, and reversible approach to manage intractable headache disorders. It has been used successfully in the treatment of occipital neuralgia, migraine, cluster headache, and other headache disorders.[1-3]

S.N. Narouze (✉)
Center for Pain Medicine, Summa Western Reserve Hospital,
1900 23rd Street, Cuyahoga Falls, OH 44223, USA
e-mail: narouzs@hotmail.com

S.N. Narouze (ed.), *Atlas of Ultrasound-Guided Procedures in Interventional Pain Management*,
DOI 10.1007/978-1-4419-1681-5_27, © Springer Science+Business Media, LLC 2011

Limitations of the Current ONS Technique

The major technical problem with ONS other than lead migration is stimulation-induced neck muscle spasm, which is very uncomfortable and painful.[4] This depends on the level as well as the depth of the implanted lead, which cannot be controlled by fluoroscopy. On the contrary, the author found that ultrasonography is very valuable in identifying subcutaneous tissue, various muscle layers, and the GON can be easily seen at the C1-2 level between the inferior oblique muscle (IOM) and the semispinalis capitis (SSC)[5] (Figure 27.1).

Anatomy of the GON

The GON arises from C2 dorsal ramus and curves around the inferior border of the IOM to ascend on its superficial surface. Then it penetrates the SSC and invariably the splenius muscle to end subcutaneously near the nuchal line by penetrating the trapezius muscle or the fascia.[6–8]

The classical technique for occipital nerve stimulation describes lead placement in the subcutaneous tissues at C1 level.[1] Traditionally, the lead is placed with fluoroscopy and if the lead is too superficial one may experience unpleasant dysthesias in the overlying skin area, and if placed deep, it may invariably penetrate the occipital muscles, which usually leads to painful muscle spasms upon stimulation (Figure 27.2).

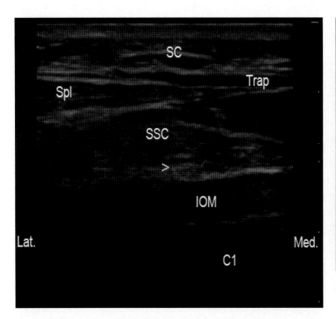

Figure 27.1. Short-axis sonogram at C1 level showing the greater occipital nerve (*arrow head*). *IOM* inferior oblique muscle, *SSC* semispinalis capitis, *Spl* splenius muscle, *Trap* trapezius muscle, *SC* subcutaneous tissue, *Med.* medial, *Lat.* lateral. Note at this level, the GON is more than 1 cm deep to the subcutaneous tissue (the semispinalis capitis muscle is inbetween). Reprinted with permission, Cleveland Clinic Center for Medical Art & Photography© 2009–2010. All rights reserved.

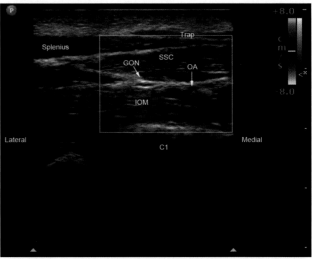

Figure 27.2. Another short axis sonogram at C1 level showing the greater occipital nerve (*arrow*) and an occipital artery branch (OA). *IOM* inferior oblique muscle, *SSC* semispinalis capitis. Note at C1 level, the GON is separated from the subcutaneous tissue by the semispinalis capitis (SSC) muscle.

Occipital Field Stimulation vs. Peripheral Nerve Stimulation

Ultrasound-guided technique will enable the lead to be placed subcutaneously near the nuchal line where the GON is superficial without intervening muscle. As one cannot reliably visualize the GON at the nuchal line level and the lead is placed subcutaneously, we refer to this approach as "occipital field stimulation." On the other hand, the GON can be recognized and the lead can be placed intentionally between the inferior oblique and semispinalis muscle (where the nerve runs) at C1-2 level. In the latter case, the GON can be stimulated with minimal settings and this can save the life of the battery; however, any attempt at increasing the stimulation will result in muscle stimulations and spasms. We refer to this latter approach as "occipital PNS" (Figure 27.3).

Technique of US-Guided ONS Lead Implant

The procedure is performed with the patient in the prone position (for bilateral leads) or lateral decubitus (for unilateral leads), using a high-frequency ultrasound transducer (low-frequency transducer may be used depending on body habitus). A transverse short axis view is obtained by applying the transducer in the midline over the occiput and then scanning caudally to identify C1-2 level. C1 lacks a spinous process and the first bifid spinous process encountered is C2.

Then the transducer is moved laterally to identify the various layers of the suboccipital muscles and the GON can be easily visualized between the SSC and the IOM (Figures 27.1 and 27.2). The needle is then introduced in-plane and the lead is navigated in the plane between the SSC and IOM (Figure 27.2). This can be confirmed with fluoroscopy if needed (Figure 27.4). On stimulation, the patient will feel paresthesias in the

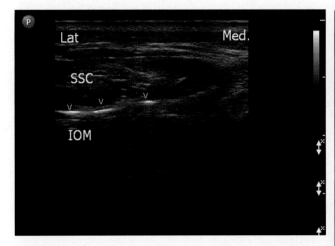

Figure 27.3. Short axis sonogram at C1 level showing the lead (*arrow heads*) placed between the semispinalis capitis (SSC) muscle and the inferior oblique muscle (IOM). *Med.* medial, *Lat.* lateral. Reprinted with permission, Cleveland Clinic Center for Medical Art & Photography© 2009–2010. All rights reserved.

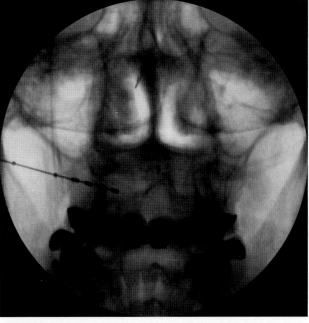

Figure 27.4. Fluoroscopic confirmation of the lead placement for greater occipital nerve stimulation. Reprinted with permission, Ohio Pain and Headache Institute.

distribution of the GON at minimal settings (PNS stimulation) compared to the subcutaneously placed lead (field stimulation), which usually require much higher settings that deplete the battery sooner.

REFERENCES

1. Weiner RL, Reed KL. Peripheral neurostimulation for control of intractable occipital neuralgia. *Neuromodulation*. 1999;2:217–221.
2. Kapural L, Mekhail N, Hayek SM, Stanton-Hicks M, Malak O. Occipital nerve electrical stimulation via the midline approach and subcutaneous surgical leads for treatment of severe occipital neuralgia: a pilot study. *Anesth Analg*. 2005;101:171–174.
3. Schwedt TJ, Dodick DW, Hentz J, Trentman TL, Zimmerman RS. Occipital nerve stimulation for chronic headache: long-term safety and efficacy. *Cephalalgia*. 2007;27:153–157.
4. Hayek SM, Jasper J, Deer TR, Narouze S. Occipital neurostimulation-induced muscle spasms: implications for lead placement. *Pain Physician*. 2009;12(5):867–876.
5. Narouze S. Ultrasonography in pain medicine: future directions. *Tech Reg Anesth Pain Manag*. 2009;13(3):198–202.
6. Mosser SW, Guyuron B, Janis JE, Rohrich RJ. The anatomy of the greater occipital nerve: implications for the etiology of migraine headaches. *Plast Reconstr Surg*. 2004;113:693–697.
7. Becser N, Bovim G, Sjaastad O. Extracranial nerves in the posterior part of the head. Anatomic variations and their possible clinical significance. *Spine*. 1998;23:1435–1441.
8. Bovim G, Bonamico L, Fredriksen TA, Lindboe CF, Stolt-Nielsen A, Sjaastad O. Topographic variations in the peripheral course of the greater occipital nerve. Autopsy study with clinical correlations. *Spine*. 1991;16:475–478.

28

Ultrasound-Guided Groin Stimulation

Samer N. Narouze

Introduction

Groin neurostimulation or ilioinguinal, iliohypogastric, and genitofemoral nerve stimulation offers the potential for a minimally invasive, low risk, and reversible approach to manage intractable neuropathic pain in the groin and pelvic areas.[1] Recently, the author has been using groin neurostimulation successfully in the treatment of postherniorrhaphy neuropathic pain.

S.N. Narouze (✉)
Center for Pain Medicine, Summa Western Reserve Hospitals,
1900 23rd Street, Cuyahoga Falls, OH 44223, USA
e-mail: narouzs@hotmail.com

S.N. Narouze (ed.), *Atlas of Ultrasound-Guided Procedures in Interventional Pain Management*,
DOI 10.1007/978-1-4419-1681-5_28, © Springer Science+Business Media, LLC 2011

Limitations of the Current Technique

The procedure is performed either blindly with the help of surface landmarks or under fluoroscopy. In both techniques, the depth of the lead placement cannot be reliably determined. If superficial, the patient will feel unpleasant burning sensations in the skin, and if deep in the muscles, the patient will have painful muscle contractions and lack of efficacy from the stimulation.

Anatomy of the Ilioinguinal and Iliohypogastric Nerves

Please refer to Chapter 16 on ultrasound-guided blocks for pelvic pain.

Groin Field Stimulation vs. Peripheral Nerve Stimulation

Ultrasound-guided technique will enable the lead to be placed subcutaneously superficial to the abdominal muscles; this technique is called "groin field stimulation." In this case, the patient usually feels paresthesias only in the groin area and this may help in cases with neuroma formation in the surgical scar after herniorrhaphy.

On the other hand, the plane between the internal oblique muscle (IOM) and transversus abdominis muscle (TAM) (the IL and IH nerves run in this plane) can be recognized and the lead can be placed intentionally in this plane between the two muscle layers; this is called "ilioinguinal/iliohypogastric peripheral nerve stimulation (PNS)." In this latter scenario, upon stimulation, the patient will feel paresthesias along the territory of the nerves and down into the testicle. We prefer this approach in cases of ilioinguinal entrapment neuropathy with testicular pains.

Technique of Ultrasound-Guided IL/IH PNS Lead Implant

The procedure is performed with the patient in the supine position, using a high-frequency linear ultrasound transducer (low-frequency curved transducer may be used depending on body habitus). A transverse short-axis view is obtained by applying the transducer over the groin area just medial to the anterior superior iliac spine.

Then the transducer is moved medially to identify the various layers of the abdominal wall muscles (Figure 28.1). Sometimes the ilioinguinal and iliohypogastric nerves can be recognized between the IOM and the TAM (see Chap. 21). The needle is then introduced in-plane and the lead is navigated in the plane between the IOM and TAM (Figure 28.2). This can also be confirmed with fluoroscopy (Figure 28.3). On stimulation, the patient will feel paresthesias in the distribution of the IL/IH at minimal settings "PNS stimulation" compared to the subcutaneously placed lead "field stimulation" (Figure 28.2).

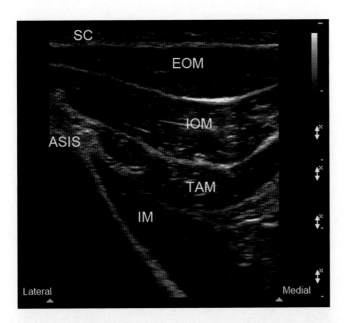

Figure 28.1. Short-axis sonogram of the right groin at the level of the anterior superior iliac spine (ASIS). *SC* subcutaneous tissue, *EOM* external oblique muscle, *IOM* internal oblique muscle, *TAM* transversus abdominus muscle, *IM* iliacus muscle. Reproduced with permission from Ohip pain and Headache Institute. Reprinted with permission, Ohio Pain and Headache Institute.

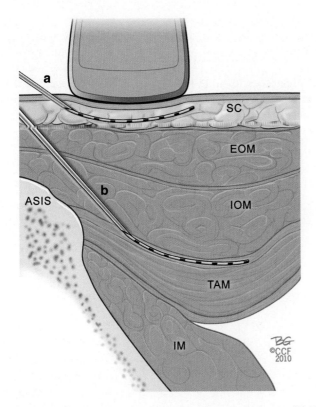

Figure 28.2. (a) Subcutaneous lead placement for groin "field" stimulation. (b) "PNS" lead placement in the plane between the internal oblique muscle (IOM) and the transversus abdominus muscle (TAM). *ASIS* anterior superior iliac spine, *SC* subcutaneous tissue, *EOM* external oblique muscle, *IM* iliacus muscle. Reprinted with permission, Cleveland Clinic Center for Medical Art & Photography© 2010. All rights reserved.

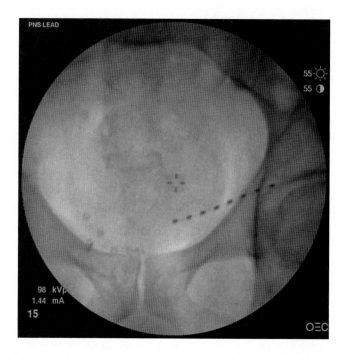

Figure 28.3. Fluoroscopic confirmation of the lead placement for ilioinguinal and iliohypogastric nerve stimulation. Reprinted with permission, Ohio Pain and Headache Institute.

REFERENCE

1. Rauchwerger JJ, Giordano J, Rozen D, Kent JL, Greenspan J, Closson CW. On the therapeutic viability of peripheral nerve stimulation for ilioinguinal neuralgia: putative mechanisms and possible utility. *Pain Pract.* 2008;8(2):138–143.

29

Ultrasound-Guided Atlanto-Axial and Atlanto-Occipital Joint Injections

Samer N. Narouze

Introduction

The atlanto-axial joint accounts for up to 16% of patients with occipital headache. In human volunteers, distending the lateral atlanto-axial joint with contrast agent produces occipital pain and injection of local anesthetic into the joint relieves the headache.[1,2]

The clinical presentation of atlanto-axial joint pain is not specific and therefore cannot be used alone to establish the diagnosis. The only means of establishing a definite diagnosis is a diagnostic block with intra-articular injection of local anesthetic.[1]

Intra-articular steroids are effective in short-term relief of pain originating from the lateral atlanto-axial joint.[3]

S.N. Narouze (✉)
Center for Pain Medicine, Summa Western Reserve Hospital,
1900 23rd Street, Cuyahoga Falls, OH 44223, USA
e-mail: narouzs@hotmail.com

S.N. Narouze (ed.), *Atlas of Ultrasound-Guided Procedures in Interventional Pain Management*,
DOI 10.1007/978-1-4419-1681-5_29, © Springer Science+Business Media, LLC 2011

Anatomy of the Atlanto-Axial and Atlanto-Occipital Joints

Atlanto-axial and atlanto-occipital joint intra-articular injections have the potential for serious complications; so it is imperative to be familiar with the anatomy of those joints in relation to the surrounding vascular and neural structures. The vertebral artery lies lateral to the atlanto-axial joint as it courses through the C2 and C1 foramina. Then it curves medially to go through the foramen magnum crossing the medial posterior aspect of the atlanto-occipital joint.

The C2 dorsal root ganglion and nerve root with its surrounding dural sleeve cross the posterior aspect of the middle of the joint. Therefore, during atlanto-axial joint injection, the needle should be directed toward the posterolateral aspect of the joint. This will avoid injury to the C2 nerve root medially or the vertebral artery laterally. On the other hand, the atlanto-occipital joint should be accessed from the most superior posterior lateral aspect to avoid the vertebral artery medially. Meticulous attention should be paid to avoid intravascular injection as the anatomy may be variable. Inadvertent puncture of the C2 dural sleeve with CSF leak or high spinal spread of the local anesthetic may occur with atlanto-axial joint injection if the needle is directed only few millimeters medially.[4]

Ultrasound allows visualization of soft tissues, nerves, and vessels (abnormal anatomy), which has the potential to improve the safety of atlanto-axial and atlanto-occipital joint injections by decreasing the incidence or by avoiding injury of nearby structures.[5]

Ultrasound-Guided Atlanto-Axial and Atlanto-Occipital Joint Injection Technique

The procedure is performed with the patient in the prone position, using a high-frequency ultrasound transducer (low-frequency transducer may be used depending on body habitus). A transverse short-axis view is obtained by applying the transducer in the midline over the occiput and then scanning caudally to identify C1-2 level. C1 lacks a spinous process and the first bifid spinous process encountered is C2.

Then the transducer is moved laterally till the C2 nerve root and dorsal root ganglion (DRG) is seen, more laterally the C1-2 joint (AA joint) appears in the image between the C2 DRG medially and the vertebral artery laterally (Figures 29.1–29.3). The transducer is adjusted so that the AA joint is in the middle of the picture and a 22-gauge blunt-tip needle is advanced usually out-of-plane under real-time ultrasound guidance to target the AA joint just medial to the vertebral artery (Figure 29.4). The transducer is then shifted to obtain a longitudinal scan at the C1-2 joint and the needle tip may need to be adjusted slightly to enter the joint cavity under vision.[6]

Alternatively, a longitudinal midline scan can be obtained by applying the transducer vertically in the midline over the occiput and cervical spinous processes and C1-2 level is identified as above. Then the transducer is moved laterally till the C1-2 joint (AA joint) appears in the image, slightly laterally one can identify the vertebral artery. The needle is introduced just caudal to the transducer and advanced in-plane under real-time ultrasound guidance to target the AA joint just medial to the vertebral artery (the same approach described for cervical facet intra-articular injection, Chap. 7).

The author prefers the short-axis view (although, it is out of plan approach) as in the same image one can see the needle advancement – with real time ultrasonography – into the joint between the C2 DRG medially and the vertebral artery laterally.

To image the atlanto-occipital joint (AO), in the short-axis view, the vertebral artery is followed cranially as it curves medially to enter the foramen magnum. The artery curves posterior and medial to the AO joint, so the joint can be accessed just lateral to the

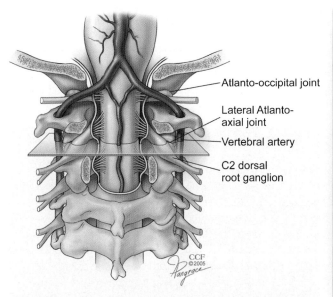

Figure 29.1. Illustration showing the ultrasound transducer in the transverse plane over the atlanto-axial joint to obtain a short-axis view. (Reprinted with permission from Cleveland Clinic).

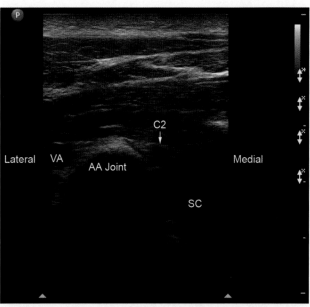

Figure 29.2. Short-axis sonogram at the level of AA joint. *VA* vertebral artery, *C2* C2 nerve root and dorsal root ganglion, *AA joint* atlanto-axial joint, *SC* spinal cord. (Reprinted with permission from Ohio Pain and Headache Institute).

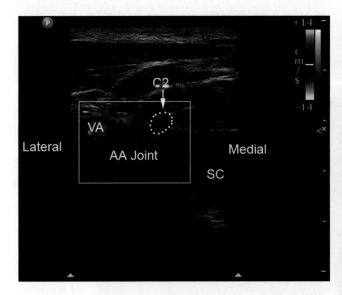

Figure 29.3. Short-axis sonogram with Doppler to show the vertebral artery (VA) just lateral to the atlanto-axial joint (AA joint). *C2* C2 nerve root and dorsal root ganglion, *SC* spinal cord. (Reprinted with permission from Ohio Pain and Headache Institute).

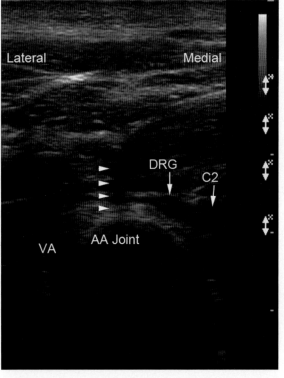

Figure 29.4. Short-axis sonogram showing the needle (out of plane) inside the atlanto-axial joint (*arrowheads*). *VA* vertebral artery, *C2* C2 nerve root, *DRG* C2 dorsal root ganglion, *AA joint* atlanto-axial joint. (Reprinted with permission from Cleveland Clinic).

vertebral artery at this point (Figure 29.5). However, in some patients the vertebral artery crosses along the whole extend of the posterior aspect of the AO joint from lateral to medial, makes it extremely difficult and unsafe to access the joint. If this is the case, the procedure is usually abandoned (Figures 29.6 and 29.7).

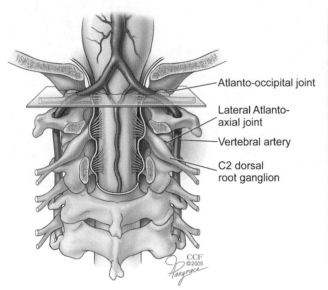

Figure 29.5. Illustration showing the ultrasound transducer in the transverse plane over the atlanto-occipital joint to obtain a short-axis view. (Reprinted with permission from Cleveland Clinic).

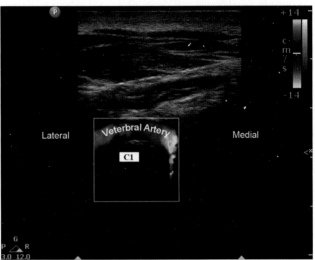

Figure 29.6. Short-axis sonogram showing the vertebral artery as it crosses medially posterior to the C1 lateral mass in its way to the foramen magnum. Note the change in the flow direction as the artery curves. Reprinted with permission from Ohio Pain and Headache Institute.

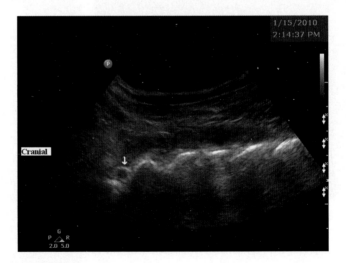

Figure 29.7. Long-axis sonogram showing a cross section of the vertebral artery (*arrow*) as it crosses medially posterior to the C1 lateral mass/atlanto-occipital (AO) joint level. (Reprinted with permission from Ohio Pain and Headache Institute).

REFERENCES

1. Aprill C, Axinn MJ, Bogduk N. Occipital headaches stemming from the lateral atlanto-axial (C1-2) joint. *Cephalalgia*. 2002;22(1):15–22.
2. Busch E, Wilson PR. Atlanto-occipital and atlanto-axial injections in the treatment of headache and neck pain. *Reg Anesth*. 1989;14(Suppl 2):45.
3. Narouze SN, Casanova J, Mekhail N. The longitudinal effectiveness of lateral atlanto-axial intra-articular steroid injection in the management of cervicogenic headache. *Pain Med*. 2007;8:184–188.
4. Narouze S. Complications of head and neck procedures. *Tech Reg Anesth Pain Manag*. 2007;11: 171–177.
5. Narouze S. Ultrasonography in pain medicine: future directions. *Tech Reg Anesth Pain Manag*. 2009;13:198–202.
6. Narouze S. Ultrasound-guided lateral atlanto-axial joint injection for the treatment of cervicogenic headache (abstract). *Pain Med*. 2009;10:222.

30

Ultrasound-Assisted Cervical Diskography and Intradiskal Procedures

Samer N. Narouze

Introduction

The role of diagnostic cervical diskography in the evaluation of patients with neck pain and degenerative disk disease remains controversial.[1] However, provocative cervical diskography is performed in an effort to identify the origin of cervical pain and hence help directing appropriate intervention. Ultrasound will play a pivotal role in performing cervical diskography and percutaneous intradiskal cervical procedures as it will allow us to accurately visualize the various relevant nearby soft tissue structures and avoid their injury.[2]

S.N. Narouze (✉)
Center for Pain Medicine, Summa Western Reserve Hospital,
1900 23rd Street, Cuyahoga Falls, OH 44223, USA
e-mail: narouzs@hotmail.com

S.N. Narouze (ed.), *Atlas of Ultrasound-Guided Procedures in Interventional Pain Management*,
DOI 10.1007/978-1-4419-1681-5_30, © Springer Science+Business Media, LLC 2011

Limitations of the Fluoroscopically Guided Cervical Diskography

Cervical diskography is traditionally performed with fluoroscopy. It can be associated with significant potential for morbidity and mortality. Diskitis, spinal cord injury, vascular injury, prevertebral abscess, and subdural empyema have all been reported as complications of diagnostic cervical diskography.[1,3,4] In a retrospective analysis of 4,400 cervical disk injections in 1,357 patients, significant complications occurred in about 0.6% of the patients and 0.16% of cervical disk injections.[1]

Inadvertent esophageal perforation associated with improper needle placement may be a leading cause for the development of diskitis.[3] The organisms typically cultured are the indigenous mouth and oropharyngeal flora, implicating an esophageal source, transmitted by the diskography needle rather than a skin source. Epidural, subdural, or retropharyngeal abscesses may occur as sequelae of fulminant disk infection or as the primary infection after penetration of the esophagus.[4]

Diskography is routinely performed with fluoroscopy which is unable to identify the esophagus and neck vessels and feared of the disastrous complications of diskitis and vascular injury; practitioners tend to abandon this procedure. Others recommend either using barium swallow to delineate the esophagus with fluoroscopy or using CT guidance which is not widely available, more expensive, and carries the risk of high radiation exposure.

Technique of Ultrasound-Assisted Cervical Diskography

Ultrasonography is an invaluable tool in identifying the esophagus as well as neck vessels (carotid, vertebral, inferior thyroid, ascending cervical, deep cervical, and other neck vessels), nerves, and other soft tissue structures while performing cervical diskography and accordingly a safe needle path can be planned (Figures 30.1 and 30.2).

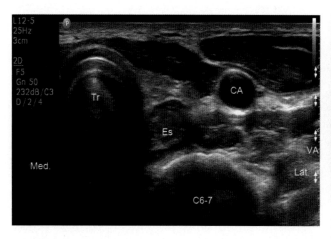

Figure 30.1. Short-axis sonogram at C6-7 disk showing the relevant anatomical structures. *Es* esophagus, CA internal carotid artery, *VA* vertebral artery, *Tr* trachea, *Med.* medial, *Lat.* lateral.

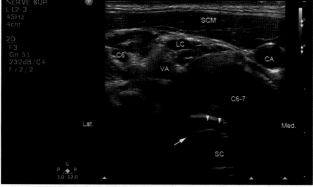

Figure 30.2. Short-axis sonogram at C6-7 disk showing the relevant anatomical structures. CA internal carotid artery, *VA* vertebral artery, C6 C6 nerve root, C6-7 C6-7 disk, SC spinal cord. *Arrowheads* pointing at the anterior epidural space posterior to the disk, and *solid arrow* pointing at the origin of C7 nerve root.

The procedure is performed with the patient in the supine position with the head slightly turned to the opposite site. High-frequency ultrasound transducer is used to obtain a short-axis view of the right neck. As the esophagus is usually slightly deviated to the left (Figure 30.1), a right-sided approach is usually preferred unless otherwise contraindicated.

The appropriate cervical spine level is identified based on the morphology of the transverse process of C6 and C7 as well by following the vertebral artery as described in Chap. 8. Scout scanning is then performed to identify a safe trajectory of the needle and to make sure that the nerve roots, esophagus, carotid artery, vertebral artery, and other neck vessels are not in the path of the needle. The patient may be asked to turn his/her head to the other side under dynamic ultrasonography to create more space between the carotid artery anteriorly and the vertebral artery posteriorly to allow room for the needle (Figure 30.2). The needle is then introduced in-plane from posterior to anterior along the safe predetermined trajectory toward the appropriate disk (Figure 30.3). Once the needle is in the disk, the procedure can be completed with fluoroscopy to monitor the spread of the contrast agent, which is not reliably detected with ultrasonography at such depth (Figure 30.4). That is why it is an ultrasound-assisted procedure rather than an ultrasound-guided one.

Alternatively, depending on body habitus, the procedure can be performed with fluoroscopy and once the radiological target and the needle puncture site are identified, ultrasound is used to verify the safe trajectory of the needle and to make sure that the esophagus, nerve roots, carotid artery, vertebral artery, and other vessels are not in the path of the needle.

In conclusion, ultrasound is a very important adjunct to fluoroscopy in performing cervical diskography. It allows for safer procedure as it may avoid injury to the relevant soft tissue structures. Ultrasound may even play a more important role with the introduction of relatively larger cooled radiofrequency needles for disk ablation (cervical biacuplasty) or with other intradiskal procedures, which require larger introducers.

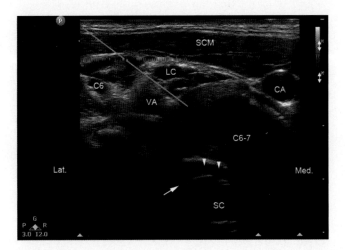

Figure 30.3. Short-axis sonogram showing the trajectory of the needle for C6-7 diskogram. CA internal carotid artery, VA vertebral artery, C6 C6 nerve root, C6-7 C6-7 disk, SC spinal cord. *Arrowheads* pointing at the anterior epidural space posterior to the disk, and *solid arrow* pointing at the origin of C7 nerve root. (Reprinted with permission from Ohio Pain and Headache Institute).

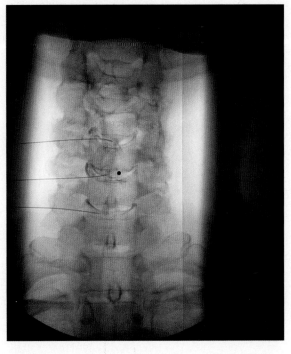

Figure 30.4. Fluoroscopic confirmation of the contrast spread for cervical diskography. (Reprinted with permission from Ohio Pain and Headache Institute).

REFERENCES

1. Zeidman SM, Thompson K, Ducker TB. Complications of cervical discography: analysis of 4400 diagnostic disc injections. *Neurosurgery*. 1995;37(3):414–417.
2. Narouze S. Ultrasonography in pain medicine: future directions. *Tech Reg Anesth Pain Manag*. 2009;13(3):198–202.
3. Cloward R. Cervical discography: technique, indications, and use in diagnosis of ruptured cervical discs. *AJR Am J Roentgenol*. 1958;79:563–574.
4. Lownie SP, Ferguson GG. Spinal subdural empyema complicating cervical discography. *Spine*. 1989;14:1415–1417.

Index

Printed in the United States of America